Pediatric Prevention

Editor

EARNESTINE WILLIS

PEDIATRIC CLINICS
OF NORTH AMERICA

www.pediatric.theclinics.com

Consulting Editor
BONITA F. STANTON

October 2015 • Volume 62 • Number 5

ELSEVIER

1600 John F. Kennedy Boulevard • Suite 1800 • Philadelphia, Pennsylvania, 19103-2899

http://www.theclinics.com

THE PEDIATRIC CLINICS OF NORTH AMERICA Volume 62, Number 5
October 2015 ISSN 0031-3955, ISBN-13: 978-0-323-40098-5

Editor: Kerry Holland
Developmental Editor: Casey Jackson

The Pediatric Clinics of North America (ISSN 0031-3955) is published bimonthly by Elsevier Inc., 360 Park Avenue South, New York, NY 10010-1710. Months of issue are February, April, June, August, October, and December. Periodicals postage paid at New York, NY and additional mailing offices. Subscription prices are $200.00 per year (US individuals), $493.00 per year (US institutions), $270.00 per year (Canadian individuals), $657.00 per year (Canadian institutions), $325.00 per year (international individuals), $657.00 per year (international institutions), $100.00 per year (US students and residents), and $165.00 per year (international and Canadian residents and students). To receive students/resident rare, orders must be accompanied by name of affiliated institution, date of term, and the signature of program/residency coordinator on institution letterhead. Orders will be billed at individual rate until proof of status is received. Foreign air speed delivery is included in all *Clinics* subscription prices. All prices are subject to change without notice. **POSTMASTER:** Send address changes to *The Pediatric Clinics of North America*, Elsevier Health Sciences Division, Subscription Customer Service, 3251 Riverport Lane, Maryland Heights, MO 63043. **Customer Service: 1-800-654-2452 (US and Canada). From outside of the US and Canada: 1-314-447-8871. Fax: 1-314-447-8029. For print support, E-mail: JournalsCustomerService-usa@elsevier.com. For online support, E-mail: JournalsOnlineSupport-usa@elsevier.com.**

Reprints. For copies of 100 or more, of articles in this publication, please contact the Commercial Reprints Department, Elsevier Inc., 360 Park Avenue South, New York, NY 10010-1710. Tel.: 212-633-3874; Fax: 212-633-3820; E-mail: reprints@elsevier.com.

The Pediatric Clinics of North America is also published in Spanish by McGraw-Hill Inter-americana Editores S.A., Mexico City, Mexico; in Portuguese by Riechmann and Affonso Editores, Rua Comandante Coelho 1085, CEP 21250, Rio de Janeiro, Brazil; and in Greek by Althayia SA, Athens, Greece.

The Pediatric Clinics of North America is covered in *MEDLINE/PubMed (Index Medicus)*, *Excerpta Medica*, *Current Contents*, *Current Contents/Clinical Medicine*, *Science Citation Index*, *ASCA*, *ISI/BIOMED*, and *BIOSIS*.

PROGRAM OBJECTIVE
The goal of the *Pediatric Clinics of North America* is to keep practicing physicians and residents up to date with current clinical practice in pediatrics by providing timely articles reviewing the state-of-the-art in patient care.

TARGET AUDIENCE
All practicing pediatricians, physicians and healthcare professionals who provide patient care to pediatric patients.

LEARNING OBJECTIVES
Upon completion of this activity, participants will be able to:
1. Review strategies for the prevention of negative social issues such as childhood obesity, youth violence, and tobacco use.
2. Discuss how genetics, epigenetics, and environmental factors all contribute to health and development in the child.
3. Recognize the impact of the Affordable Care Act on breastfeeding and other important health and social issues for children, parents, and families.

ACCREDITATION
The Elsevier Office of Continuing Medical Education (EOCME) is accredited by the Accreditation Council for Continuing Medical Education (ACCME) to provide continuing medical education for physicians.

The EOCME designates this enduring material for a maximum of 15 *AMA PRA Category 1 Credit*(s)™. Physicians should claim only the credit commensurate with the extent of their participation in the activity.

All other health care professionals requesting continuing education credit for this enduring material will be issued a certificate of participation.

DISCLOSURE OF CONFLICTS OF INTEREST
The EOCME assesses conflict of interest with its instructors, faculty, planners, and other individuals who are in a position to control the content of CME activities. All relevant conflicts of interest that are identified are thoroughly vetted by EOCME for fair balance, scientific objectivity, and patient care recommendations. EOCME is committed to providing its learners with CME activities that promote improvements or quality in healthcare and not a specific proprietary business or a commercial interest.

The planning committee, staff, authors and editors listed below have identified no financial relationships or relationships to products or devices they or their spouse/life partner have with commercial interest related to the content of this CME activity:
Cynthia Bearer, MD, PhD; Iris Wagman Borowsky, MD, PhD, FAAP; Callie L. Brown, MD; Tina L. Cheng, MD, MPH; Michelle M. Cloutier, MD; Gail M. Cohen, MD, MS; Sarah Dow-Fleisner, MA; Benard P. Dreyer, MD; Naomi Nichele Duke, MD, MPH, FAAP; Dina El Metwally, MD, PhD; William Douglas Evans, PhD; Alison J. Falck, MD; Anjali Fortna; Cesar Gonzalez, DDS, MS; Aimee M. Grace, MD, MPH; Tiffany Gray, MPH; Veronica L. Gunn, MD, MPH; Neal Halfon, MD, MPH; Robert Hall, JD, MPAff; Elizabeth E. Halvorson, MD; Summer Sherburne Hawkins, PhD, MS; Brian Hodgson, DDS; Kerry Holland; Jessica P. Hollenbach, PhD; Ivor Horn, MD, MPH; Sheri L. Johnson, PhD; Shiv S. Kapoor, MD; Indu Kumari; Ellen M. Lawton, JD; Suzanne Lazorick, MD, MPH; Lolita M. McDavid, MD, MPA; Colter Mitchell, PhD; Sandra Mooney, PhD; Johnna S. Murphy, MPH; Dipesh Navsaria, MPH, MSLIS, MD; Alice.Noble, JD, MPH; Daniel A. Notterman, MD, FAAP; Christopher Okunseri, BDS, MSc, DDPHRCSE, FFDRCSI; Svapna S. Sabnis, MBBS; Megan Sandel, MD, MPH; Lee M. Sanders, MD, MPH; Adam Schickedanz, MD; Joseph A. Skelton, MD, MS; Bonita F. Stanton, MD; Megan Suermann; Kimberly M.R. White, MS; Earnestine Willis, MD, MPH.

The planning committee, staff, authors and editors listed below have identified financial relationships or relationships to products or devices they or their spouse/life partner have with commercial interest related to the content of this CME activity:
James H. Conway, MD is a consultant/advisor for Merck & Co., Inc and GlaxoSmithKline plc, and has stock ownership in Sanofi Pasteur SA.
Kimberly A. Horn, EdD is a consultant/advisor for the American Lung Association in Colorado, and receives research support from the National Institutes of Health and the U.S. Food and Drug Administration.

UNAPPROVED/OFF-LABEL USE DISCLOSURE

The EOCME requires CME faculty to disclose to the participants:

1. When products or procedures being discussed are off-label, unlabelled, experimental, and/or investi-gational (not US Food and Drug Administration [FDA] approved); and

2. Any limitations on the information presented, such as data that are preliminary or that represent ongoing research, interim analyses, and/or unsupported opinions. Faculty may discuss information about phar-maceutical agents that is outside of FDA-approved labelling. This information is intended solely for CME and is not intended to promote off-label use of these medications. If you have any questions, contact the medical affairs department of the manufacturer for the most recent prescribing information.

TO ENROLL

To enroll in the *Pediatric Clinics of North America* Continuing Medical Education program, call customer service at 1-800-654-2452 or sign up online at http://www.theclinics.com/home/cme. The CME program is available to subscribers for an additional annual fee of USD 290.

METHOD OF PARTICIPATION

In order to claim credit, participants must complete the following:

1. Complete enrolment as indicated above.

2. Read the activity.

3. Complete the CME Test and Evaluation. Participants must achieve a score of 70% on the test. All CME Tests and Evaluations must be completed online.

CME INQUIRIES/SPECIAL NEEDS

For all CME inquiries or special needs, please contact elsevierCME@elsevier.com.

Contributors

CONSULTING EDITOR

BONITA F. STANTON, MD
Vice Dean for Research and Professor of Pediatrics, School of Medicine, Wayne State University, Detroit, Michigan

EDITOR

EARNESTINE WILLIS, MD, MPH
Kellner Professor in Pediatrics, Department of Pediatrics; Director, Center for the Advancement of Underserved Children, Medical College of Wisconsin, Milwaukee, Wisconsin

AUTHORS

CYNTHIA BEARER, MD, PhD
Mary Gray Cobey Endowed Professor of Pediatrics, University of Maryland School of Medicine, Baltimore, Maryland

IRIS WAGMAN BOROWSKY, MD, PhD, FAAP
Associate Professor; Director of the Division of General Pediatrics and Adolescent Health, Department of Pediatrics, University of Minnesota, Minneapolis, Minnesota

CALLIE L. BROWN, MD
Clinical Instructor, Department of Pediatrics, University of North Carolina at Chapel Hill, Chapel Hill, North Carolina

TINA L. CHENG, MD, MPH
Division Chief, General Pediatrics and Adolescent Medicine, Johns Hopkins School of Medicine; Professor of Pediatrics and Public Health, Department of Population, Family and Reproductive Health, Bloomberg School of Public Health, Baltimore, MD

MICHELLE M. CLOUTIER, MD
Professor of Pediatrics and Medicine, Director, Asthma Center, The Children's Center for Community Research, Connecticut Children's Medical Center, University of Connecticut Health Center, Hartford, Connecticut

GAIL M. COHEN, MD, MS
Associate Professor, Department of Pediatrics, Wake Forest School of Medicine; Brenner FIT (Families in Training) Program, Brenner Children's Hospital, Winston-Salem, North Carolina

JAMES H. CONWAY, MD, FAAP
Professor of Pediatrics, Division of Pediatric Infectious Diseases, University of Wisconsin School of Medicine and Public Health, Madison, Wisconsin

SARAH DOW-FLEISNER, MA
Boston College, School of Social Work, Chestnut Hill, Massachusetts

BENARD P. DREYER, MD, FAAP
Professor of Pediatrics, Director of Developmental-Behavioral Pediatrics, NYU School of Medicine, Director of Pediatrics, Bellevue Hospital Center, New York, New York

NAOMI NICHELE DUKE, MD, MPH, FAAP
Assistant Professor, Division of General Pediatrics and Adolescent Health, Department of Pediatrics, University of Minnesota, Minneapolis, Minnesota

DINA EL METWALLY, MD, PhD
Assistant Professor of Pediatrics, University of Maryland School of Medicine, Baltimore, Maryland

WILLIAM DOUGLAS EVANS, PhD
The Milken Institute School of Public Health, The George Washington University, Washington, DC

ALISON J. FALCK, MD
Assistant Professor of Pediatrics, University of Maryland School of Medicine, Baltimore, Maryland

CESAR GONZALEZ, DDS, MS
Associate Professor and Director, Predoctoral Program in Pediatric Dentistry, Department of Developmental Sciences, School of Dentistry, Marquette University, Milwaukee, Wisconsin

AIMEE M. GRACE, MD, MPH
Legislative Assistant, Office of US Senator Brian Schatz, Hart Senate Office Building; Adjunct Assistant Professor in Pediatrics, George Washington University School of Medicine and Health Sciences, Washington, DC

TIFFANY GRAY, MPH
The Milken Institute School of Public Health, The George Washington University, Washington, DC

VERONICA L. GUNN, MD, MPH
Assistant Clinical Professor, Department of Pediatrics, Medical College of Wisconsin; VP Population Health Management, Children's Hospital of Wisconsin, Milwaukee, Wisconsin

NEAL HALFON, MD, MPH, FAAP
Professor of Pediatrics, Public Policy, and Health Policy and Management, Professor of Community Health Sciences, Director of the Center for Healthier Children, Families, and Communities, UCLA Schools of Medicine, Public Health, and Public Policy, Los Angeles, California

ROBERT HALL, JD, MPAff
Associate Director, Department of Federal Affairs, American Academy of Pediatrics, Washington, DC

ELIZABETH E. HALVORSON, MD
Assistant Professor, Department of Pediatrics, Wake Forest School of Medicine, Winston-Salem, North Carolina

SUMMER SHERBURNE HAWKINS, PhD, MS
Boston College, School of Social Work, Chestnut Hill, Massachusetts

BRIAN HODGSON, DDS
Associate Professor, Department of Developmental Sciences, School of Dentistry, Marquette University, Milwaukee, Wisconsin

JESSICA P. HOLLENBACH, PhD
Assistant Professor, Department of Pediatrics; Director of Asthma Programs, Asthma Center, Children's Center for Community Research, CT Children's Medical Center, University of Connecticut School of Medicine, Hartford, Connecticut

IVOR HORN, MD, MPH
Medical Director, Center for Diversity and Health Equity, Seattle Children's Hospital; Professor, Department of Pediatrics, University of Washington School of Medicine, Seattle, WA

KIMBERLY A. HORN, EdD
The Milken Institute School of Public Health, The George Washington University, Washington, DC

SHERI L. JOHNSON, PhD
Assistant Professor, Department of Pediatrics, Center for the Advancement of Underserved Children, Medical College of Wisconsin, Milwaukee, Wisconsin

SHIV S. KAPOOR, MD
Assistant Professor of Pediatrics, University of Maryland School of Medicine, Baltimore, Maryland

ELLEN M. LAWTON, JD
National Center for Medical-Legal Partnership, Washington, DC

SUZANNE LAZORICK, MD, MPH
Associate Professor, Department of Pediatrics, Brody School of Medicine, East Carolina University; Department of Public Health, East Carolina University, Greenville, North Carolina

LOLITA M. McDAVID, MD, MPA
Medical Director, Child Advocacy and Protection, Rainbow Babies and Children's Hospital, Professor of Pediatrics, Case Western Reserve University School of Medicine, Cleveland, Ohio

COLTER MITCHELL, PhD
Research Assistant Professor, Institute of Social Research, University of Michigan-Ann Arbor, Ann Arbor, Michigan

SANDRA MOONEY, PhD
Associate Professor of Pediatrics, University of Maryland School of Medicine, Baltimore, Maryland

JOHNNA S. MURPHY, MPH
Boston Medical Center, Boston, Massachusetts

DIPESH NAVSARIA, MPH, MSLIS, MD
Department of Pediatrics, University of Wisconsin School of Medicine and Public Health, Madison, Wisconsin

ALICE NOBLE, JD, MPH
Boston College, Law School, Newton Centre, Massachusetts

DANIEL A. NOTTERMAN, MD, FAAP
Professor, Department of Molecular Biology, Princeton University, Princeton, New Jersey

CHRISTOPHER OKUNSERI, BDS, MSc, DDPHRCSE, FFDRCSI
Professor and Director, Predoctoral Program in Dental Public Health, Department of
Clinical Services, School of Dentistry, Marquette University, Milwaukee, Wisconsin

SVAPNA S. SABNIS, MBBS
Associate Clinical Professor, Department of Pediatrics, Downtown Health Center,
Medical College of Wisconsin, Milwaukee, Wisconsin

MEGAN SANDEL, MD, MPH
Boston University School of Medicine, Boston, Massachusetts

LEE M. SANDERS, MD, MPH
Department of Pediatrics, Stanford University School of Medicine, Stanford, California

ADAM SCHICKEDANZ, MD, FAAP
Clinical Instructor and Robert Wood Johnson Clinical Scholar, Departments of Pediatrics
and Internal Medicine, UCLA David Geffen School of Medicine, Los Angeles, California

JOSEPH A. SKELTON, MD, MS
Associate Professor, Department of Pediatrics, Wake Forest School of Medicine;
Brenner FIT (Families in Training) Program, Brenner Children's Hospital; Department of
Epidemiology and Prevention, Wake Forest School of Medicine, Winston-Salem,
North Carolina

KIMBERLY M.R. WHITE, MS
University of Maryland School of Medicine, Baltimore, Maryland

Contents

A framework is presented for child poverty prevention and its consequences for lifelong health and success on a national scale.

Violence involvement remains a leading cause of morbidity and mortality for youth and young adults in the United States. The impact of adverse childhood experiences on violence involvement can be translated to the cellular level, including alterations in brain structure and function responsible for stress reactivity and coping. This knowledge is counterbalanced by a growing understanding of what works in the realm of youth violence prevention. Incorporating a resilience framework, with its focus on building developmental assets and resources at individual, family, and community levels, offers a renewed approach to fostering healthy behaviors and coping strategies.

With more tobacco products now available and heavily marketed, dual tobacco use is increasing among youth. We systematically reviewed literature on dual tobacco use interventions, with an emphasis on mass health communication strategies. The review identified 46 articles meeting initial criteria and ultimately included 8 articles. Included studies reported a mix of health communication and social marketing techniques. Although there is a body of research on dual tobacco use, there is limited literature describing interventions aimed at controlling it. Design and evaluation of such interventions showing reductions in dual use of cigarettes, smokeless, and alternative products would advance the field.

Children interact with the physical environment differently than adults, and are uniquely susceptible to environmental toxicants. Routes of absorption, distribution, metabolism, and target organ toxicities vary as children grow and develop. This article summarizes the sources of exposure and known adverse effects of toxicants that are ubiquitous in our environment, including tobacco smoke, ethanol, solvents, heavy metals, volatile organic compounds, persistent organic pollutants, and pesticides. Preventive strategies that may be used in counseling children and their families are highlighted.

Asthma is the most common chronic disease among children. It cannot be prevented but can be controlled. Industrialized countries experience high lifetime asthma prevalence that has increased over recent decades. Asthma has a complex interplay of genetic and environmental triggers.

Studies have revealed complex interactions of lung structure and function genes with environmental exposures such as environmental tobacco smoke and vitamin D. Home environmental strategies can reduce asthma morbidity in children but should be tailored to specific allergens. Coupled with education and severity-specific asthma therapy, tailored interventions may be the most effective strategy to manage childhood asthma.

This article provides a brief introduction to various aspects of oral health care in children, with emphasis on the epidemiology, risk assessment, prevention, and treatment modalities for dental caries. In addition, barriers to dental care and the involvement of pediatricians in advocating for and providing preventive dental care for children are reviewed. Oral health care is one of the most prevalent unmet needs among infants, toddlers, and adolescents in the United States. Routine or preventive dental visits are important for early diagnosis, prevention, and treatment of oral diseases, and for establishing and maintaining good oral health and overall well-being.

Recently, a new research agenda emphasizing interactions between social factors and health has emerged. The term social determinant of health often refers to any nonmedical factor directly influencing health. Health across the life span is strongly and adversely affected by social disadvantage. Research in epigenetics indicates that alterations in DNA methylation may provide a causal link between social adversity and health disparity. Likewise, accelerated loss of telomeres is correlated with chronic stress. Research is still required to develop an understanding of the role of epigenetics and perturbed telomere function in linking social adversity with health outcome.

The overweight and obesity epidemic among children and adolescents in the United States continues to worsen, with notable racial, ethnic, and socioeconomic disparities. Risk factors for pediatric obesity include genetics; environmental and neighborhood factors; increased intake of sugar-sweetened beverages (SSBs), fast-food, and processed snacks; decreased physical activity; shorter sleep duration; and increased personal, prenatal, or family stress. Pediatricians can help prevent obesity by measuring body mass index at least yearly and providing age- and development-appropriate anticipatory guidance to families. Public policies and environmental interventions aim to make it easier for children to make healthy nutrition and physical activity choices. Interventions focused on family habits and parenting strategies have also been successful at preventing or treating childhood obesity.

> Many of the social determinants of health are rooted in legal problems. Medical-legal partnerships (MLPs) have the potential to positively change clinical systems. This change can be accomplished by integrating legal staff into health care clinics to *educate* staff and residents on social determinants of health and their legal origins. When the MLP team works *directly* with patients to identify and address legal needs that improve health outcomes, and incorporate legal insights and solutions into health care practice where the patient population is overwhelmingly impacted by social conditions, outcomes are beneficial to children and families.

> School readiness and educational success is strongly mediated by early literacy skills. In both exam-room and community-based settings, child-health providers can affect the trajectory of early literacy by implementing evidence-based, culturally appropriate interventions that support child development, parenting skills, and child-caregiver interaction. Despite limited research on the subject, these interventions should also attend to the evolving role of digital-media exposure (both positive and negative) on the developmental health of children.

> The Affordable Care Act has caused and continues to cause sweeping changes throughout the health system in the United States. Poorly explained, complex, controversial, confusing, and subject to continuous legal and regulatory definition, the law stands as a hallmark piece of legislation that will change the health sector in America forever. This article summarizes the Affordable Care Act with a focus on children, families, and disparities. Also provided is the context of the current system of health care coverage in the United States.

> In restructuring the delivery of primary care to improve the wellness of a community, every community must review its own circumstances for factors such as resources and capacities, health concerns, social and political perspectives, and competing priorities. Strengthening the health care team with community health workers to create a patient-centered medical home can enhance health care access and outcomes. Community health workers can serve as critical connectors between health systems and communities; they facilitate access to and improve quality and culturally sensitive medical care, emphasizing preventive and primary care.

Foster Care and Child Health   1329

Lolita M. McDavid

> Children in foster care need more from health providers than routine well-child care. The changes in legislation that were designed to prevent children from languishing in foster care also necessitate a plan that works with the child, the biological family, and the foster family in ensuring the best outcome for the child. This approach acknowledges that most foster children will return to the biological family. Recent research on the effect of adverse childhood experiences across all socioeconomic categories points to the need for specifically designed, focused, and coordinated health and mental health services for children in foster care.

PEDIATRIC CLINICS OF NORTH AMERICA

ISSUE OF RELATED INTEREST

Child and Adolescent Psychiatric Clinics
July 2015 (Vol. 24, Issue 3)
Family-Based Treatment in Child & Adolescent Psychiatry
Michelle L. Rickerby and Thomas A. Roesler, *Editors*

THE CLINICS ARE AVAILABLE ONLINE!
Access your subscription at:
www.theclinics.com

Foreword

Pediatric Prevention

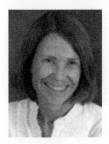

Bonita F. Stanton, MD
Consulting Editor

The goals of prevention in pediatrics and the mechanisms for achieving it are constantly evolving.

Expectations for childhood outcomes have radically changed over time and by nation. When infant and childhood mortality approached 150-300/1000 live births, survival was the main focus. As vaccines and antibiotics became available, followed by oral rehydration solution, many nations began to enjoy rapidly decreasing rates of mortality and could focus on major morbidities such as malnutrition. The role of education in improving health outcomes became accepted in many—and then most—nations. During much of the twentieth century, efforts focusing on psychosocial development seemed to be limited to wealthier nations and populations, but over the past two to three decades, there has been an expanded focus among nations across the globe on prevention and early treatment in this area.

In recent years, we have begun to understand the long-term consequences of early childhood diseases, conditions, and exposures. We now understand that such disorders or exposures in childhood can permanently impact metabolic and structural pathways, rendering (for example) weight loss or learning substantially more difficult and/or greatly increasing the risk of cardiovascular disease in adulthood, even when the childhood morbidity is overcome.

The ever-increasing evidence regarding the contributions of perinatal adversity—and even prenatal stressors—on long-term outcomes remind us of the long reach of environment and the need to constantly have a lifespan approach to growth and development.

In this issue, the authors provide a superb collection of state-of-the-art conditions for which effective primary and/or secondary prevention are now available. Consistent with the epidemiology of chronic illness, this issue has a particular emphasis on at-risk populations. Several articles also address how changes in the systems of health care delivery can make the goal of healthy children more attainable, regardless of demographic and/or socioeconomic factors. In some cases, the updates reaffirm

http://dx.doi.org/10.1016/j.pcl.2015.07.001
0031-3955/15/$ – see front matter © 2015 Published by Elsevier Inc.
pediatric.theclinics.com

earlier studies and understandings of disease causation and prevention, but in many others, our knowledge and understanding have advanced greatly in the new millennium. Today, major goals for childhood throughout the world must include happiness and optimal growth and development, leading to successful and healthy adult status.

Pediatricians have long accepted responsibility for the health of children; it is time that we also accept responsibility for the health of the adults that our children will become.

Bonita F. Stanton, MD
School of Medicine
Wayne State University
1261 Scott Hall
540 East Canfield, Suite 1261
Detroit, MI 48201, USA

E-mail address:
bstanton@med.wayne.edu

Preface

Preventive Pediatrics Issues for Child Health Care Providers

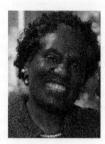

Earnestine Willis, MD, MPH
Editor

Preventive pediatrics has been defined as the prevention of diseases and the promotion of physical, mental, and social well-being for children to reach optimal growth and development. Why Preventive Pediatrics? Because it is essential that pediatricians and other child health care providers continuously examine their approach to keeping children well and thriving in order for them to develop into productive adults. Recognizing the changing needs of children in our society, pediatricians and other child health care providers must become knowledgeable of the most current and emerging issues impacting children's health in order to effectively coordinate preventive services into their medical practices. These emerging needs may include higher prevalence of childhood poverty, obesity, exposures to environmental toxins, children entering out-of-home placement (foster care), and other conditions occurring within complex health care delivery and social service systems which requires the integration of preventive services for children.

Social determinants of health have long been recognized as circumstances in which individuals are born, grow up, play, live, work, pray, and age, all influencing health status. Repeatedly, experts have acknowledged that health status is shaped by forces such as gene-environmental interactions, limited social capital, community resources, social policies, as well as families' economic conditions. This issue conveys a contemporary perspective for common health conditions highlighting social burdens that underresourced children and families face. The 15 topics reviewed in this issue are just a few of the conditions that child health care providers should be up-to-date on regarding health conditions and promising preventive interventions among children. Authors have been requested to discuss the benefits of several interventions that child health care providers must consider in serving children. Those include the benefits of breastfeeding; immunizations; medical legal partnerships; early literacy promotion; community health workers as an expansion to the health care team; and oral health risk assessments. The prevalence of health conditions, including oral health disease,

Pediatr Clin N Am 62 (2015) xvii–xviii
http://dx.doi.org/10.1016/j.pcl.2015.07.002
0031-3955/15/$ – see front matter © 2015 Published by Elsevier Inc.

asthma, childhood maltreatment, and obesity, must be prevented and/or controlled. In the meantime, pediatricians and other child health care providers must become familiar with the Affordable Care Act and provisions impacting children. Preventive interventions need to be incorporated into every primary care setting to enable population health improvement for children. In other words, system-level interventions require community-level collaborations to improve health outcomes.

Child health care providers such as pediatricians and family medicine physicians are in pivotal positions to be strong advocates in preventive health services for children and families by broadening their understanding of service systems, unique population characteristics, and social factors acting favorably or unfavorably on children's health. Robert Haggerty, MD stated years ago that pediatricians must recognize that children and their health needs are best understood and attended to within the interlinking context of their biology, family, and the community. In fact, the life course theory posits that understanding how to prevent threats to childhood and youth growth and development is essential for preventing adult onset diseases. This would suggest that we need to explore greater understanding of the latest theories proposed in the field of epigenetics that could offer promising interventions and could contribute to a reduction of existing and future health disparities. Future research that incorporates epigenetics might illuminate the mechanisms that result in the manifestation of health disparities experienced across generations by far too many children in this nation.

Earnestine Willis, MD, MPH
Department of Pediatrics
Center for the Advancement
of Underserved Children
Medical College of Wisconsin
8701 Watertown Plank Road
Milwaukee, WI 53226, USA

E-mail address:
ewillis@mcw.edu

Breastfeeding and the Affordable Care Act

Summer Sherburne Hawkins, PhD, MS[a],*, Sarah Dow-Fleisner, MA[a],
Alice Noble, JD, MPH[b]

KEYWORDS

- Breastfeeding • Affordable Care Act • WIC • Preventative care • Medicaid

KEY POINTS

- Mothers who receive or qualify for the Special Supplemental Nutrition Program for Women, Infants, and Children (WIC) or have lower income are less likely to start and continue breastfeeding than their more advantaged counterparts.
- As of March 23, 2010, the Patient Protection and Affordable Care Act (ACA) required employers to provide reasonable break time and space to express breast milk.
- As of January 1, 2013, the ACA required insurance companies to cover breastfeeding support, supplies, and counseling at no cost to new mothers.
- This ACA preventive care benefit does not generally extend to all Medicaid recipients or women in the WIC program.
- State and federal legislative and regulatory efforts will be needed to provide comprehensive coverage for all women and reduce disparities in breastfeeding.

INTRODUCTION

Increasing breastfeeding rates is a national priority because of the health, psychosocial, and economic benefits accrued by families and society.[1–3] The American Academy of Pediatrics recommends that infants are exclusively breastfed for approximately the first 6 months of life, after which complementary foods can be introduced, and to continue breastfeeding for 1 year or longer.[2] The most recent data from 2011 demonstrate that 79.2% of infants started to breastfeed and 18.8% were exclusively breastfed for the

All authors have no conflicts of interest to declare.

Research reported in this publication was supported by the Eunice Kennedy Shriver National Institute of Child Health & Human Development of the National Institutes of Health under award number R00HD068506 to Dr S.S. Hawkins.

[a] Boston College, School of Social Work, McGuinn Hall, 140 Commonwealth Avenue, Chestnut Hill, MA 02467, USA; [b] Boston College, Law School, 885 Centre Street, Newton Centre, MA 02459, USA

* Corresponding author.

E-mail address: summer.hawkins@bc.edu

first 6 months, whereas 49.4% of infants received some breast milk at 6 months.[4] The Healthy People 2020 target is to increase the proportion of infants who are ever breastfed to 81.9%, those who are exclusively breastfed at 6 months to 25.5%, and those who receive any breast milk at 6 months to 60.6%.[3] Although more-advantaged mothers have already met and often exceed the Healthy People 2020 breastfeeding targets, groups of women with lower levels of education or income or who are receiving benefits from the Special Supplemental Nutrition Program for Women, Infants, and Children (WIC) are far from achieving these goals.[1,5,6]

The *2011 US Surgeon General's Call to Action to Support Breastfeeding* identified returning to work as an important barrier to breastfeeding for many women.[7] Research has found that women who return to work soon after birth or return full-time are less likely to start breastfeeding than women who are not employed.[7–9] Mothers who work full-time also have a shorter duration of breastfeeding than nonemployed mothers.[7,9,10] Guendelman and colleagues[7] examined the role of maternity leave and occupational characteristics on breastfeeding among women who were employed full-time in California, one of only a few states that provides paid family leave. They found that women with maternity leave of 12 weeks or less were less likely to start breastfeeding and more likely to stop after successfully beginning than women who did not return to work. Women with short maternity leave who were nonmanagers or had inflexible jobs had poorer breastfeeding outcomes than their more advantaged counterparts.[7] In addition, a study of low-income mothers found that those in administrative and manual occupations quit breastfeeding earlier than other women.[11] Taken together, this evidence suggests that, in order to achieve national breastfeeding targets,[3] additional support in the workplace is needed to promote breastfeeding.

Thus despite progress toward achieving the Healthy People 2020 breastfeeding targets,[4] socioeconomic status and the workplace create barriers to breastfeeding for many women. The recent implementation of the Patient Protection and Affordable Care Act (ACA),[12] and its highly publicized provisions in support of breastfeeding, provides an opportune time to consider current legislation and its potential to address the socioeconomic disparities associated with breastfeeding. To that end, the authors first review the reported benefits of breastfeeding and current data on breastfeeding among US women, identifying disparities in breastfeeding rates based on income and employment status. The authors then analyze and compare the breastfeeding provisions of the major statutory programs designed to support breastfeeding, including the ACA, Medicaid, and WIC.[13] The authors examine whether such measures adequately address the socioeconomic disparities in breastfeeding rates and consider how well they assist working mothers who choose to breastfeed. The authors conclude with a set of recommendations.

DISPARITIES IN BREASTFEEDING

The population-level benefits of breastfeeding are well established.[1,2,14,15] Full-term infants who are breastfed are at reduced risk for sudden infant death syndrome, ear infections, gastrointestinal infections, and respiratory infections, as well as chronic conditions, including asthma, obesity, and type 2 diabetes mellitus.[1,2,14,15] Preterm infants who are not breastfed have higher rates of necrotizing enterocolitis.[14] Mothers who breastfeed are at lower risk for type 2 diabetes mellitus and breast and ovarian cancers.[1,2,14,15] The benefits of breastfeeding also extend to the economy and environment. If 90% of US mothers meet the recommendation of exclusive breastfeeding for 6 months, Bartick and Reinhold[16] estimate that 911 deaths would be averted and the US economy would save nearly $13 billion. The largest impact would be on reductions in sudden infant death syndrome ($4.7 billion; 447 deaths), necrotizing enterocolitis ($2.6 billion; 249 deaths), and lower respiratory tract infections ($1.8 billion; 172 deaths).[16] Furthermore, 90% compliance would save the US economy $3.7 billion in direct and indirect pediatric health costs, $10.1 billion in premature death from pediatric disease, and $3.9 billion on infant formula.[17] Breast milk is a renewable food and does not have an environmental footprint. In contrast, infant formulas and other human milk substitutes have packaging, shipping, and fuel costs required for the manufacture and transporting of these products.[1]

Despite these benefits and steady improvement in breastfeeding rates over recent decades,[4,18] significant disparities persist. Mothers' socioeconomic circumstances remain one of the strongest indicators of breastfeeding. Mothers who receive or qualify for WIC or who have lower levels of education are less likely to start and continue breastfeeding than their more-advantaged counterparts.[1,5] **Table 1** illustrates these socioeconomic disparities in breastfeeding rates using 2011 data from the National Immunization Survey.[6] Regardless of whether the indicator is education, income, or WIC eligibility, there is approximately a 20 percentage point gap in rates of breastfeeding initiation between the most disadvantaged mothers and those who are better off. The gap extends to almost 30 percentage points for mothers reporting any

Table 1
Healthy People 2020 breastfeeding targets and rates of any and exclusive breastfeeding by sociodemographics among children born in 2011

	Any Breastfeeding			Exclusive Breastfeeding[a]
	Ever Breastfed (%)	Breastfed at 6 mo (%)	Breastfed at 12 mo (%)	Through 6 mo (%)
Healthy People 2020 target[3]	81.9	60.6	34.1	25.5
US National	79.2	49.4	26.7	18.8
Maternal education				
Less than high school	69.1	34.4	19.7	13.5
High school graduate	69.2	38.2	19.6	15.8
Some college or technical school	81.0	46.1	23.6	16.5
College graduate	91.2	68.3	38.1	25.5
Poverty income ratio[b]				
<100	70.5	37.8	20.3	14.2
100–199	77.9	45.5	24.7	18.0
200–399	85.8	57.7	32.1	22.0
400–599	87.1	61.9	34.9	25.2
600 or greater	90.6	67.9	33.5	23.1
Receiving WIC				
Yes	71.8	37.8	19.7	13.9
No but eligible	83.4	56.1	32.8	26.5
Ineligible	89.9	66.0	36.2	24.9

Data from Breastfeeding rates based on samples from the 2012 and 2013 National Immunization Survey, Centers for Disease Control and Prevention, Department of Health and Human Services.[6]
[a] Exclusive breastfeeding is defined as only breast milk.
[b] Poverty income ratio is defined as the ratio of self-reported family income to the federal poverty threshold value depending on the number of people in the household.

breastfeeding at 6 months. For example, 72% of women who receive WIC initiated breastfeeding and 38% breastfed to 6 months, whereas comparable rates for women who were ineligible for WIC were 90% and 66%, respectively.[6]

Breastfeeding rates decrease rapidly within a few weeks after birth. Data from the Pregnancy Risk Assessment Monitoring System, a representative survey of US mothers, illustrates that in 2009, 79% of mothers initiated breastfeeding, whereas only 58% were breastfeeding at 4 weeks post partum.[19] This 20 percentage point drop in breastfeeding rates suggests that women are experiencing significant challenges to continue breastfeeding beyond their hospital stay. A study of low-income mothers also found that the highest risk of quitting breastfeeding occurred during the first month post partum followed by the time period around when women returned to work.[11]

Returning to work presents significant challenges for many women to start and continue breastfeeding. In 2013, 57% of mothers worked outside the home during their infant's first year, increasing to 61% with 1 year olds and 65% with 2 year olds.[20] Approximately 71% of these mothers worked full-time regardless of their child's age.[20] Mothers who return to work full-time are less likely to start breastfeeding and continue for a shorter amount of time than those who are not employed.[7-10] Healthy People 2020 has a target to increase the proportion of employers that report providing an on-site lactation room to 38%.[3] However, a survey by the Society for Human Resource Management in 2014 found that 28% of companies reported having an on-site lactation room down from 34% in 2013.[21] Six percent of companies offered lactation support services, defined as lactation consulting and education, also down from 8% the prior year.[21] Follow-up research is needed to help determine whether the decrease in lactation rooms and support services is really going down or an artifact of the survey or study sample. There may be additional obstacles for women who wish to continue breastfeeding after returning to work. Employment may have inflexible work hours, insufficient break times, and lack of private and clean facilities to express and store breast milk.[1]

ROLE OF LEGISLATION

Legislation can help reduce socioeconomic disparities in breastfeeding rates and the related barriers to breastfeeding for working mothers.[22] Historically, such laws were promulgated at the state level.[23] In general, state laws create a patchwork of regulation of variable significance depending on where the breastfeeding woman lives. In fact, research demonstrates that the proportion of women protected by comprehensive breastfeeding policies in the workplace varied widely between states.[23,24] Only a minority of state-level laws address the need of breastfeeding employees for break time and private space or prohibit discrimination against breastfeeding employees. As of January 2015, only 25 states and Washington, DC had any law related to breastfeeding in the workplace.[25]

A federal law holds greater promise for a uniform and comprehensive breastfeeding policy. The ACA provides the first nationwide approach to promote breastfeeding in the workplace and to increase access to breastfeeding supplies, counseling, and support among insured women.[12] However, despite some gains as a result of these federal efforts, incomplete coverage remains.

PATIENT PROTECTION AND AFFORDABLE CARE ACT

Passed in 2010, the ACA contains 2 provisions that directly affect breastfeeding mothers. The first provision requires certain employers to provide reasonable break time and a private space to express breast milk.[26] The second provision requires insurers to provide coverage of breastfeeding supplies and support services.[27] Although these provisions are indeed a breakthrough in many respects for promotion of breastfeeding, the provisions are not without limitations that may moderate their effectiveness in supporting breastfeeding and decreasing breastfeeding disparities.

Section 4207 of the ACA, amending Section 7 of the Fair Labor Standards Act (FLSA), with certain limitations, requires employers to provide employees a reasonable amount of time to express milk for 1 year after a child's birth each time that she needs to express milk and to provide a location to express breast milk, that is not a bathroom, that is shielded from view, and is free from intrusion from coworkers and the public.[26] Such employers are not required to compensate nursing mothers during breaks to express milk; but if an employee has compensated breaks and she uses them to express milk, then she must be compensated in a similar way.

The FLSA, however, does not apply to all employees and employers. As an amendment to the FLSA, the ACA provision is similarly limited in its applicability. The FLSA covers employees that are subject to the overtime pay requirements in Section 7, which requires an employer to compensate the employee with premium pay for work in excess of 40 hours in a workweek.[28] As a result, the ACA provision generally covers hourly workers but not salaried employees. Although this limit to the application of the breastfeeding requirement of §4207 is not insignificant, it should be noted that hourly workers face greater barriers to breastfeeding compared with salaried workers as they have less control in their schedules and may face possible pay reductions if they take breaks to breastfeed.[1] Like the FLSA, §4207 also provides an undue hardship exemption for certain employers that employ fewer than 50 employees. An undue hardship will be found if the requirement imposes on the small employer significant difficulty or expense when considered in relation to the size, financial resources, nature, or structure of the employer's business.[26]

Importantly, the ACA provision provides a floor not a ceiling for regulation in this area: states remain free to adopt laws that provide additional protections beyond those provided in the ACA. For example, states could require employers to pay women during break times to express milk even though this is not mandated by the ACA.[26]

Although this provision in the ACA provides those mothers covered by it the necessary time and space to either breastfeed or use a breast pump, only 4% of companies offer a subsidized or nonsubsidized child care center on site or near site.[21] This fact suggests that most women who continue breastfeeding after returning to work use a breast pump. For certain breastfeeding mothers, a second provision of the ACA related to breastfeeding may provide greater access to such pumps and, therefore, increase the rate of breastfeeding in the workplace. As noted later, however, some significant limitations apply that may temper the impact of this provision.

The ACA requires all new insurance policies in both the individual and group markets, and including the state and federal health insurance marketplaces, to (1) provide coverage for certain preventive services, including comprehensive prenatal and postnatal lactation support, counseling, and equipment rental for the duration of breastfeeding, as recommended by the Health Resources and Services Administration (HRSA),[29] and (2) to provide that coverage with no cost sharing by the individual insured.[27] The requirement, referred to herein as §2713, became effective for all non-grandfathered health insurance plans or policies issued on or after August 1, 2012. Grandfathered plans (ie, those in existence on the date of passage of the ACA) are not included in this requirement.[30]

Although scores of preventive items and services are now covered under §2713,[31] this requirement for coverage of breastfeeding items and services has garnered substantial attention in the popular press, if not yet in the peer-reviewed literature. Because most policies follow a calendar year, the media firestorm started within days after January 1, 2013 when most women were affected by these health insurance changes:

The Breast Pump Industry Is Booming, Thanks to Obamacare.
—Sarah Kliff, The Washington Post (January 4, 2013)[32]

Through anecdotal evidence of newspaper articles and blog posts, it seemed that medical suppliers and shops were getting bombarded with inquiries for breast pumps.

However, only a few weeks later, the potential gaps and limitations of the law were becoming apparent:

Breast Pump Coverage Under New Law Varies in Practice.
—Ann Carrns, The New York Times (January 28, 2013)[33]

The ACA requirements for coverage of breastfeeding support, supplies, and counseling are not detailed, leaving room for coverage variation among insurance policies. Moreover, insurers may generally determine the frequency, method, treatment, or setting for the provision of the required items or services recommended, consistent with reasonable medical management techniques. The specific recommendations for breastfeeding provided by the HRSA include "comprehensive lactation support and counseling by a trained provider during the pregnancy and/or in the postpartum period, and costs for renting breastfeeding equipment."[29] The requirement was later clarified to state that insurers may also cover the purchase of equipment, but no particular equipment is specified.[34] Thus, some plans may cover only a manual breast pump rather than the costlier electric pump. **Table 2** provides more details on what the legislation covers and what is left to the discretion of insurers. This provision poses significant challenges for lactating mothers returning to work and impacts low-income mothers who will be unable to obtain the costlier pumps absent insurance coverage. Indeed, insurance companies are given latitude in terms of what is covered and interpret the requirements differently.[35]

Also, with regard to the counseling requirement, guidance is not offered as to what constitutes a trained lactation counseling provider or how frequently lactation counseling and education services are to be made available. The regulations do provide that coverage with no cost sharing is only required under §2713 of in-network providers, unless, however, there are no in-network counselors. In that case, counseling by an out-of-network provider must be covered with no cost sharing. How such services are to be reimbursed is left to the insurers; as a result, reimbursement of lactation consultations and support services varies across insurance companies, providing further inconsistencies in coverage.[34] Costs will likely influence what an insurer will cover, given the lack of detailed requirements. Here, too, the popular press has chronicled numerous problems women are facing because of the lack of clear guidance with respect to coverage of these services under §2713:

Breast-Feeding Services Lag Behind the Law.
—Catherine Saint Louis, The New York Times (September 30, 2013)[36]

Madden and Curtis[35] emphasize that, despite the good intentions of the law, without more detailed regulations for-profit insurance companies may interpret the requirements as narrowly (ie, as economically) as possible in determining coverage of these

Table 2
Select elements of the breastfeeding support, supplies, and counseling provision provided through the ACA for both nongrandfathered plans and Medicaid coverage through alternative benefit plans (includes coverage of individuals enrolled through the ACA's Medicaid expansion)

What Is Covered at No Cost Sharing?	Requirements for Coverage	Within Discretion of Each Insurer
Breastfeeding education and lactation consultation provided in network	• They are available both before and after birth and for the duration of breastfeeding. • If such services are not available within the insurer's network, out-of-network services must be provided with no cost sharing.	• Subject to reasonable medical management to determine frequency, method, treatment, or setting • Reimbursement policy outside the scope of the HRSA guidelines and regulations
Breast pump	• It is available for the duration of breastfeeding and in conjunction with each birth. • Over-the-counter items and services recommended under the preventive services provision are covered without cost sharing as long as prescribed by a health care provider.	• Subject to reasonable medical management to determine frequency, method, treatment, or setting • Type of pump covered[a] • Whether pump is rented or purchased • Whether provider preauthorization or prescription is required • Whether provided before or after birth
Breast pump supplies	• They are available for the duration of breastfeeding and in conjunction with each birth. • Note: The specific supplies required to be covered are not stated.	• Subject to reasonable medical management to determine frequency, method, treatment, or setting

[a] Over-the-counter products, such as breast pumps, recommended under the preventive services provision are covered without cost sharing when prescribed by a health care provider.

Data from United States Department of Labor. FAQS about Affordable Care Act implementation part XII. Available at: http://www.dol.gov/ebsa/faqs/faq-aca12.html. Accessed February 5, 2015.

items and services.[35] The government has yet to issue more specific guidelines for this provision and seems unwilling to further constrain insurers under this provision.

As the earlier discussion makes clear, despite the introduction of a national standard for breastfeeding promotion, many women will remain outside the reach of the ACA provisions. Certain women in the workplace do not fit the criteria for coverage under §4207, or their employer may qualify for an undue hardship exemption. In terms of the preventive care requirements, the regulations leave significant wiggle room for insurers to provide less-than-optimal equipment and counseling for breastfeeding mothers. To a certain extent, however, the ACA does reach into the lower-income population. The preventive care provision applies to all private insurance, including insurance obtained through the state and federal marketplaces. Also, all insurance plans available through the marketplace must provide coverage for certain benefits that the

ACA and its implementing regulations identify as "essential health benefits."[37] These benefits include all of the preventive care requirements of §2713, at no cost sharing. Lower-income individuals, those living at more than 100% of the federal poverty level (FPL), are eligible for subsidized health insurance through state or federal marketplaces.[38] Such subsidies, depending on income, can cover the total cost of insurance.

MEDICAID PROGRAM

Medicaid is a means-tested, individual entitlement program that finances the delivery of primary, preventive, and acute medical care services and long-term care services for certain low-income individuals. Medicaid is jointly funded by the federal and state governments.[39] Traditionally, Medicaid covered only certain categories of low-income individuals, such as children and pregnant women, among others. One of the significant changes wrought by the ACA is the expansion of Medicaid beyond these categories to all individuals up to 133% of the FPL.[40] States may opt into or decline the expansion. As noted later, whether a state expands pursuant to the ACA has implications for access to breastfeeding supports, supplies, and services. Within the Medicaid program, coverage for breastfeeding-related benefits, like that provided in the ACA, does not come as one-size-fits-all coverage. Two main categories of coverage under Medicaid largely determine access to breastfeeding services and supplies: traditional Medicaid and the so-called Medicaid Alternative Benefit Plans (ABPs), the latter authorized more recently through the Deficit Reduction Act of 2008.[41] With respect to breastfeeding-related benefits, the Medicaid ABPs are more closely aligned to the benefits available to individuals through the insurance plans from the marketplace. All Medicaid expansion coverage will be through ABPs.

Traditional Medicaid

Eligibility for most groups in the traditional program is calculated based on a percentage of the FPL, which was $24,250 for a family of 4 in 2015.[42] States provide a basic set of mandated services determined by the federal government but can choose to offer optional benefits. Medicaid coverage of pregnancy-related services does not explicitly state that breastfeeding or other lactation services are covered but is considered broad enough to include lactation services.[43] The Centers for Medicare and Medicaid Services recommend that states include lactation services as separately reimbursed pregnancy-related services rather than only coordinating and referring women to WIC.[43] Given that under the traditional program there is no minimum Medicaid statute or federal Medicaid regulations on standards for provisions of breast pumps or lactation services, states are responsible for determining policy; the coverage of services varies widely across states.[30] A survey by the Kaiser Family Foundation in 2007/2008 found that Medicaid programs cover breastfeeding equipment rental in 31 of 44 states, breastfeeding education in 25 of 44 states, and individual lactation consultation in 15 of 44 states.[44] Furthermore, 9 of the states that responded to the survey did not cover any of these breastfeeding support services.[19] The survey was performed before passage of the ACA and Deficit Reduction Act and may produce different results after 2014 when the requirement for breastfeeding preventive services for state ABP plans took effect.

For traditional Medicaid programs, the ACA did not change the provision of breastfeeding support, supplies, and counseling among Medicaid recipients. Section 4106 of the ACA, however, does provide a 1% permanent increase in federal Medicaid matching rates for preventive services recommended by the US Preventive Services Task Force at a level A or B.[45] These services includes the level B recommendation on breastfeeding counseling during pregnancy and post partum.[46] This incentive is consistent with the overall goal of the ACA to increase access to preventive care. It is unclear what, if any, impact the 1% increase incentive will have on the provision of counseling services by state Medicaid programs. The ACA has a more direct impact on breastfeeding women covered by Medicaid ABPs, including all newly covered by the ACA's Medicaid expansion.

Medicaid Expansion and Alternative Benefit Plans

Rather than providing the traditional set of Medicaid benefits, states may choose to offer an alternative set of benefits (also known as benchmark or benchmark-equivalent plans) for certain Medicaid beneficiaries. States must, however, enroll all individuals newly covered as a result of the expansion in ABPs. Significantly, under the ACA, all ABPs are required to cover essential health benefits, which include all preventive services provided under §2713.[47] As a result, women who gain Medicaid coverage through the Medicaid expansion will be entitled to coverage consistent with the HRSA recommendation, including comprehensive prenatal and postnatal lactation support, counseling, and equipment rental for the duration of breastfeeding.[29,34] This benefit must be provided with no cost sharing.[48] Thus coverage of Medicaid for this group will be aligned with the coverage available through the marketplace. At the same time, the failure of regulators, discussed earlier, to specify what exactly must be covered to satisfy these breastfeeding-related requirements will likewise create (or exacerbate) a lack of uniformity in coverage across state Medicaid programs. Those women who move between Medicaid expansion coverage and marketplace coverage as their income changes, the churn effect, noted earlier, will have the same benefit entitlement (preventive care under §2713 as an essential health benefit at no cost sharing, but the insurer in the marketplace may interpret the breastfeeding-related requirement differently than the state Medicaid program), revealing another aspect of the patchwork nature of coverage.

Moreover, for those states that have not expanded Medicaid coverage, low-income individuals may have fewer options for health care. If the household income is more than 100% of the FPL, individuals or families will be able to purchase a private health insurance plan through the marketplace and may qualify for subsidies, in some cases covering 100% of the cost. In states that do not expand Medicaid, individuals or families may not meet the financial requirements for coverage through Medicaid and may also make too little to afford coverage through the marketplace, creating a health care coverage gap.[49] As of January 2015, 28 states and Washington, DC adopted the Medicaid expansion, 7 states are under discussion, and 15 states chose not to adopt the expansion.[50]

WOMEN, INFANTS, AND CHILDREN PROGRAM

The US Department of Health and Human Services recommends that if a state's Medicaid program does not cover breast pumps, then women should check their eligibility for a free one through the WIC program.[30] The WIC program is supported by the US Department of Agriculture to protect the health of low-income pregnant, postpartum, and breastfeeding women, infants, and children up to 5 years of age by providing foods to supplement their diet, education, and breastfeeding promotion and support.[51] Women are eligible for WIC whose income is between 100% and 185% of the FPL. Unlike Medicaid, which is an entitlement program, WIC is a block grant program funded primarily by the federal government. Grants are awarded to states through annual appropriations. Individuals who meet eligibility requirements receive benefits subject to the availability of funds. Women are automatically income eligible if they are eligible for other government-funded programs, including Medicaid. However, approximately 17% of women may be eligible for WIC but not enrolled.[52] Research has shown that WIC participants and eligible nonparticipants are more disadvantaged and have higher health risks than ineligible women (ie, women with private health insurance).[52]

The WIC program promotes breastfeeding to all pregnant women, unless medically contraindicated. Each state has a WIC breastfeeding coordinator who oversees and organizes available breastfeeding services. Mothers who choose to breastfeed are provided information through counseling and breastfeeding educational materials, provided support through peer counselors, and eligible to participate in WIC longer than nonbreastfeeding mothers; those who exclusively breastfeed receive an enhanced food package and can receive breast pumps, breast shells, or nursing supplementers to help support the initiation and duration of breastfeeding.[53] Breast pumps are not distributed prenatally; before a pump is issued, WIC staff determine whether mothers can obtain a pump from the hospital, through private insurance, or Medicaid.

Because WIC funds are limited, states need to prioritize which mothers receive a breast pump and what type because of the variability in cost. Breast pump programs should include an evaluation of the mother and infant to determine the type of pump required, a triage system for distribution if need exceeds supply, and criteria for issuance of each type of pump.[54] When deciding whether and which pump to provide, some of the additional factors that WIC staff are encouraged to consider are the number of hours of separation, frequency of separation, amount of formula provided by WIC, and the mother's breastfeeding goals.[54]

COMPARISON OF COVERAGE OF BREASTFEEDING ITEMS AND SERVICES

The authors now turn to a comparison of the breastfeeding education, lactation consultation, breast pumps, and breast pump supplies provided through Medicaid and WIC. As the authors noted earlier, the ACA breastfeeding preventive services requirements of §2713 apply to women receiving coverage through the Medicaid expansion. Also, the population of low-income women who are covered through insurance is not stagnant; but individuals may churn through the private insurance sector and Medicaid program as their income fluctuates. Medicaid coverage for breastfeeding items and services has changed in some states and for some populations as a result of the ACA Medicaid expansion. No deadline has been set for states that decide to join the expansion, so coverage of the Medicaid populations is in flux.

The authors conducted a survey of the Medicaid and WIC programs of all 50 states and Washington, DC (51 states) to determine what items and services are provided for breastfeeding mothers. State Medicaid breastfeeding provisions were identified through a Web search of the Centers for Medicare and Medicaid Services, and state WIC breastfeeding resources were identified through a Web search of the WIC program. If a search function was available, the following terms were used: breastfeeding, breast pump, lactation, lactation consultation, lactation services, durable medical equipment breast pump, pregnancy-related services. Medicaid generally covers items defined as durable medical equipment, and coverage varies by state.[55] For each state, breast pump codes were searched in the durable medical equipment manual. The Web search focused on locating information on coverage of breastfeeding educational classes or materials related to breastfeeding, lactation consultation, and breast pumps and supplies. Overall, state Web sites varied widely in the accessibility and completeness of information related to breastfeeding provisions.

For each state, the breastfeeding coordinator or program director from WIC and a Medicaid state contact or public frequently asked questions (FAQ) forum were contacted via e-mail to confirm the accuracy of the Web search. If the initial Web search did not yield information and a confirmation was not received by the state contact, no information for that state is presented. For Medicaid, findings from the pre-ACA Kaiser report[44] were included if no other information was available.

Table 3 provides definitions of breastfeeding items and services for purposes of determining coverage based on those provided by the National WIC Association.[54] The ACA and its implementing regulations do not provide detailed definitions of the items and services required to be covered under §2713.

Medicaid and WIC distribute breast pumps in one of 2 ways: Mothers are (1) permitted to keep the breast pump or (2) required to return it to the agency or supplier. For the first method of distribution, mothers may either be provided with a pump at no cost or reimbursed for the cost of a breast pump after purchase through an authorized supplier and are allowed to keep the pump indefinitely. For the second

Table 3
Definitions of breastfeeding items and services based on those provided by the National WIC Association

Breastfeeding Items and Services	Definition	Notes
Breastfeeding education	Group or individual classes, peer support, breastfeeding support lines, and educational materials	—
Lactation consultation	Includes individuals with the following certifications: IBCLC, CLC, CLE, and CLS	—
Breast pump	Electrically or manually controlled device used to remove milk from a mother's breast	• Manual: single-user breast pump powered by the user, often by hand; least efficient and durable type of breast pump; provided to mother to keep • Single-user electric: electronically powered breast pump[56]; provided to mother to keep • Multiple-user electric: electronically powered breast pump with a closed system that requires the use of a collection kit (parts of the pump that touch the breast and collect milk); hospital-grade (type of multi-user electric pump that operates on a closed system) most durable and efficient type of multi-user electric pump; loaned to mother to return
Breast pump supplies	Collection kit, tubing, extra tubing or bottles, or flanges	—

Abbreviations: IBCLC, International Board Certified Lactation Consultant; CLC, Certified Lactation Counselor; CLE, Certified Lactation Educator; CLS, Certified Lactation Specialist.

Data from National WIC Association. Position paper: guidelines for WIC agencies providing breast pumps, #08-002. Available at: https://s3.amazonaws.com/aws.upl/nwica.org/Guidelines_for_WIC_Agencies_Providing_Breast_Pumps.pdf. Accessed January 20, 2015.

method, mothers are loaned a pump at no cost or reimbursed for the rental of a pump through an authorized supplier and then are required to return the pump after breast-feeding has concluded. These distribution methods differ slightly between WIC and Medicaid. For WIC, breast pumps are purchased by the WIC agency using federal funds.[57] The pump is then given to the mother to keep or is loaned to the mother then returned to the WIC agency. With Medicaid, the pump is purchased from an authorized supplier and reimbursed by Medicaid or the pump is rented from an autho-rized supplier and Medicaid pays the rental cost and the mother then returns the pump after use.[55] As such, provided/reimbursed indicates that the mother retains posses-sion of the breast pump, whereas loan/rental indicates the mother borrows the pump while breastfeeding and returns it afterward.

Breast pumps vary in cost (ie, manual is least expensive) and efficiency (ie, manual is least efficient). Therefore, the type of breast pump provided is a balance between cost and efficiency. As a grant-based program, WIC must work with resources that may be limited, particularly when demand for services increases. The main criteria used by Medicaid and WIC to determine which type of breast pump include separation of breastfeeding dyad caused by work or school and infant or maternal medical neces-sity.[54] In some states, Medicaid may also require prior authorization or physician pre-scription for durable medical equipment.[58]

Medicaid Breastfeeding Items and Services

For Medicaid, some Web resources were available for 43 states; 13 states confirmed the information regarding breastfeeding items and services. Of the remaining 8 states, the pre-ACA Kaiser report[44] indicated that 5 states reported no services, 1 state had no data, and 2 states did not respond. **Table 4** provides more detailed information on Medicaid breastfeeding items and services. Medicaid programs may provide addi-tional breastfeeding resources or include additional restrictions that are not listed on the state Web site.

- Fourteen states cover breastfeeding education.
- Twelve states cover lactation consultation.
- Thirty-nine states include the provision of a breast pump.
  - Twenty-four states provide or reimburse a manual pump.
  - Twenty-five states provide or reimburse a single-user electric pump.
    - Of those, 17 states provide a single-user pump for medical necessity or because of separation of the breastfeeding dyad and require documentation.
  - Twenty-eight states cover rental costs for a multi-user/hospital-grade pump.
    - Of those, 23 states provide a multi-user/hospital-grade pump for medical necessity or because of separation of the breastfeeding dyad and require documentation.
  - Eight states indicate Medicaid did not cover breast pumps, and 7 states did not include breast pumps as durable medical equipment.
- Sixteen states cover breast pump supplies and 3 states for hospital-grade pumps only.

Women, Infants, and Children Breastfeeding Items and Services

For WIC, some Web resources were available for all 51 states, and 34 states confirmed the information regarding breastfeeding items and services. **Table 5** provides more detailed information on breastfeeding items and services for the WIC program. WIC programs may provide additional breastfeeding resources or include additional restrictions that are not listed on the state Web site.

Table 4
State breastfeeding items and services provided through Medicaid

State	Breastfeeding Education[e]	Lactation Consultation[f]	Breast Pump	Breast Pump Supplies[g]
Alabama[c,h]	—	—	—	—
Alaska[b]	—	—	L(E)[d]	—
Arizona[b]	Yes	—	L(E)[d]	—
Arkansas[b,h]	Yes	Yes	—	—
California[b]	Yes	Yes	P(M) P(S)[d] L(E)[d]	Yes
Colorado[a]	No	No	P(M) P(S)[d] L(E)[d]	Yes
Connecticut[b]	—	—	P(M) P(S)[d] L(E)[d]	—
Delaware[b]	—	—	L(E)[d]	—
Washington, DC[b]	Yes	Yes	P(M) P(S)[d] L(E)[d]	—
Florida[c,h]	—	—	—	—
Georgia[b]	—	—	L(E)[d]	—
Hawaii[a]	—	Yes	P(M) P(S)[d] L(E)[d]	No
Idaho[a]	Yes	Yes	P(M) P(S)[d] L(E)[d]	Yes
Illinois[b]	—	—	P(S)[d]	—
Indiana[b]	Yes	—	Y[d]	—
Iowa[a,h]	No	Yes	No	Yes
Kansas[b]	—	—	P(M)[d] P(S)[d]	—
Kentucky[a]	No	No	L(E)[d]	No
Louisiana[c,h]	—	—	—	—
Maine[c,h]	—	—	—	—
Maryland[a]	No	No	L(E)[d]	Yes
Massachusetts[b]	—	—	P(M) P(S) L(E)	—
Michigan[b]	—	—	P(M) P(S) L(E)[d]	—
Minnesota[a]	Yes	Yes	P(M) P(S) L(E)	H only
Mississippi[a]	No	No	P(M) P(S)[d]	Yes
Missouri[b]	Yes	—	Yes	—
Montana[b]	—	—	L(E)[d]	Yes
Nebraska[b]	—	—	L(E)[d]	Yes
Nevada[a]	No	No	No	No
New Hampshire[b]	—	—	P(M)	—
New Jersey[h]	—	—	—	—
New Mexico[b]	—	—	P(S)[d]	—
New York[b]	Yes	Yes	P(M) P(S) L(E)[d]	Yes
North Carolina[c,h]	—	—	—	—
North Dakota[a]	No	No	P(M) P(S) L(E)[d]	Yes
Ohio[b]	—	—	P(M) P(S)[d] L(E)[d]	H only
Oklahoma[a,h]	No	Yes	No	No
Oregon[b]	—	—	P(M) P(S)[d] L(E)[d]	Yes
Pennsylvania[b]	Yes	Yes	P(M) P(S)	—
Rhode Island[b]	Yes	Yes	P(M) P(S) L(E)	Yes
South Carolina[b]	—	—	Yes	—

(continued on next page)

Table 4
(*continued*)

State	Breastfeeding Education[e]	Lactation Consultation[f]	Breast Pump	Breast Pump Supplies[g]
South Dakota	—	—	—	—
Tennessee[a]	Yes	Yes	L(E)[d]	No
Texas[a]	No	No	P(M) P(S)[d] L(E)[d]	Yes
Utah[a]	No	No	P(M) P(S)	No
Vermont[b]	Yes	—	L(E)[d]	—
Virginia[c]	—	—	—	—
Washington[a]	No	No	P(M) P(S)[d] L(E)[d]	Yes
West Virginia[b]	—	—	P(M)[d] P(S)[d]	Yes
Wisconsin	—	—	P(M) P(S)[d] L(E)[d]	Yes
Wyoming[a]	Yes	No	P(M) P(S) L(E)	H only

Em dash indicates no information available via Web search, state contact, or pre-ACA Kaiser report.

Abbreviations: E, multi-user or hospital-grade electric pump; H only, only hospital-grade pumps; L, loaned to or rented by the mother and returned after use; M, manual pump; P, provided at no cost or reimbursed and retained by the mother; S, single-user electric pump.

[a] Information confirmed by state contact.

[b] Information from Web search only.

[c] Information from the pre-ACA Kaiser report.[44]

[d] Pump type determined by following: separation of breastfeeding dyad because of work or school, infant or maternal medical necessity, and/or requires prior authorization or physician prescription required for pump.

[e] Education includes group or individual classes, breastfeeding call lines, educational materials, and peer support.

[f] Lactation consultation includes consultation from the International Board Certified Lactation Consultant, Certified Lactation Counselor, Certified Lactation Educator, and Certified Lactation Specialist.

[g] Breast pumps supplies include tubing, flanges, and other additional supplies and are available with electric single-user or multi-user pumps.

[h] Breast pump not listed as durable medical equipment.

- All states cover breastfeeding education.
- All states cover lactation consultation.
- All states include the provision of a breast pump.
  - Forty-six states provide a manual pump.
  - Thirty-nine states provide a single-user electric pump.
    - Of those, 15 states provide a single-user pump for medical necessity or because of separation of the breastfeeding dyad following breastfeeding assessment and based on availability.
  - Forty-two states loan a multi-user/hospital-grade pump.
    - Of those, 21 states provide a multi-user/hospital-grade pump for medical necessity or because of separation of the breastfeeding dyad following breastfeeding assessment and based on availability.
- All states cover some breast pump supplies, although the type of supplies may vary.

Among those states that confirmed the information on breastfeeding provisions, WIC staff noted that individual agency funding and the population served impact the services provided, including the quantity and type of pump available, education services, and lactation consultation. WIC programs are trying to maximize the breastfeeding provisions offered to mothers within a limited budget.

Table 5
State breastfeeding items and services provided through the WIC program

State	Breastfeeding Education[d]	Lactation Consultation[e]	Breast Pump	Breast Pump Supplies[f]
Alabama[a]	Yes	Yes	P(M) L(E)	Yes
Alaska[a]	Yes	Yes	P(M) P(S) L(E)	Yes
Arizona[a]	Yes	Yes	P(M) L(E)	Yes
Arkansas[a]	Yes	Yes	P(M) P(S)	Yes
California	Yes	Yes	P(M) P(S) L(E)[c]	Yes
Colorado[a]	Yes	Yes	P(M) P(S) L(E)	Yes
Connecticut[b]	Yes	Yes	P(M) P(S)[c]	Yes
Delaware[b]	Yes	Yes	P(M) P(S)	Yes
Washington, DC[b]	Yes	Yes	P(M) L(E)[c]	Yes
Florida[a]	Yes	Yes	P(M) P(S) L(E)[c]	Yes
Georgia[b]	Yes	Yes	P(M) L(E)	Yes
Hawaii[a]	Yes	Yes	P(M) P(S) L(E)	Yes
Idaho[a]	Yes	Yes	P(M) P(S) L(E)	Yes
Illinois[b]	Yes	Yes	P(S)	Yes
Indiana[a]	Yes	Yes	P(M) P(S) L(E)	Yes
Iowa[b]	Yes	Yes	Yes[c]	Yes
Kansas[a]	Yes	Yes	P(M) P(S)[c] L(E)[c]	Yes
Kentucky[b]	Yes	Yes	P(M) P(S)[c] L(E)[c]	Yes
Louisiana[b]	Yes	Yes	P(M) P(S)[c] L(E)[c]	Yes
Maine[a]	Yes	Yes	P(M) P(S) L(E)	Yes
Maryland[a]	Yes	Yes	P(M) P(S)[c] L(E)[c]	Yes
Massachusetts[a]	Yes	Yes	P(M) P(S) L(E)	Yes
Michigan[a]	Yes	Yes	P(M) P(S)[c] L(E)[c]	Yes
Minnesota[a]	Yes	Yes	P(M) L(E)[c]	Yes
Mississippi[b]	Yes	Yes	Yes	Yes
Missouri[a]	Yes	Yes	P(M) P(S)[c] L(E)[c]	Yes
Montana[a]	Yes	Yes	P(M) P(S) L(E)	Yes
Nebraska[b]	Yes	Yes	P(M) P(S) L(E)[c]	Yes
Nevada[b]	Yes	Yes	L(E)[c]	Yes
New Hampshire[a]	Yes	Yes	P(M) P(S)[c] L(E)[c]	Yes
New Jersey[a]	Yes	Yes	P(M) P(S)[c] L(E)[c]	Yes
New Mexico[b]	Yes	Yes	P(M) P(S)[c] L(E)[c]	Yes
New York[b]	Yes	Yes	P(M) P(S)[c] L(E)[c]	Yes
North Carolina[b]	Yes	Yes	P(M) P(S)[c] L(E)[c]	Yes
North Dakota[a]	Yes	Yes	P(M) L(E)	Yes
Ohio[b]	Yes	Yes	P(M) P(S) L(E)	Yes
Oklahoma[b]	Yes	Yes	P(M) P(S)	Yes
Oregon[b]	Yes	Yes	P(S)[c]	Yes
Pennsylvania[a,g]	Yes	Yes	P(M) P(S) L(E)	Yes
Rhode Island[a,g]	Yes	Yes	P(M) P(S)[c] L(E)[c]	Yes
South Carolina[a]	Yes	Yes	P(M) P(S) L(E)	Yes

(continued on next page)

Table 5
(continued)

State	Breastfeeding Education[d]	Lactation Consultation[e]	Breast Pump	Breast Pump Supplies[f]
South Dakota[a]	Yes	Yes	P(M) P(S) L(E)	Yes
Tennessee[a]	Yes	Yes	P(M) L(E)[c]	Yes
Texas[a]	Yes	Yes	P(M) P(S) L(E)	Yes
Utah[a]	Yes	Yes	P(M) P(S) L(E)	Yes
Vermont[a]	Yes	Yes	P(M) P(S) L(E)	Yes
Virginia[a]	Yes	Yes	P(M) P(S) L(E)	Yes
Washington[a]	Yes	Yes	P(M) L(E)[c]	Yes
West Virginia[b]	Yes	Yes	P(M) P(S)[c]	Yes
Wisconsin[a]	Yes	Yes	P(M) P(S) L(E)	Yes
Wyoming[a]	Yes	Yes	P(M) L(E)[c]	Yes

Abbreviations: E, multi-user or hospital-grade electric pump; H only, only hospital-grade pumps; L, loaned to or rented by the mother and returned after use; M, manual pump; P, provided at no cost or reimbursed and retained by the mother; S, single-user electric pump.

[a] Information confirmed by state contact.

[b] Information from Web search only.

[c] Pump type determined by the following: separation of breastfeeding dyad because of work or school, infant or maternal medical necessity, and/or certification as exclusively breastfeeding following assessment by WIC staff.

[d] Education includes group or individual classes, breastfeeding call lines, educational materials, and peer support.

[e] Lactation consultation includes consultation from the International Board Certified Lactation Consultant, Certified Lactation Counselor, Certified Lactation Educator, and Certified Lactation Specialist.

[f] Breast pumps supplies include tubing, flanges, and other additional supplies and are available with electric single-user or multi-user pumps.

[g] Only for those who do not qualify through Medicaid or other insurance.

GAPS IN COVERAGE

Breastfeeding rates vary widely by women's socioeconomic circumstances. Women with more advantaged circumstances are more likely to start and continue breastfeeding than women with more disadvantaged circumstances, as measured by WIC status, education, or income.[1,5,6] Legislation can be a valuable tool in reducing socioeconomic disparities in breastfeeding rates. The authors began this review with an observation that states provide a patchwork of provisions that support breastfeeding mothers in a variety of ways and that a more uniform and comprehensive approach was needed consistent with the status of breastfeeding as a national priority. The ACA goes far in some areas in providing that comprehensive and consistent national support of breastfeeding mothers. Breastfeeding workers may find a more welcoming workplace, including break time and a private space for expressing milk; working and nonworking mothers may have other supports, such as lactation counseling, and supplies, such as breast pumps, provided through the §2713 preventive care provisions at no cost.

Despite the national reach of the ACA, gaps persist: workplace rules do not apply to all workplaces and preventive items and services at no cost sharing is limited to those individuals who receive their health care coverage through (nongrandfathered) private insurance. For breastfeeding women whose income is more than 100% of the FPL, new subsidized coverage through the marketplaces may be available and will include the breastfeeding-related preventive items and services. This ACA preventive care benefit does not generally extend to all Medicaid recipients. Individuals enrolled in Medicaid ABPs, including those individuals in 28 states who qualify for the new expansion coverage, are entitled to the ACA preventive care items and services at no cost sharing. Traditional Medicaid recipients may face less generous breastfeeding-related benefits and, in some states, no such benefits at all.

Unfortunately some women will continue to fall through the cracks between insurance coverage and Medicaid. Although the WIC program is a safety net for low-income women and provides many of the same breastfeeding provisions as through the ACA, resources are limited. State Medicaid programs are referring women to their WIC programs if breastfeeding provisions are not provided.[43] WIC is not an entitlement program, and its support to breastfeeding women eligible for its services is limited by the amount of the block grant received. WIC staff must prioritize who receives breast pumps, and the preferred type of pump and extra supplies are not always available.

Even within programs, a lack of uniformity of benefits will likely result. For example, insurers have little guidance or oversight in what benefits are actually due in order to comply with the requirements of §2713. The same uncertainty exists for §2713 coverage for those enrolled in Medicaid expansion coverage.

In light of the designation of breastfeeding as a national priority, the present mix of state and federal law, even after historic health reform, presents an unacceptable patchwork rather than a unified commitment to eliminating breastfeeding disparities. At the same time, the new coverage through the ACA is a step forward from the earlier legislation limited to states. To keep the trend of broadening coverage continuing, both state and federal legislative and regulatory efforts, along with a commitment by insurers to effective implementation of the law, will be needed.

RECOMMENDATIONS

- Although this review has focused on state and federal legislation as a means of reducing disparities, health care providers should become familiar with the benefits available under the various health care coverage options and provide information to patients who may be unaware of their rights both in the workplace and with regard to access to lactation counseling, education, and supplies related to breastfeeding.
- As noted, there are several gaps in the ACA provisions related to workplace break time and private space to express milk. Given that the House of Representatives has recently voted to repeal the ACA, the 56th such vote, it is unlikely that gaps in the coverage of this provision will be filled in by Congress anytime soon.[59] It can, however, provide a starting point for states to create similar workplace rights. States should finish the work begun by the ACA and pass legislation protecting all women in the workplace.
- States should continue to evaluate participation in the Medicaid expansion. Certainly, much is to be gained for breastfeeding women. Over time more states will likely sign on. A better understanding of what is at stake for breastfeeding mothers, and other low-income groups, may accelerate the rate of state adoption.
- Additional research is needed with regard to insurance and state Medicaid compliance with the preventive care requirements of §2713. How do insurers vary in terms of services and supplies provided to breastfeeding mothers, and

what services and supplies are optimal for the breastfeeding mother both in and out of the workplace?

- Similarly, research concerning Medicaid coverage is needed. For most states, information on the availability of breastfeeding resources is either not easily accessible or programs do no provide these provisions. Greater transparency via the Internet should be a priority for these state programs. Such measures should include improved Web sites to provide easily accessible and up-to-date information on breastfeeding provisions federally and for each state.
- Armed with such research findings, advocates should seek out state and federal regulators and press the case for more detailed guidance as to specific services and supplies insurers and state programs should provide breastfeeding mothers consistent with the law. Enforcement should be made a priority.

Considering the benefits of breastfeeding,[1,2,14–17] growing disparities could have important short- and long-term consequences for child health. The ACA's reform of breastfeeding coverage in the United States is a significant but insufficient step to ease the impacts of such disparities.

REFERENCES

1. US Department of Health and Human Services. The Surgeon General's call to action to support breastfeeding. Washington, DC: US Department of Health and Human Services; 2011.
2. Section on Breastfeeding. Breastfeeding and the use of human milk. Pediatrics 2012;129:e827–41.
3. US Department of Health and Human Services. Healthy people 2020: maternal, infant, and child health objectives. 2011. Available at: http://www.healthypeople. gov/2020/topics-objectives/topic/maternal-infant-and-child-health/objectives. Accessed January 10, 2015.
4. Centers for Disease Control and Prevention. Breastfeeding report card: United States, 2014. Available at: http://www.cdc.gov/breastfeeding/pdf/2014breast feedingreportcard.pdf. Accessed December 2, 2014.
5. Centers for Disease Control and Prevention. Racial and ethnic differences in breastfeeding initiation and duration, by state - National Immunization Survey, United States, 2004-2008. MMWR Morb Mortal Wkly Rep 2010;59:327–34.
6. Centers for Disease Control and Prevention. Rates of any and exclusive breastfeeding by socio-demographics among children born in 2011. Available at: http://www. cdc.gov/breastfeeding/data/nis_data/rates-any-exclusive-bf-socio-dem-2011.htm. Accessed January 17, 2015.
7. Guendelman S, Kosa JL, Pearl M, et al. Juggling work and breastfeeding: effects of maternity leave and occupational characteristics. Pediatrics 2009;123:e38–46.
8. Hawkins SS, Griffiths LJ, Dezateux C, et al. Maternal employment and breastfeeding initiation: findings from the Millennium Cohort Study. Paediatr Perinat Epidemiol 2007;21:242–7.
9. Mandal B, Roe BE, Fein SB. The differential effects of full-time and part-time work status on breastfeeding. Health Policy 2010;97:79–86.
10. Hawkins SS, Griffiths LJ, Dezateux C, et al. The impact of maternal employment on breast-feeding duration in the UK Millennium Cohort Study. Public Health Nutr 2007;10:891–6.
11. Kimbro RT. On-the-job moms: work and breastfeeding initiation and duration for a sample of low-income women. Matern Child Health J 2006;10:19–26.

12. US Government. Patient Protection and Affordable Care Act, Pub. Law 111-148, as amended by the Health Care and Education Reconciliation Act (HCERA), Pub. Law 111–152.
13. Child Nutrition Act, Section 17, 42 U.S.C. 1786, reauthorized in 2010, Healthy Hunger-Free Kids Act, Pub. Law 111–296.
14. Ip S, Chung M, Raman G, et al. Breastfeeding and maternal and infant health outcomes in developed countries. Evid Rep Technol Assess 2007;153:1–186.
15. Dieterich CM, Felice JP, O'Sullivan E, et al. Breastfeeding and health outcomes for the mother-infant dyad. Pediatr Clin North Am 2013;60:31–48.
16. Bartick M, Reinhold A. The burden of suboptimal breastfeeding in the United States: a pediatric cost analysis. Pediatrics 2010;125:e1048–56.
17. Bartick M. Breastfeeding and the US economy. Breastfeed Med 2011;6:313–8.
18. Grummer-Strawn LM, Shealy KR. Progress in protecting, promoting, and supporting breastfeeding: 1984-2009. Breastfeed Med 2009;4:S31–9.
19. Centers for Disease Control and Prevention. Breastfeeding initiation and duration at 4 weeks. Available at: http://www.cdc.gov/prams/pdf/snapshot-report/breast feeding.pdf. Accessed January 15, 2015.
20. US Bureau of Labor Statistics. Table 6. Employment status of mothers with own children under 3 years old by single year of age of youngest child and marital status, 2011-2012 annual averages. Available at: http://data.bls.gov/cgi-bin/print.pl/news.release/famee.t06.htm. Accessed March 27, 2014.
21. Society for Human Resource Management. 2014 Employee benefits: an overview of employee benefits offerings in the US. Alexandria (VA): Society for Human Resource Management; 2014.
22. Raju TN. Reasonable break time for nursing mothers: a provision enacted through the Affordable Care Act. Pediatrics 2014;134:423–4.
23. Nguyen TT, Hawkins SS. Current state of US breastfeeding policies. Matern Child Nutr 2013;9:350–8.
24. Murtagh L, Moulton AD. Working mothers, breastfeeding, and the law. Am J Public Health 2011;101:217–23.
25. National Conference of State Legislatures. Breastfeeding state laws. Available at: http://www.ncsl.org/research/health/breastfeeding-state-laws.aspx. Accessed January 29, 2015.
26. US Department of Labor. Break time for nursing mothers. Available at: http://www.dol.gov/whd/nursingmothers/. Accessed January 20, 2015. ACA §4207, amending Section 7 of the Fair Labor Standards Act by adding §29 U.S.C. § 207(r).
27. ACA §1001, adding §2713 to the Public Health Service Ac; 42 U.S.C. §300gg-12.
28. US Department of Labor. Wage and hour division: overtime pay. Available at: http://www.dol.gov/whd/overtime_pay.htm. Accessed January 25, 2015.
29. US Department of Health and Human Services. Women's preventive services guidelines. Available at: http://www.hrsa.gov/womensguidelines/. Accessed March 25, 2014.
30. US Department of Health and Human Services. Breast pumps and insurance coverage: what you need to know. Available at: http://www.hhs.gov/healthcare/prevention/breast-pumps/. Accessed January 25, 2015.
31. Institute of Medicine. Clinical preventive services for women: closing the gaps. Washington, DC: The National Academies Press; 2011.
32. Kliff S. The breast pump industry is booming, thanks to Obamacare. Wash Post 2013.
33. Carrns A. Breast pump coverage under new law varies in practice. The New York Times 2013.

34. United States Department of Labor. FAQS about Affordable Care Act implementation part XII. Available at: http://www.dol.gov/ebsa/faqs/faq-aca12.html. Accessed February 5, 2015.

35. Madden S, Curtis B. The case for creating a model insurance policy: payer coverage of breastfeeding counseling services, pumps, and supplies. Breastfeed Med 2013;8:450–2.

36. Saint Louis C. Breast-feeding services lag behind the law. The New York Times 2013.

37. ACA §1302; 42 U.S.C. §18022.

38. Centers for Medicare & Medicaid Services. Income levels that qualify for lower health coverage costs. Available at: http://www.healthcare.gov/lower-costs/qualifying-for-lower-costs/. Accessed February 10, 2015.

39. Available at: http://www.medicaid.gov/medicaid-chip-program-information/by-topics/eligibility/eligibility.html. Accessed January 30, 2015.

40. ACA §2001; 42 U.S.C. §1396a.

41. Public Law 109–171.

42. Centers for Medicare & Medicaid Services. 2015 Federal poverty level standards. Available at: http://www.medicaid.gov/federal-policy-guidance/downloads/cib-01-29-2015.pdf. Accessed January 30, 2015.

43. Centers for Medicare & Medicaid Services. Medicaid coverage of lactation services. 42 C.F.R. §440.210. Available at: http://www.medicaid.gov/Medicaid-CHIP-Program-Information/By-Topics/Quality-of-Care/Downloads/Lactation_Services_IssueBrief_01102012.pdf. Accessed January 20, 2015.

44. Ranji U, Salganicoff A, Stewart AM, et al. State Medicaid coverage of perinatal services: summary of state findings. Washington, DC: Henry J. Kaiser Family Foundation and George Washington University School of Public Health and Health Services; 2009.

45. ACA §4106; 42 U.S.C. §1396(a)(13).

46. US Preventive Services Task Force. Breastfeeding: counseling. Available at: http://www.uspreventiveservicestaskforce.org/uspstf/uspsbrfd.htm. Accessed February 6, 2015.

47. 45 C.F.R. §156.115(a)(4).

48. US Department of Health and Human Services, Centers for Medicare & Medicaid Services. Medicaid, children's health insurance programs: essential health benefits in alternative benefit plans, eligibility notices, fair hearing and appeal processes for Medicaid and exchange eligibility appeals and other provisions related to eligibility and enrollment for exchanges Medicaid and CHIP, and Medicaid premiums and cost sharing. Final Rule. 78 Fed. Reg. 42159, 42224 (July 15, 2013).

49. Centers for Medicare & Medicaid Services. Medicaid expansion and what it means for you. Available at: http://www.healthcare.gov/medicaid-chip/medicaid-expansion-and-you/. Accessed January 30, 2015.

50. The Henry J. Kaiser Family Foundation. State decisions on health insurance marketplaces and the Medicaid expansion. Available at: http://kff.org/health-reform/state-indicator/state-decisions-for-creating-health-insurance-exchanges-and-expanding-medicaid/. Accessed January 30, 2015.

51. US Department of Agriculture. Women, Infants, and Children (WIC). Available at: http://www.fns.usda.gov/wic/women-infants-and-children-wic. Accessed January 5, 2015.

52. Centers for Disease Control and Prevention. Eligibility and enrollment in the Special Supplemental Nutrition Program for Women, Infants, and Children (WIC)–27

states and New York City, 2007-2008. MMWR Morb Mortal Wkly Rep 2013;62: 189–93.

53. US Department of Agriculture. Women, Infants and Children (WIC): breastfeeding promotion and support in WIC. Available at: http://www.fns.usda.gov/wic/breastfeeding-promotion-and-support-wic. Accessed January 5, 2015.

54. National WIC Association. Position paper: guidelines for WIC agencies providing breast pumps, #08–002. Available at: http://s3.amazonaws.com/aws.upl/nwica.org/Guidelines_for_WIC_Agencies_Providing_Breast_Pumps.pdf. Accessed January 20, 2015.

55. The Henry J. Kaiser Family Foundation. Medicaid benefits: medical equipment and supplies. Available at: http://kff.org/medicaid/state-indicator/medical-equipment-and-supplies/. Accessed February 7, 2015.

56. US Food and Drug Administration. Buying and renting a breast pump. Available at: http://www.fda.gov/MedicalDevices/ProductsandMedicalProcedures/HomeHealthandConsumer/ConsumerProducts/BreastPumps/ucm061952.htm. Accessed February 7, 2015.

57. US Department of Agriculture. Women, Infants and Children (WIC): breastfeeding promotion in WIC: current federal requirements. Available at: http://www.fns.usda.gov/wic/breastfeeding-promotion-wic-current-federal-requirements. Accessed January 29, 2015.

58. Centers for Medicare & Medicaid Services. The basics of durable medical equipment, prosthetics, orthotics, and supplies. Available at: http://www.cms.gov/Outreach-and-Education/Medicare-Learning-Network-MLN/MLNProducts/downloads/DMEPOS_Basics_FactSheet_ICN905710.pdf. Accessed February 6, 2015.

59. Pear R. House GOP against votes to repeat the health care law. The New York Times 2015.

Overcoming Challenges to Childhood Immunizations Status

Svapna S. Sabnis, MBBS[a],*, James H. Conway, MD[b]

KEYWORDS

- Childhood immunization • Vaccines • Health disparities • Missed opportunities
- Vaccine hesitancy • Immunization information systems

KEY POINTS

- Multiple strategies should be considered to address improving immunization rates and decreasing disparities.
- These may be at a physician or patient level, practice or health systems level, community level, as well as at a state and national level.
- Use of immunization information systems is vital in effectively implementing these strategies.

INTRODUCTION

Vaccines are one of the greatest public health achievements and are one of most cost-effective ways to prevent diseases and advance global welfare.[1] Although immunization coverage rates have been steadily increasing in the United States, overall rates are still less than the 90% target for Healthy People 2020. In 2013, vaccination coverage for children 19 to 35 months old reached the 90% national Healthy People 2020 target for measles, mumps, and rubella vaccine (MMR), hepatitis B vaccine (Hep B), poliovirus vaccine, and varicella vaccine. However, coverage rates were below target levels for diphtheria, tetanus, and pertussis vaccine (DTaP), pneumococcal conjugate vaccine (PCV), *Haemophilus influenzae* type b vaccine (Hib), hepatitis A

Disclosures: Dr S.S. Sabnis has nothing to disclose. Dr J.H. Conway has received financial support for research from Sanofi Pasteur (IRB protocol M-2009-1222, Award #PRJ31GT), and has served as a consultant for Merck Vaccines. Neither of these associations has influenced any of the materials or information in this article.

[a] Department of Pediatrics, Downtown Health Center, Medical College of Wisconsin, 1020 North 12th Street, Milwaukee, WI 53233, USA; [b] Division of Pediatric Infectious Diseases, University of Wisconsin School of Medicine & Public Health, 600 Highland Avenue, H4/450 CSC, Madison, WI 53792, USA
* Corresponding author.
E-mail address: ssabnis@mcw.edu

vaccine (Hep A), rotavirus, and the hepatitis B birth dose.[2] For the combined series recommended for children aged 19 to 35 months (4:3:1:3*:3:1:4)[1] national rates were 70.4%.

Increasing rates have led to dramatic declines in illness and mortality related to vaccine-preventable illness[3] (**Table1**). Routine childhood vaccinations also significantly decrease costs to society.[4] However, disparities remain with significantly less vaccination coverage for black children (65%) and children living below the federal poverty level (64.4%).[2] DTaP, PCV, Hib, and rotavirus in particular had lower immunization rates, suggesting that these children had difficulty in maintaining regular and on-time well-child visits.

Adolescent immunization rates have also increased for routinely recommended vaccines to 86.0% for greater than or equal to 1 tetanus toxoid, reduced diphtheria toxoid, and acellular pertussis (TdaP) vaccine; 77.8% for greater than or equal to 1 meningococcal conjugate vaccine for serotypes A, C, Y and W (MenACWY) vaccine;

Table 1
Estimated numbers of illnesses, hospitalizations, and deaths prevented by routine childhood immunization for selected vaccine-preventable diseases among children born during the Vaccines for Children era in the United States, 1994 to 2013

Vaccine-preventable Disease[a]	Cases Prevented (in Thousands)		
	Illnesses	Hospitalizations	Deaths
Diphtheria	5073	5073	507.3
Tetanus	3	3	0.5
Pertussis	54,406	2697	20.3
Hib	361	334	13.7
Polio	1244	530	14.8
Measles	70,748	8877	57.3
Mumps	42,704	1361	0.2
Rubella	36,540	134	0.3
Congenital rubella syndrome	12	17	1.3
Hep B	4007	623	59.7
Varicella	68,445	176	1.2
Pneumococcus-related diseases[b]	26,578	903	55.0
Rotavirus	11,968	327	0.1
Total	322,089	21,055	731.7

[a] Vaccines were considered as preventing disease for birth cohorts born in all years during 1994 to 2013 except for the following, which were only in use for part of the 20-year period: varicella, 1996 to 2013; 7-valent and 13-valent pneumococcal conjugate vaccines, 2001 to 2013; and rotavirus, 2007 to 2013.
[b] Includes invasive pneumococcal disease, otitis media, and pneumonia.
From Whitney CG, Zhou F, Singleton J, et al. Benefits from immunization during the vaccines for children program era - United States, 1994–2013. MMWR Morb Mortal Wkly Rep 2014;63(16):354.

---

[1] Combined vaccine series for 19 to 35 months includes greater than or equal to 4 doses of DTaP, greater than or equal to 3 doses of poliovirus vaccine, greater than or equal to 1 dose of measles-containing vaccine, full series of Hib vaccine (≥3 or ≥4 doses, depending on product type), greater than or equal to 3 doses of Hep B, greater than or equal to 1 dose of varicella vaccine, and greater than or equal to 4 doses of PCV.

57.3% human papillomavirus (HPV) vaccine dose among female patients, and 34.6% for greater than or equal to 1 HPV dose among male patients. Completion rates for 3 doses of HPV vaccine are only 37.6% for girls and 13.9% for boys.[5] Lower vaccination rates for HPV compared with TdaP and MenACWY are concerning. For children living below the poverty level and for black adolescents, TdaP and MenACWY vaccination rates were similar, and rates for an initial dose of HPV were higher for boys and girls, but completion rates for the HPV series were lower. Coverage for Hispanic adolescents was generally higher. However, rates for all groups are still below the goals for Healthy People 2020 of greater than 90%.

Despite overall increases in immunization rates, there remain significant disparities in childhood immunization rates between racial/ethnic groups and among economically disadvantaged populations.[6] In these areas of underimmunization (pockets of need), which are often poor urban areas with significant barriers to immunization and limited health care resources, disease introduction could have vast impact because of low herd immunity and opportunity for widespread outbreaks.[7,8] Pediatricians can play a vital role in helping to narrow the gap in immunization coverage rates.

Broader immunization coverage results in decreased prevalence of vaccine-preventable disease. With less experience with these infections, there is both less fear of the diseases and a gradual devaluing of the importance of vaccines in the public consciousness. As real or perceived concerns about vaccine side effects are perpetuated by media, or spread in communities through word of mouth, there is the emergence of vaccine hesitation. Although this may be seen more commonly in a different demographic group, in which parents may be more educated and more affluent, similar issues of fear and misinformation can emerge in any setting. Under immunization rates and vaccine refusals have been noted to occur in geographic clusters.[9] Children living in these clusters are at higher risk for individual disease, and the community at risk for disease outbreaks.

BARRIERS TO IMMUNIZATION
Provider/System Barriers

Financial barriers
Vaccine costs and copays are potential barriers to vaccination. Vaccine costs have increased dramatically with the development of new vaccines and expansion of the vaccine schedule. In 1987, the entire vaccine series cost $37 for an individual in the public sector and $116 in the private sector.[10] According to prices updated in January 2015, the series from birth to adulthood costs approximately $1452 per individual in the public sector and $2012 in private sector.[11]

As a means to help provide vaccines for underserved groups, in 1963 Section 317 of the Public Service Act was launched. This program provided discretionary grants to states, select large cities, and territories to conduct routine childhood and adult immunization programs in a partnership model with local health departments. However, following the measles outbreak of 1989 to 1991, it was clear that there were large populations who were still underserved by immunization programs. In 1994, Congress passed the Omnibus Reconciliation Act, which created the Vaccines for Children program. This federal entitlement program was designed to address these issues by providing vaccines free of cost to uninsured and underinsured children 18 years of age and younger (**Fig. 1**).

More recently, the Affordable Care Act (ACA) requires that vaccines recommended by the Advisory Committee on Immunization Practices (ACIP) before September 2009 be administered without copayments or other cost-sharing requirements when those

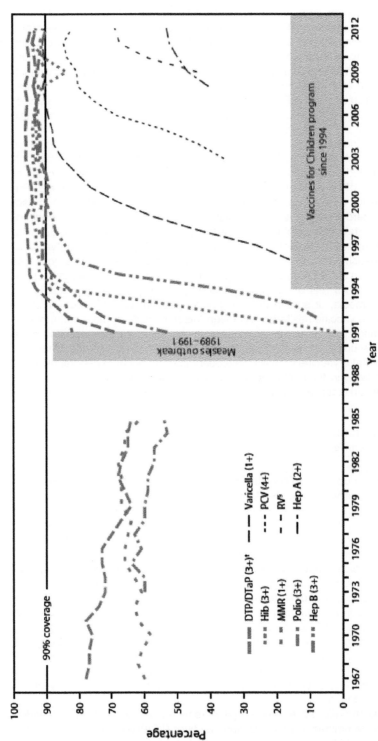

Fig. 1. Vaccine coverage rates among preschool-aged children in the United States, 1967 to 2012. Since 1996, coverage with 1 dose of a measles-containing vaccine has exceeded Healthy People targets of 90%, up from less than 70% before the 1989 to 1991 outbreak. DTP/DTaP, diphtheria tetanus pertussis/diphtheria tetanus acellular pertussis; Hep A, hepatitis A; Hep B, hepatitis B; Hib, Haemophilus influenzae type b; MMR, measles mumps and rubella; PCV, pneumococcal conjugate vaccine; RV, rotavirus vaccine. (*From* Whitney CG, Zhou F, Singleton J, et al. Benefits from immunization during the vaccines for children program era - United States, 1994–2013. MMWR Morb Mortal Wkly Rep 2014;63(16):353.)

services are delivered by an in-network provider.[12] However, health plans are not required to cover vaccinations delivered by an out-of-network provider, which may place a cost-sharing burden on families. Pharmacists and health departments may be considered out of network, thus preventing families from being able to use these as immunization sites.[13]

Access to immunization

At present, the US Centers for Disease Control and Prevention (CDC) recommends vaccination against 16 different vaccine-preventable diseases for children. The vaccine schedule was intended to be coordinated with the well-child visit.[14] In the past, vaccines have been administered in a primary care physician's office and usually during scheduled appointments. This approach may affect the parents' ability to bring a child in for vaccinations because of parent work schedules and inability to take time off from work.

Missed opportunities for immunization

Missed opportunities for immunizations are a well-documented cause for underimmunization.[15,16] They occur when a child who is eligible for a vaccine and has no medical contraindications to vaccination fails to be immunized during a provider visit.[17] These missed opportunities may occur because the physician does not immunize at acute care visits or because of misunderstandings about contraindications, such as during mild illness. It may occur because of providers' reluctance to give multiple shots at 1 visit, or simply from oversight. Vaccine shortages, which occur intermittently, also contribute to underimmunizations or delayed immunizations by missed opportunities. During a shortage of Hib vaccine (December 2007 to September 2009) there was an interim recommendation to defer the booster dose, but to continue the primary series. This recommendation resulted in a decrease in the percentage of fully vaccinated children from 66% to 39.5%. Despite interim recommendations, the primary series coverage was also affected and was reduced by 7 percentage points.[18] Similar national shortages have occurred with PCV (2001 and 2003–2004), varicella vaccine (2002), and influenza vaccine (2004–2005).[19–21] The impact of local or clinic-level vaccine shortages are not well measured but are also likely to be significant.

Family/Social Barriers

Socioeconomic barriers

Children living below the poverty level and black children are documented to consistently have lower vaccination coverage rates.[2] Factors associated with underimmunization include having public or no insurance, belonging to a family with 2 or more children living in the household, and having parents who are unmarried.[22] Children who were enrolled in Women, Infants, and Children (WIC) during the first year of life, and children who were not eligible for WIC, tended to have higher vaccination coverage than those who were WIC eligible but not enrolled. Younger maternal age, history of fewer maternal prenatal care visits, higher birth order, and receiving care at public health clinics were also associated with late initiation of immunizations.[23]

Vaccine hesitancy

In contrast with the families described earlier, a growing group of parents are refusing vaccines. These families refuse or defer vaccines for a growing variety of reasons.[24–27] Many parents are worried about unsubstantiated vaccine side effects such as autism. Concerns also include a fear of overwhelming the child's immune system with too many antigens, leading to parents' requests for an alternate or delayed vaccination schedule (eg, the Dr Sears[28] schedule). Parents may have objections to a specific vaccine because of personal beliefs or certain components of the vaccine (eg, adjuvants). Other reasons include distrust toward vaccine manufacturers, the government, and health care providers, and a preference for natural immunity.[29,30]

Vaccine exemptions are a growing problem. Allowable reasons for exemption vary from state to state, with all states allowing medical exemptions. Religious exemptions to vaccination are granted in 48 states and Washington, DC. In addition, 20 states allow philosophic, or personal-belief, exemptions. Only Mississippi and West Virginia do not allow either type of nonmedical exemption.[31] The ease of obtaining exemptions can also vary (**Fig. 2**). Personal-belief exemptions in particular, when easily obtained, are predictive of increased disease risk among exempt children and in their communities.[32–35] Parents of children with exemptions are more likely to perceive low susceptibility to vaccine-preventable disease, low vaccine efficacy and safety, and less trust in the government compared with parents who have vaccinated their children.[36] Although parents who vaccinate their children may have similar concerns, these tend to be less frequent or manageable. Parents of children with exemptions are less likely to consider medical and public health authorities to be trusted sources for vaccine information and were more likely to trust and use practitioners of complimentary or alternative medicine.

There have been recent resurgences noted across the United States in vaccine-preventable diseases, including measles, pertussis, and mumps, which have been attributed to importation by unvaccinated individuals and transmission among under-vaccinated communities.

Box 1
Recommendations

Provider/system barriers

Addressing financial barriers

- Decrease out-of-pocket costs
- Vaccines for Children Program
- State health insurance programs

Improving access to immunizations

- In the medical home
- Expanding the immunization neighborhood
  - School-based health centers
  - WIC program offices
  - Child care centers
  - Pharmacies

Decrease missed opportunities to vaccinate

- AFIX
- Standing orders

Reminder recall strategies

- Population-based recall
- Clinic-based recall

Expanded use of immunization information systems

Legal requirements for immunizations for school or daycare

Family/social barriers

Community-based strategies

• Target high-risk communities

• Integration with existing community programs

Promoting WIC

Addressing vaccine hesitancy

• Gain parents' trust

• Parent education

• Effective communication

Abbreviation: AFIX, assessment, feedback, incentives, exchange.

RECOMMENDATIONS
Provider/System Barriers

Addressing financial barriers
The Institute of Medicine has made the following suggestions to address financial barriers that impede universal uptake of vaccines recommended by the ACIP.[10] These suggestions include an insurance mandate that applies to all private and public health plans, and a federal subsidy to cover vaccine costs and administration fees, combined with a government subsidy and voucher plan. They have also suggested that a process be developed to determine societal benefits of the vaccines as a means to calculate subsidy levels for different vaccines based on estimated benefits.

Out-of-pocket costs such as copays or office visit fees have been shown to be correlated with lower immunization levels.[37] Eleven studies reviewed by the Community Guide show a 22% (16- 33%) median increase in immunization rates by reducing out-of-pocket costs for vaccinations.[38,39] They recommend broader promotion of the Vaccines for Children Program and Medicaid/state children's health insurance programs to decrease immunization costs, especially among children of low-income families.

It is important that all financial barriers to vaccines be removed, to enable equal access and improved immunization rates.[40,41] The impact of the ACA on decreasing financial barriers for patients remains to be seen. The benefits of the ACA requiring no copays or cost sharing for vaccinations should apply at all sites, including those considered out of network, such as pharmacies. In addition, there are many exceptions that need to be addressed, such as exempting some employer plans from these requirements (**Box 1**).

Improving access to immunization
The Standards for Child and Adolescent Immunization Practices recommend that immunizations should be provided in a medical home whenever possible.[42] Although this recommendation is ideal for providing continuity, stable medical responsibility, maintaining a child's medical records, and providing other relevant information, this is not always feasible. More recent recommendations suggest identifying other venues for vaccinations if children in a community do not have convenient access to a medical home.[44] Suggested venues include public health department clinics; WIC program

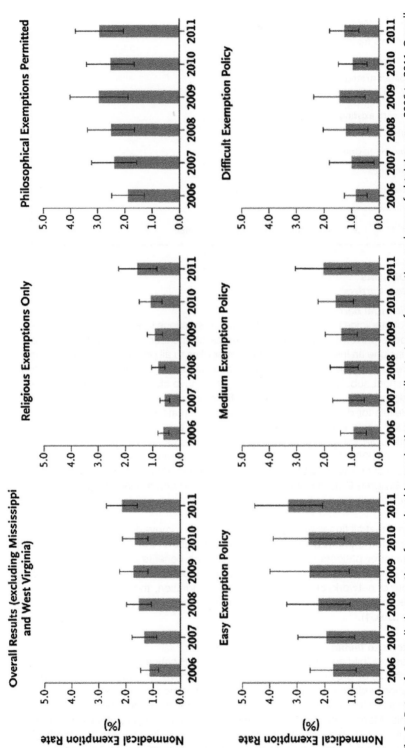

Fig. 2. Rates of nonmedical exemptions from school immunization, according to type of exemption and ease of obtaining one, 2006 to 2011. Overall mean rates of nonmedical exemptions per year for 48 states and the District of Columbia (excluding Mississippi and West Virginia, which do not allow nonmedical exemptions), as well as the rates for the types of exemptions allowed (religious reasons only and philosophic reasons permitted), are shown for the years 2006 to 2011 (top row of graphs). Mean rates of nonmedical exemptions per year according to the level of difficulty (easy, medium, or difficult, as modified from the criteria described by Rota et al.[43]) of the exemption policies are also shown (bottom row of graphs). I bars represent 95% confidence intervals. (*From* Omer SB, Richards JL, Ward M, et al. Vaccination policies and rates of exemption from immunization, 2005–2011. N Engl J Med 2012;367(12):1170; with permission.)

offices; child care centers; school-based health clinics (SBHCs); and, in those states that allow it, pharmacies.

SBHCs are particularly advantageous for adolescent immunizations. Compared with community health centers within a single system, children and adolescents seen in SBHCs were significantly more likely to be up to date and have higher completion rates for vaccines that required multiple doses.[45] Advantages of SBHCs are that patients can be seen over time for multiple visits, which is a benefit especially for older children and adolescents, because follow-up visits are often challenging, disrupting school or parent work schedules, and are often complicated by transportation issues. It is generally simpler to conduct reminder recall for vaccinations in this setting because regular communication to parents is part of the system. In general, SBHCs see patients regardless of their insurance status or ability to pay, potentially removing cost as a barrier. However, many SBHCs lack adequate funding, and many private and public patients do not pay for services received at SBHCs. However, some insurers are now partnering with such groups and providing financial support to ease the strain on busy offices, especially for periodic immunizations such as influenza.

We support policies to help support SBHCs, allowing them to deliver immunizations and other care to underserved children and adolescents. Insurers and other providers should consider supporting such programs as a means to ease congestion in their own offices and promote routine immunizations.

Pharmacists and other ancillary health care providers may also play an important role in improving immunization access. Pharmacists as immunizers have been shown to improve immunization rates in adult populations.[46,47] In the state of Wisconsin, pharmacists can immunize children aged 6 years and older. They serve as additional vaccination sites and provide support for parents whose work hours make it difficult to seek care for their children during clinic hours. A survey of family physicians showed that 95% of physicians were willing to collaborate with nonphysicians to provide out-of-office immunizations. Concerns included being informed about immunizations received outside of their offices, training of nonphysicians to administer immunizations and to respond to potential complications of immunization, and potential loss of preventive health opportunities.[48]

We recommend using alternate sites and expanding the immunization neighborhood.[49] An important component of the success of this method is access to immunization records and the ability to update these in real time. Alternate sites should have access to up-to-date immunization information and also be required to update the child's immunization information at the time of delivery of the vaccine. Use of immunization information systems (immunization registries) is a highly recommended.

Decreasing missed opportunities for immunization

AFIX (assessment, feedback, incentives, exchange) is a CDC quality-improvement program shown by systematic review to increase vaccination rates by a median of 9.4%.[50,51] This dynamic strategy has 4 parts: (1) assessment of the health care provider's vaccination coverage levels and immunization practices, to identify opportunities for improvement of vaccination coverage levels and decrease missed vaccination opportunities; (2) feedback of results to the provider (and ideally other staff, including nurses, clerical staff, and office managers) along with recommended quality-improvement strategies to improve processes, immunization practices, and coverage levels; (3) incentives to recognize and reward improved performance; (4) exchange of information with providers to follow up on their progress toward quality improvement in immunization services and improvement in immunization coverage levels. AFIX visits are expected to address the Healthy People 2020's objectives by increasing the proportion of providers who have had vaccination coverage levels among children in their practice population measured within the past year to 50%, for both public health and private providers.

Provider vaccine education to improve knowledge or change attitudes may include written materials, computerized modules and videos, lectures, and other continuing medical education programs. Used along with feedback (AFIX) they are effective, but significant improvement in rates has not been shown when used alone.[52]

Standing orders are an extremely effective and simple way to increase vaccination rates. They authorize nurses, pharmacists, and other health care personnel (as allowed by state law) to assess a client's immunization status and administer vaccinations according to a protocol approved by an institution or provider without the need for examination or direct order from the provider at the time of the visit. Systematic review of 24 studies showed a 24% (14%–37%) increase in vaccination rates when providers use standing orders.[53]

Reminder recall interventions

Reminder interventions involve communicating to members of a target population that vaccinations are due. Recall actions involve notifying the target population that they are late or overdue for vaccinations. These reminders have typically been delivered by telephone, letters, or postcard, but other newer technologies, such as social media or short message service (SMS) text messages show considerable promise.[54] These communications may be accompanied by educational messages regarding the importance of vaccination, which may also activate other members of these social networks. Multiple studies have shown these interventions to be effective.[55–57] A systematic review by the Task Force on Community Preventive Services showed 6.1% median increase in vaccination coverage with the use of reminder recall interventions.[58]

Although reminder recall interventions have been shown in multiple studies to be highly effective, implementation is challenging for busy pediatric practices, and these tools are underused by clinicians.[59,60] Population-based recalls for immunizations using centralized immunization information systems have been shown to be more effective and cost-effective than practice-based interventions.[61,62] As access to immunization registries has increased, and combined with the broad use of electronic health records (EHRs) required by the ACA, these recall activities may also be conducted by larger health care systems. Although this method seems more cost-effective than the practice-based recall, population-based reminder/recall would still require additional resources. In the future, as technological advancements continue, centralized computer-based reminder systems could be integrated with registries in order to decrease costs.

Provider reminders that individual clients are due for specific vaccinations are also very effective; studies show a median increase in vaccination rates of 10%.[63] Although labor intensive, techniques by which providers can be reminded vary widely, but can include notes posted in client charts, alerts in electronic medical records, and letters sent by post or email.

Expanded use of immunization information systems

Immunization Information Systems (IISs) are an important tool in improving immunization rates and can be effective through multiple capabilities. They are population-based computerized databases that record or collect immunization data from vaccine providers and can interoperate with EHR systems.[64] They are highly effective in increasing vaccination rates and were recommended after systematic review by the Task Force on Community Preventive Services.[65] They can generate vaccination coverage reports and support patient reminder recall systems, as well as provider assessment and feedback (AFIX) and provider reminders. In addition, they offer the capability for providers to determine the vaccination status of children at any location with access to the system (eg, clinics, health departments, schools, pharmacists, and emergency rooms). Other capabilities include identifying missed vaccination opportunities and disparities in vaccination coverage. A Healthy People 2020 target is to increase the proportion of children aged less than 6 years whose immunization records are in fully operational, population-based IIS to 95%.

Legal requirements for immunizations: school requirements, vaccine mandates, and vaccine exemptions

School entry requirements have been used for many years as an effective intervention for improving immunization rates, and offer broad protection for potentially vulnerable populations. Although vaccine mandates (allowing only medical exemptions) have been upheld by courts and have been recommended by professional societies such as the American Medical Association, the American Academy of Pediatrics, the Pediatric Infectious Diseases Society, and the Infectious Diseases Society of America, states in general are wary of mandating a medical intervention without accommodating personal or religious beliefs.

State requirements for school or daycare entry vary. Studies have shown them to be associated with higher immunization rates among preschool-aged children independently of other individual and household factors.[66,67] Thirty-four states currently have middle school requirements for immunization with TdaP.[68] Twelve states have similar requirements for at least 1 dose of meningococcal vaccine and not surprisingly, none have yet to enact a requirement for Human Papilloma Virus (HPV) vaccine. These mandates can potentially generate public discord when the community has not been adequately informed or engaged in the planning of new mandates. Poor community engagement and communication potentially lead to higher rates of nonmedical exemptions, even when there is minimal public disapproval or concern about a vaccine.

Blank and colleagues[31] recommend tightening the process for obtaining nonmedical exemptions and adding a vaccine education component in order to decrease exemption rates. In view of the high costs generated to society by disease outbreaks, related to people who were intentionally unvaccinated, some experts have recommended stronger measures.[69] Constable and colleagues[70] discussed possible solutions for discouraging vaccine exemptions, including penalties (taxes on underimmunized individuals) or incentives (tax cuts for vaccinators, vouchers). These measures have been used in various forms for tobacco use and could be applied at a state level or by insurance companies.

Family/Social Barriers

Socioeconomic barriers

Various strategies have been proposed to address socioeconomic barriers. Case management can be effective but is not necessarily cost-effective.[71] It may be considered for very-high-risk cases but is difficult to implement on a large scale. Community-based strategies, which may be more effective, target certain high-risk communities with low immunization rates and involve integration of immunization promotion into existing community service programs. These strategies identify eligible parents, providing education and reminders about their child's needed immunizations.[72,73]

The ACIP has long recommended that Special Supplemental Nutrition Program for WIC settings should promote vaccination strategies for eligible children at risk for undervaccination.[74] Effective strategies include assessment of a child's immunization status and referral to a provider if underimmunized. Other effective supplemental strategies include monthly vouchers, other parental incentives, outreach, and compliance tracking.[75,76]

Eligible children enrolled in WIC tend to have higher immunization coverage, comparable with more affluent children. However, not all eligible children are benefiting from WIC. A study comparing WIC and non-WIC (but eligible) children estimated that 8% of eligible children never made use of the program and, among disenrolled children, most still met income eligibility requirements. The benefits of WIC participation have been clearly shown to be effective in improving immunization disparities.[77] Strong efforts must be made to identify, enroll, and retain eligible children in WIC in order to benefit from vaccination promotion strategies.

Box 2
Resources

Physician resources

Assessing evidence to improve immunizations:

  http://www.thecommunityguide.org/vaccines/index.html

Talking to parents about immunizations:

  http://www.immunize.org/concerns/comm_talk.asp

  http://shotbyshot.org/

  http://www.voicesforvaccines.org/

  http://www2.aap.org/immunization/pediatricians/refusaltovaccinate.html

Parents' resources for questions about immunization

  http://www.pbs.org/wgbh/nova/body/vaccines-calling-shots.html

  http://www2.aap.org/immunization/multimedia/soundadvice.html

  http://www.vaccinateyourbaby.org/faq/index.cfm

Vaccine hesitancy

Trust in physicians and in medical professionals is central in parent decisions on vaccination. A qualitative study of maternal decision making on vaccines found that factors promoting vaccination included trusting the pediatrician, feeling satisfied by the pediatrician's discussion about vaccine, and not wanting to diverge from the cultural norms. Factors inhibiting a decision to vaccinate were feeling unable to trust the pediatrician, having a trusting relationship with an alternate health care provider or other person who did not believe in vaccinating, anxiety about side effects, beliefs that vaccine-preventable diseases are not serious, and thinking that high vaccination rates decrease children's risk of disease.[30]

Parent education, effective communication, and gaining parental trust are all critical in convincing hesitant parents to immunize. In order to effectively communicate with vaccine-hesitant parents, providers must understand parents' immunization concerns and the influences leading to misinformation (**Box 2**). They should have an open discussion at an early stage and provide clear, easily comprehensible answers about known vaccine side effects, as well as accurate information about vaccine-preventable disease. It is thought that personal stories and images of those affected by vaccine-preventable diseases might be helpful reminders of the importance of immunization. It is thought that these discussions and provider recommendations may reassure some vaccine-hesitant parents about the safety and benefits of vaccines and, more importantly, the risks of vaccine-preventable diseases.[78]

The providers' manner of recommending vaccines may influence parent acceptance as well. An observational study involving videotaped provider-parent vaccine discussions during health supervision visits showed that most providers used a presumptive manner when recommending vaccines (eg, saying, "Well, we have to do some shots") rather than participatory manner (eg, "What do you want to do about shots?"). Parents were more likely to resist vaccine recommendations if the provider used a participatory format.[79]

More research is needed to understand how to individualize these findings effectively. A systematic review in 2012 by Sadaf and colleagues[80] concluded that there is a need for randomized controlled trials to evaluate interventions to address parental vaccine refusal and hesitancy, assessing their impact on vaccination rates among refusing parents. Parents of children considering exemptions should be targeted with extra effort to provide them with accurate information from sources that they trust.[36]

SUMMARY/DISCUSSION

No single strategy is sufficient to improve immunization rates and decrease disparities; multiple strategies are needed. Vaccines need to be accessible, and available at multiple sites, including the medical home as well as alternate providers such as pharmacies, WIC settings, and schools. They should be provided with no financial burden to families. Vaccine status should be assessed and vaccines given in a timely fashion at all possible opportunities. All efforts should be made for reminder and recall of children due for vaccines, not only at a clinic level but also by the use of IIS at a state level.

It should be recognized that pockets of underimmunization can still occur, not just in poor urban areas but in geographic clusters of vaccine hesitancy and refusal. Further research is needed to effectively address the concerns of vaccine-hesitant parents and communicate effectively with these families. In addition, state legal immunization requirements for daycares and schools should be encouraged and strengthened, and nonmedical exemptions discouraged. The role of IIS in these efforts is vital because broad use of IIS makes it possible to access immunization information at multiple sites, conduct reminder recall, and assess vaccination rates at various levels to identify areas of need. At present IIS are state based; a national system would enable sharing of immunization data across state borders.

REFERENCES

1. Centers for Disease Control and Prevention. Ten great public health achievements–United States, 2001-2010. MMWR Morb Mortal Wkly Rep 2011;60(19): 619–23.
2. Elam-Evans LD, Yankey D, Singleton JA, et al. National, state, and selected local area vaccination coverage among children aged 19–35 months—United States, 2013. MMWR Morb Mortal Wkly Rep 2014;63(34):741–8.
3. Roush SW, Murphy TV, Vaccine-Preventable Disease Table Working Group. Historical comparisons of morbidity and mortality for vaccine preventable diseases in the United States. JAMA 2007;298(18):2155–63.
4. Zhou F, Santoli J, Messonnier ML, et al. Economic evaluation of the 7-vaccine routine childhood immunization schedule in the United States, 2001. Arch Pediatr Adolesc Med 2005;159(12):1136–44.

5. Elam-Evans LD, Yankey D, Jeyarajah J, et al. National, regional, state, and selected local area vaccination coverage among adolescents aged 13–17 years—United States, 2013. MMWR Morb Mortal Wkly Rep 2014;63(29):625–33.

6. Findley SE, Irigoyen M, Stockwell MS, et al. Changes in childhood immunization disparities between central cities and their respective states, 2000 versus 2006. J Urban Health 2009;86(2):183–95.

7. Santoli JM, Setia S, Rodewald LE, et al. Immunization pockets of need: science and practice. Am J Prev Med 2000;19(suppl 3):89–98.

8. Rosenthal J, Raymond D, Morita J, et al. African-American children are at risk of a measles outbreak in an inner-city community of Chicago, 2000. Am J Prev Med 2002;23(3):195–9.

9. Lieu TA, Ray GT, Klein NP, et al. Geographic clusters in underimmunization and vaccine refusal. Pediatrics 2015;135:280–9.

10. Hinman AR, Orenstein WA, Rodewald L. Financing immunizations in the United States. Clin Infect Dis 2004;38(10):1440–6.

11. Available at: http://www.cdc.gov/vaccines/programs/vfc/awardees/vaccine-management/price-list/index.html. Accessed January 12, 2015.

12. Available at: http://www.hhs.gov/healthcare/facts/factsheets/2010/09/The-Affordable-Care-Act-and-Immunization.html. Accessed January 12, 2015.

13. Available at: http://www.immunize.org/presentations/tan_impact_ACA_immunizations.pdf. Accessed January 12, 2015.

14. Available at: http://www.cdc.gov/vaccines/schedules/downloads/child/0-18yrs-child-combined-schedule.pdf. Accessed January 12, 2015.

15. Wood D, Pereyra M, Halfon N, et al. Vaccination levels in Los Angeles public health centers: the contribution of missed opportunities to vaccinate and other factors. Am J Public Health 1995;85:850–3.

16. Fu LY, Zook K, Gingold J, et al. Frequent vaccination missed opportunities at primary care encounters contribute to underimmunization. J Pediatr 2015;166:412–7.

17. Holt E, Guyer B, Hughart N, et al. The contribution of missed opportunities to childhood underimmunization in Baltimore. Pediatrics 1996;97(4):474–80.

18. Santibanez TA, Shefer A, Briere EC, et al. Effects of a nationwide Hib vaccine shortage on vaccination coverage in the United States. Vaccine 2012;30(5):941–7.

19. Fairbrother G, Donauer S, Staat MA, et al. Cincinnati pediatricians' measured and reported immunizing behavior for children during the national shortages of pneumococcal conjugate vaccine. Vaccine 2013;31(17):2177–83.

20. Zimmerman RK, Tabbarah M, Bardenheier B, et al. The 2002 United States varicella vaccine shortage and physician recommendations for vaccination. Prev Med 2005;41(2):575–82.

21. Kempe A, Daley MF, Stokley S, et al. Impact of a severe influenza vaccine shortage on primary care practice. Am J Prev Med 2007;33(6):486–91.

22. Bardenheier BH, Yusuf HR, Rosenthal J, et al. Factors associated with underimmunization at 3 months of age in four medically underserved areas. Public Health Rep 2004;119(5):479–85.

23. Feemster KA, Spain CV, Eberhart M, et al. Identifying infants at increased risk for late initiation of immunizations: maternal and provider characteristics. Public Health Rep 2009;124(1):42–53.

24. Wheeler M, Buttenheim AM. Parental vaccine concerns, information source, and choice of alternative immunization schedules. Hum Vaccin Immunother 2013;9(8):1782–9.

25. Fredrickson DD, Davis TC, Arnould CL, et al. Childhood immunization refusal: provider and parent perceptions. Fam Med 2004;36:431–9.

26. Gust DA, Woodruff R, Kennedy A, et al. Parental perceptions surrounding risks and benefits of immunization. Semin Pediatr Infect Dis 2003;14:207–12.
27. Gust DA, Darling N, Kennedy A, et al. Parents with doubts about vaccines: which vaccines and reasons why. Pediatrics 2008;122:718–25.
28. Sears RW. The vaccine book: making the right decision for your child. New York: Little, Brown; 2007.
29. Luthy KE, Beckstrand RL, Meyers CJH. Common perceptions of parents requesting personal exemption from vaccination. J Sch Nurs 2012;29(2):95–103.
30. Benin A, Wisler-Scher D, Colson E, et al. Qualitative analysis of mothers' decision making about vaccines for infants: the importance of trust. Pediatrics 2006;117:1532–41.
31. Blank NR, Caplan AL, Constable C. Exempting schoolchildren from immunizations: states with few barriers had highest rates of nonmedical exemptions. Health Aff 2013;32:1282–90.
32. Omer SB, Richards JL, Ward M, et al. Vaccination policies and rates of exemption from immunization, 2005-2011. N Engl J Med 2012;367(12):1170–1.
33. Omer SB, Pan WKY, Halsey NA, et al. Nonmedical exemptions to school immunization requirements: secular trends and association of state policies with pertussis incidence. JAMA 2006;296(14):1757–63.
34. Omer SB, Peterson D, Curran EA, et al. Legislative challenges to school immunization mandates, 2009-2012. JAMA 2014;311(6):620–1.
35. Atwell JE, Otterloo JV, Zipprich J, et al. Nonmedical vaccine exemptions and pertussis in California, 2010. Pediatrics 2013;132:624–30.
36. Salmon DA, Moulton LH, Omer SB, et al. Factors associated with refusal of childhood vaccines among parents of school-aged children: a case-control study. Arch Pediatr Adolesc Med 2005;159(5):470–6.
37. Molinari NA, Kolasa M, Messonnier ML, et al. Out-of-pocket costs of childhood immunizations: a comparison by type of insurance plan. Pediatrics 2007;120(5):e1148–56.
38. Available at: http://www.thecommunityguide.org/vaccines/RRclientoutofpocketcosts.html. Accessed January 12, 2015.
39. Briss PA, Rodewald LE, Hinman AR, et al. Reviews of evidence regarding interventions to improve vaccination coverage in children, adolescents, and adults. Am J Prev Med 2000;18(1S):97–140.
40. Lindley MC, Shen AK, Orenstein WA, et al. Financing the delivery of vaccines to children and adolescents: challenges to the current system. Pediatrics 2009;124(Suppl 5):S548–57.
41. Shortridge EF, Moore JR, Whitmore H, et al. Policy implications of first-dollar coverage: a qualitative examination from the payer perspective. Public Health Rep 2011;126(3):394–9.
42. National Vaccine Advisory Committee. Standards for child and adolescent immunization practices. Pediatrics 2003;112:958–63.
43. Rota JS, Salmon DA, Rodewald LE, et al. Processes for obtaining nonmedical exemptions to state immunization laws. Am J Public Health 2001;91:645–8.
44. American Academy of Pediatrics. Policy statement: increasing immunization coverage committee on practice and ambulatory medicine and council on community pediatrics. Pediatrics 2010;125(6):1295–304.
45. Federico SG, Abrams L, Everhart RM, et al. Addressing adolescent immunization disparities: a retrospective analysis of school-based health center immunization delivery. Am J Public Health 2010;100(9):1630–4.
46. Higginbotham S, Stewart A, Pfalzgraf A. Impact of a pharmacist immunizer on adult immunization rates. J Am Pharm Assoc 2003;2012(52):367–71.

47. Taitela M, Cohen E, Duncanc I, et al. Pharmacists as providers: targeting pneu-mococcal vaccinations to high risk populations. Vaccine 2011;29(45):8073–6.
48. Bergus GR, Ernst ME, Sorofman BA. Physician perceptions about administration of immunizations outside of physician offices. Prev Med 2001;32(3):255–61.
49. Bobo N. Increasing immunization rates through the immunization neighborhood recognizing school-located immunization programs. NASN Sch Nurse 2014; 29(5):224–8.
50. Available at: http://www.cdc.gov/vaccines/programs/afix/about/overview.html.
51. Available at: http://www.thecommunityguide.org/vaccines/providerassessment.html.
52. Available at: http://www.thecommunityguide.org/vaccines/providereducation.html.
53. Available at: http://www.thecommunityguide.org/vaccines/standingorders.html.
54. Stockwell MS, Kharbanda EO, Martinez RA, et al. Text4Health: impact of text message reminder-recalls for pediatric and adolescent immunizations. Am J Public Health 2012;102(2):e15–21.
55. Szilagyi PG, Bordley C, Vann JC, et al. Effect of patient reminder/recall interventions on immunization rates: a review. JAMA 2000;284(14):1820–7.
56. Szilagyi P, Vann J, Bordley C, et al. Interventions aimed at improving immunization rates. Cochrane Database Syst Rev 2002;(4):CD003941.
57. Jacobson Vann JC, Szilagyi P. Patient reminder and patient recall systems to improve immunization rates: edited 2009. Cochrane Database Syst Rev 2009;(3):CD003941.
58. Available at: http://www.thecommunityguide.org/vaccines/clientreminder.html. Accessed January 12, 2015.
59. Tierney CD, Yusuf H, McMahon SR, et al. Adoption of reminder and recall messages for immunizations by pediatricians and public health clinics. Pediatrics 2003;112(5):1076–82.
60. Saville AW, Albright K, Nowels C, et al. Getting under the hood: exploring issues that affect provider-based recall using an immunization information system. Acad Pediatr 2011;11(1):44–9.
61. Kempe A, Saville A, Dickinson LM, et al. Population-based versus practice-based recall for childhood immunizations: a randomized controlled comparative effectiveness trial. Am J Public Health 2013;103(6):1116–23.
62. Suh CA, Saville A, Daley MF, et al. Effectiveness and net cost of reminder/recall for adolescent immunizations. Pediatrics 2012;129(6):e1437–45.
63. Available at: http://www.thecommunityguide.org/vaccines/providerreminder.html. Accessed January 12, 2015.
64. Centers for Disease Control and Prevention. Progress in immunization information systems - United States, 2010. MMWR Morb Mortal Wkly Rep 2012;61(25):464–7.
65. Groom H, Hopkins DP, Pabst LJ, et al. Immunization information systems to increase vaccination rates: a community guide systematic review. J Public Health Manag Pract 2015;21(3):1–22.
66. Davis MM, Gaglia MA. Associations of daycare and school entry vaccination requirements with varicella immunization rates. Vaccine 2005;23(23):3053–60.
67. Wilson TR, Fishbein DB, Ellis PA, et al. The impact of a school entry law on adolescent immunization rates. J Adolesc Health 2005;37(6):511–6.
68. Available at: http://www2a.cdc.gov/nip/schoolsurv/schImmRqmt.asp. Accessed January 12, 2015.
69. Sugerman DE, Barskey AE, Delea MG, et al. Measles outbreak in a highly vaccinated population, San Diego, 2008: role of the intentionally undervaccinated. Pediatrics 2010;125:747–55.

70. Constable C, Blank NR, Caplan AL. Rising rates of vaccine exemptions: problems with current policy and more promising remedies. Vaccine 2014;32:1793–7.
71. Wood D, Halfon N, Donald-Sherbourne C, et al. Increasing immunization rates among inner-city, African American children. A randomized trial of case management. JAMA 1998;279(1):29–34.
72. Findley SE, Irigoyen M, Sanchez M, et al. Community-based strategies to reduce childhood immunization disparities. Health Promot Pract 2006;7(3 Suppl): 191S–200S.
73. Findley SE, Irigoyen M, Sanchez M, et al. Effectiveness of a community coalition for improving child vaccination rates in New York City. Am J Public Health 2008; 98(11):1959–62.
74. Centers for Disease Control and Prevention (CDC). Recommendations of the Advisory Committee on Immunization Practices: programmatic strategies to increase vaccination coverage by age 2 years—linkage of vaccination and WIC services. MMWR Morb Mortal Wkly Rep 1996;45(10):217–8.
75. George T, Shefer A, Rickert D, et al. A status report from 1996-2004: are more effective immunization interventions being used in the Women, Infants, and Children (WIC) Program? Matern Child Health J 2007;11(4):327–33.
76. Hutchins SS, Rosenthal J, Eason P, et al. Effectiveness and cost-effectiveness of linking the Special Supplemental Program for Women, Infants, and Children (WIC) and immunization activities. J Public Health Policy 1999;20(4):408–26.
77. Thomas TN, Kolasa MS, Zhang F, et al. Assessing immunization interventions in the Women, Infants, and Children (WIC) Program. Am J Prev Med 2014;47(5): 624–8.
78. Healy CM, Pickering LK. How to communicate with vaccine-hesitant parents. Pediatrics 2011;127(Suppl 1):S127–33.
79. Opel DJ, Heritage J, Taylor JA, et al. The architecture of provider-parent vaccine discussions at health supervision visits. Pediatrics 2013;132(6):1037–46.
80. Sadaf A, Richards JL, Glanz J, et al. A systematic review of interventions for reducing parental vaccine refusal and vaccine hesitancy. Vaccine 2013;31(40): 4293–304.

Childhood Poverty

Understanding and Preventing the Adverse Impacts of a Most-Prevalent Risk to Pediatric Health and Well-Being

Adam Schickedanz, MD[a,b], Benard P. Dreyer, MD[c],*,
Neal Halfon, MD, MPH[d]

KEYWORDS

- Poverty • Income • Low-income • Financial assets • Social determinants of health
- Life course

KEY POINTS

- Children living in poor households are at greater risk for worse health, less productivity, and harms to well-being far into adulthood and on into subsequent generations.
- Timing and duration of poverty matter for outcomes throughout the life course, especially for education attainment, health, and lifetime productivity.
- Attention must be focused on interventions at the levels of policy advocacy and the pediatric health delivery system on ways to protect the health and well-being of children and families in economic hardship from the dynamic disadvantages and trauma wrought by poverty.
- A framework for the prevention of child poverty and its dangerous consequences for lifelong health and success on a national scale is presented.

INTRODUCTION

Poverty is the most pervasive of risks for America's children. It routinely cuts short children's lives, ravages the health of families, and blights communities to the detriment of society as a whole. However, the hazards of poverty for child health and well-being are preventable. This has been recognized by pediatricians for more than a century. Abraham Jacobi, a founder of modern pediatrics in America, was born into poverty

Disclosure: none.
[a] Department of Pediatrics, UCLA David Geffen School of Medicine, 10833 Le Conte Ave, Los Angeles, CA 90095, USA; [b] Department of Internal Medicine, UCLA David Geffen School of Medicine, 10833 Le Conte Ave, Los Angeles, CA 90095, USA; [c] Department of Pediatrics, NYU School of Medicine, Bellevue Hospital Center, 550 First Avenue, New York, NY 10016, USA; [d] UCLA David Geffen School of Medicine, Public Health, and Public Policy, 10833 Le Conte Ave, Los Angeles, CA 90095, USA
* Corresponding author.
E-mail address: bpd1@nyumc.org

Pediatr Clin N Am 62 (2015) 1111–1135
http://dx.doi.org/10.1016/j.pcl.2015.05.008
0031-3955/15/$ – see front matter © 2015 Elsevier Inc. All rights reserved.

pediatric.theclinics.com

and was an outspoken advocate for the needs of low-income orphans. A principle area of advocacy for the American Academy of Pediatrics today continues to be elimination of child poverty and its preventable ills. Although the notion that the harms of poverty are preventable is not new, today, more than ever, pediatricians have the capability to reduce the ills that low-income children suffer. With more than 1 in 5 of the nation's children living in poverty and nearly half of families struggling to make ends meet on a low income, the pediatrician's ability to intervene could not come at a more critical time.

Decades of evidence make clear that the harms of poverty are much more than a matter of unidimensional material and financial shortage but, instead, are an encompassing and unremitting experience of disadvantage, trauma, and disease. Shortage of capital can be expected to lead to significant health harms and functional limitations in a society in which nearly every basic transaction is monetary. The reality that poverty undergirds and entrenches pediatric disease at all levels is more apparent than ever based on new evidence into the direct, indirect, and contextual effects of poverty; the lifelong harms of poverty that compound over sequential sensitive periods of child development; and the knowledge of what works to reduce the prevalence and complications of poverty.

This article reviews this evidence, presents promising programs to prevent harms of poverty, and outlines a comprehensive framework for child poverty prevention, including a vision of the ways pediatricians can protect the health of low-income children through innovation and action.

DEFINING THE EXTENT OF CHILDHOOD POVERTY

About 15 million, or 1 in 5, American children live below the federal poverty line (FPL).[1] Children are the poorest of all age groups in the United States, where the child poverty rate ranks among the very worst in the developed world.[2] Other first-world nations with similar child poverty rates, such as the United Kingdom,[3] have managed to reverse course as a result of concerted public and political leadership. Yet, in the United States the number of poor children has remained persistently high for decades.

As staggering as the nation's child poverty rate is, the standard measure of poverty used, the FPL, actually significantly underestimates the number of families in economic need. The FPL was created in the mid-1960s, when the economic demands on families were far fewer than today. At the time, food costs represented about a third of a family's budget and the pretax income poverty threshold (the FPL) was simply estimated to be the cost of the minimal adequate food intake multiplied by 3 and adjusted for family size. The FPL represented about half of the median household income when it was devised. However, because its calculation has changed little aside from adjustments for inflation, it is now equivalent to less than a third of median income.[4] Without adjustments to reflect the growth in the cost of raising children and the range of expenses facing families, changes in acceptable living standards, and place-based variation in cost of living, the FPL measure is now seen as too simplistic and too low in real dollars. Nevertheless, it continues to be the conventional needs test for myriad program eligibility, simultaneously entrenching its position as the prevailing poverty benchmark and justifying limited access to programs for many low-income families that could benefit.

Alternative poverty measures exist to address the practical and policy limitations of the FPL and delineate the population of poor children (**Fig. 1**). If the poverty line were still set at half of median income, as it was initially intended in the United States and as has become common in most developed nations, 1 in 3 American children would be

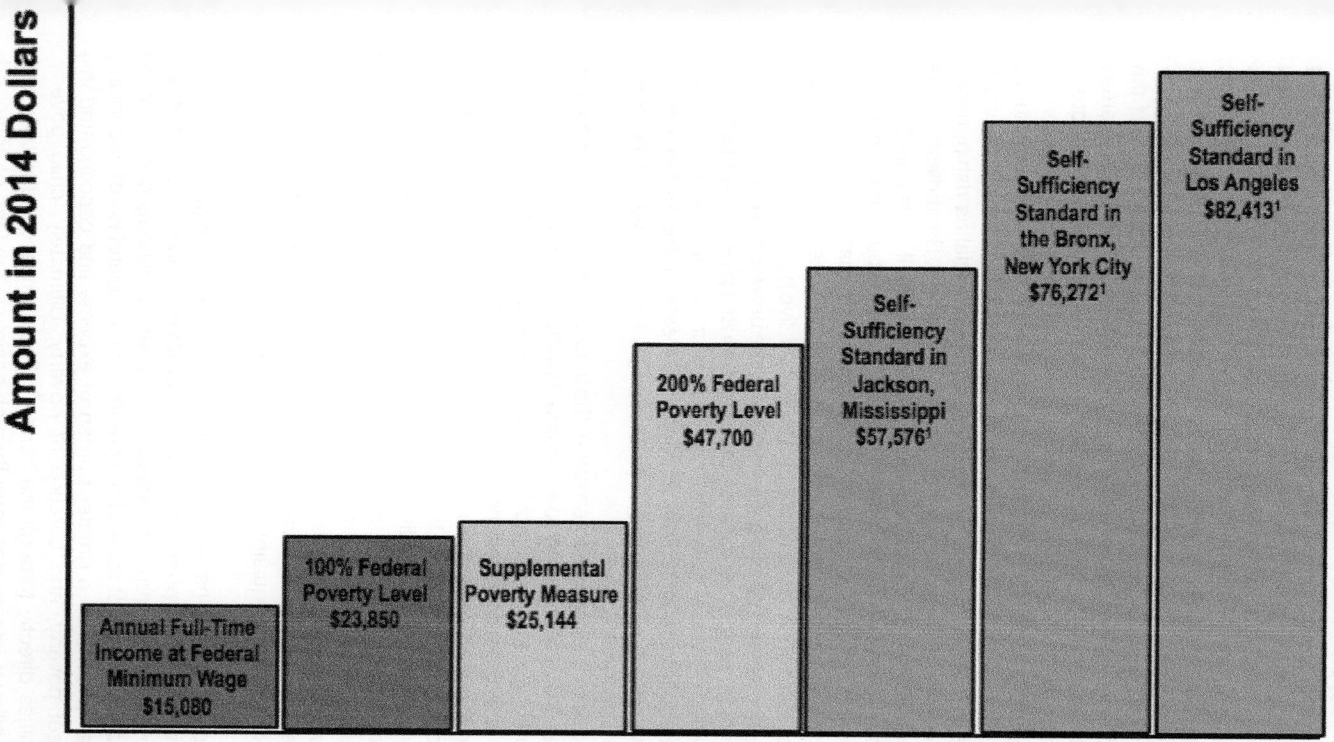

Amount in 2014 Dollars

- Self-Sufficiency Standard in Los Angeles $82,413[1]
- Self-Sufficiency Standard in the Bronx, New York City $76,272[1]
- Self-Sufficiency Standard in Jackson, Mississippi $57,576[1]
- 200% Federal Poverty Level $47,700
- Supplemental Poverty Measure $25,144
- 100% Federal Poverty Level $23,850
- Annual Full-Time Income at Federal Minimum Wage $15,080

References:

1. Cooper D. The minimum wage used to keep workers out of poverty — It's not anymore. 2013. Economic Policy Institute. http://www.epi.org/publication/minimum-wage-workers-poverty-anymore-raising/

2. Center for Women's Welfare Mississippi, New York City, and Los Angeles self-sufficiency standard calculators. http://www.selfsufficiencystandard.org/pubs.html

Fig. 1. Amount in 2014 dollars of standard and alternative poverty measures for an American family of 2 parents and 2 preschool age children renting a home. (*Data from* Cooper D. The minimum wage used to keep workers out of poverty – It's not anymore. Economic Policy Institute. December 14, 2013. Accessed: http://www.epi.org/publication/minimum-wage-workers-poverty-anymore-raising/. Accessed February 16, 2015. Data collected from self-sufficiency standard wage calculators for Jackson, MS (http://mepconline.org/self-sufficiency-standard/basic-economic-security-calculator), New York, NY (http://www.wceca.org/self_sufficiency.php), and Los Angeles, CA (http://www.insightcced.org/calculator.html) based on a 2 parent, 2 preschool child family renting a home.)

considered poor.[2] If the poverty line reflected the cost of food, clothing, shelter, medical costs, and other basics, as many economists have suggested, it would also exceed the FPL. The Supplemental Poverty Measure (SPM)[5] is a step in the right direction that defines the poverty line as the national average cost of a minimum set of basic expenses for families at the 33rd income percentile, with those earning less than the cost of those basic expenses being considered poor.[6] The SPM also counts as income those government in-kind benefits that support the family. However, this measure omits key expenses like child care and insurance premiums[7] without completely accounting for regional variation in costs of living.[8] Minimum family incomes needed to maintain an acceptable standard of living vary from 163% of the FPL in more affordable cities like Casper, Wyoming, to 338% of FPL in high-cost areas like Boston, Massachusetts.[9] The most complete measures of minimum adequate family income, such as the Self-Sufficiency Standard, include all necessary expenses found in basic family budgets, such as child care, transportation, insurance premiums, and taxes. A third to half of all families earn less than the Self-Sufficiency Standard. Considering income as well as savings needed to weather financial hardship, nearly half of American households experience liquid-asset poverty.[10] Regardless of the measure, with so many families struggling to get by economically, it is clear that financial hardship is not the exception for children in the United States but is often the rule.

Two hundred percent of the FPL is used as a conservative estimate by researchers, federal agencies, and in public polls as the lowest family income needed to make ends meet.[11] Forty-four percent of American children, nearly half, live below 200% of FPL,[12] often called the low-income standard. Families with income between 100% and 200% of the FPL are considered near-poor because they can be just a pink slip, traffic ticket, or medical bill away from financial collapse. Children in near-poor families often suffer adverse health and educational outcomes at roughly the same rates as those living below the FPL,[13] consistent with the ample evidence that these children experience comparable levels of economic stress.

As the range of poverty measures demonstrate, the impact of economic hardship is not only experienced below a particular low-income threshold but toxic stress is also meted out in proportion to a person's position along the entire length of the income gradient. When half of all children experience significant health risks as a consequence of their socioeconomic position, the notion of a threshold begins to lose meaning while the pitch of the gradient itself becomes the more salient issue. Emerging understandings of how poverty and income inequality affect population health explain how absolute income effects, relative income effects, and contextual effects of income inequality[14] contribute substantively to the risk of low birth weight, infant mortality, child injuries, abuse, teen births, obesity, and low achievement.[15,16] Accordingly, the children at highest risk live in areas with both high rates of absolute income poverty and a high degree of income inequality. Effective solutions will have to address both issues.

Child poverty and low income have effects that ripple across all segments of society. Some groups bear a disproportionate burden, however. Children younger than 5 years (1 in 4 below FPL), children in historically underserved minority communities (more than 1 in 3), and children of recent immigrants (1 in 3, regardless of documentation status)[17–19] all experience a greater burden of extreme and concentrated income poverty, asset poverty, and duration of poverty. Ultimately, child poverty affects all communities directly through the harms to impoverished individuals and indirectly through spillover effects that carry through society in the form of untapped human capital and hamstrung collective economic productivity.[20,21] One way or another, child poverty affects us all.

THE IMPACT OF POVERTY ON HEALTH AND WELL-BEING

Pediatricians are well aware of the health consequences of child poverty. The leading causes of childhood chronic disease and mortality seen in pediatrics every day, including prematurity, obesity, asthma, developmental delay, failure to thrive, accidents, and many more, are strongly linked to being poor, with rates many times higher among low-income children (**Table 1**). Equally critical are poverty's impacts on overall well-being, such as failing academic attainment and exposure to emotional trauma, because they will shape children's lifelong health trajectories well into adulthood, predisposing them to intergenerational cycles of poverty. Although the consequences of childhood illness for health into adulthood are well-recognized as targets for prevention, recent evidence describing the mechanisms through which poverty affects lifelong health trajectories and the onset and severity of disease offers new opportunities for disease prevention.

Child Health

Poverty is a dominant determinant of child health. Income-poor children are more likely to be born preterm, be chronically ill,[22] be physically impaired,[23] have greater health care needs,[24] experience physical and emotional trauma,[25] have cognitive impairment,[26] and lack resources to overcome these challenges.[27] Furthermore, the mean relative health status of children living in poverty is measurably worse from the time of birth, compared with income-sufficient children. This health gap worsens as illness burdens grow over time.[28]

Child Well-Being

Poverty affects well-being, family functioning, and a child's experience of their environment in a variety of adverse ways. Not only are poor children exposed to greater threats to lifelong well-being, they also lack protective factors available to their income-sufficient peers (**Fig. 2**). Children in poverty have the deck stacked against them from the earliest age. Indeed, research on the intrauterine environment has demonstrated a link between maternal deprivation from poverty in utero, adverse neuroendocrine exposures to the fetus, and later deficits in child health, cognition, and well-being.[29]

Learning and Development

Poverty has pervasive effects on children's experiences and environments that directly shape the developing mind and its functioning.[26] Chronic financial stress has been shown to affect integral regions of the growing brain that develop sequentially,[30,31] likely leading to cascading periods of sensitivity to poverty during critical developmental windows of childhood. Due to these early neurodevelopmental changes, diminished access to high-quality preschool, and poorer early learning environments, children growing up in poverty are more likely to fall behind their academic peers in the first years of life. By preschool, children from low-income families already lag about a year behind income-sufficient children in language development.[32] On entering kindergarten, poor children score 50% lower on common cognitive measures, on average, than high-income peers.[33] By third grade, three-quarters of the children with literacy skills in the bottom quartile are from low-income families, and this gap only grows over time.[34] These early disadvantages are reinforced by underfunded and low-performing schools in low-income areas[35] that struggle to retain well-qualified teachers.[36,37] By the end of high school, 5 times as many low-income children will have dropped out, whereas those who do graduate lag 4 grade levels

Table 1
Relative risk (unadjusted) of common pediatric conditions and diagnoses for children below 100% compared with those above 400% of the Federal Poverty Level, based on 2011-2012 National Survey of Children's Health data

	Parent-Rated Fair or Poor Child Health (%)	Developmental Delay Ages 2–17 (%)	Moderate or Severe Developmental Delay Ages 2–17 (%)	Asthma (%)	Moderate or Severe Asthma (%)	Obesity Ages 10–17 (%)	Learning Disability Ages 3–17 (%)	Behavioral or Conduct Problem (%)
Prevalence at 100% FPL	7.1	4.7	3.2	11.6	4.6	26.6	12.2	5.6
Prevalence at ≥400% FPL	0.8	2.6	1.2	7.3	1.2	9	5.6	1.3
Relative Risk	8.88	1.80	2.66	1.59	3.83	2.95	2.12	4.3

Data from the Child and Adolescent Health Measurement Initiative. Data resource center for child & adolescent health. Available at: http://www.childhealthdata.org/browse/survey/.

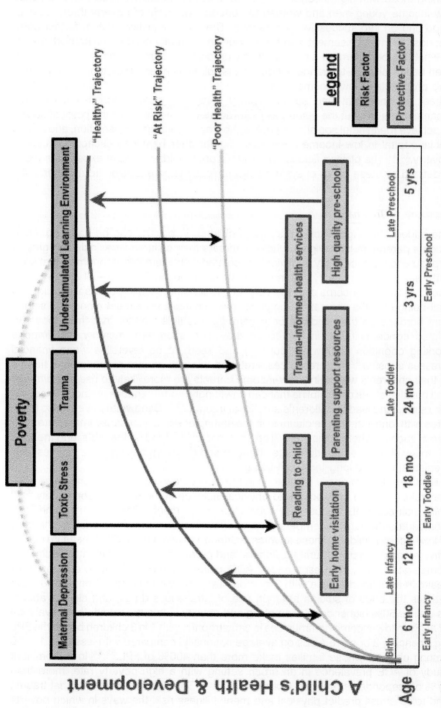

Fig. 2. Risk and protective factors in the health development of children in poverty. Healthy, at-risk, or poor health trajectories for children depending on the relative complement of risk and protective factors. Children with more protective factors will tend to enter a healthier trajectory. Poverty exerts a key risk that can create a risk cascade. (*Adapted from* Halfon N, Larson K, Lu M, et al. Lifecourse health development: past, present, and future. Matern Child Health J 2014;18:344–65.)

behind those with high-income.[38,39] These deficits in academic attainment sentence low-income young men and women to continue the cycle of poverty through adulthood and on into successive generations. The criminal justice system further compounds disenfranchisement and traps poor and minority children disproportionately in what has been termed a poverty-to-prison pipeline, criminalizing low-income children based on zero-tolerance academic discipline as a fast-track to incarceration.[40] Job prospects in low-income neighborhoods are limited by fewer opportunities for career advancement and social mobility. Stagnant local economies leave low-income areas without the resources to attract new investments or the political capital to achieve meaningful social change. Neighborhood segregation, isolation, and lack of social capital in low-income areas raise barrier after barrier to escaping cycles of poverty.[25,41] The playing field is not level for poor children, whose experience today is defined by these layers of systemic discrimination and exclusion from opportunity.

Exposure to Trauma

The added challenges facing parents of children in poverty can be daunting. Low-income parents must navigate a host of threats their children face, including greater exposure to violence, risky behaviors associated with alternative economies that arise in the setting of community material scarcity, and emotional trauma—all with fewer resources. These concerns over the very real threats that face impoverished children's well-being plus the constant struggle to make financial ends meet amount to significant burdens on the minds of poor parents. It is little wonder that these poverty-related concerns result in immediate draws on short-term memory that impede working cognition (bandwidth poverty) and seem to be reversible when financial stresses subside.[42] With resources stretched thin and greater environmental threats to their children's well-being, low-income parents are more likely to use authoritarian and punitive styles of discipline that can unwittingly model negative methods of coping with stress and lead to children's emotional trauma.[43,44] Bandwidth poverty also interferes with long-term future planning in the setting of scarcity because immediate concerns, such as whether the bus will arrive, there will be food on the table, and the walk to work will be safe, can dominate attention and decision-making more than less immediate threats to long-term well-being.

Risk of trauma is nearly ubiquitous in the lives of low-income children. These risks may take the form of exposure to physical violence in the home or community,[45,46] child maltreatment,[47] household substance use,[48] mental illness in the home,[49] or incarceration of family members,[50] all of which occur much more often in the lives of low-income children. These adverse childhood experiences (ACEs) measure cumulative emotional trauma during childhood and predict physical and mental health outcomes later in life. With each added ACE, children are more likely to develop poor health in adulthood. Those with 2 or more carry double the odds of depression and 4 times the odds of suicide attempt, use of intravenous drugs, and alcohol abuse, as well as 50% higher odds of smoking and obesity.[51] In this context, the prevalence of ACEs in low-income communities is catastrophic, with 1 in 3 children below the FPL experiencing 2 or more ACEs on average nationally, compared with less than 1 in 10 among children whose families make more than 400% of FPL.[52–54] In a prominent study of ACE prevalence in an urban setting with a high poverty rate, more than 37% of respondents reported 4 or more ACEs.[55] Through understanding that trauma and toxic stress predict physical and mental illness risk, the ways in which poverty harms childhood well-being lay the foundation for harms to physical health in childhood and later in life are becoming clear.[56]

Biochemical Mechanisms, Developmental Windows, and Adult Health

Poverty not only reduces life chances, it steals years off lives. Life expectancy for those in poverty is more than half a decade shorter than people with sufficient income.[57,58] No single mechanism accounts for all of the health harms of poverty over the life course. Instead, a host of root causes of early morbidity and mortality coalesce to disproportionately afflict low-income individuals and communities. Although deprivation of basic needs and resources (eg, nutrition, shelter, clothing, access to medical care, and safe environments for healthy living) plays a major part in precipitating premature onset of chronic disease and accelerating illness severity, this does not fully explain the income-related health disparities observed in nearly every common adult disease category.[13,59,60] Allostatic load and toxic stress, terms for poverty's adverse interpersonal and environmental exposures with resultant chronic endocrine and inflammatory effects, also play a central role to increase disease risk at the biochemical level and compound the harms of basic needs privation affecting lifelong health.[61]

The effects of poverty and toxic stress get under the skin, affecting physiologic and endocrine systems to alter health at a biochemical level. Poor children and adults have consistently higher and more reactive levels of serum cortisol,[62] the primary terminal stress hormone, resulting in impaired immune defenses,[63] aberrant cellular inflammation,[64] and dysregulation of metabolism and proper energy storage.[65] By adulthood, sympathetic dysfunction and elevated norepinephrine and epinephrine levels are often seen for individuals living under the chronic stress of poverty,[66] carrying greater risk for myocardial infarction and stroke.[67] These biochemical changes result in higher fasting glucose, triglyceride, and C-reactive protein levels[68] that correspond both in childhood and adulthood with higher rates of diabetes, obesity, and cardiovascular disease.[69,70] Consistent with cumulative cell injury from this biochemical wear-and-tear, chromosomes of individuals in with lower socioeconomic status show early shortening of telomeres, a marker of accelerated cellular senescence.[71–73]

Ample evidence suggests biochemical harms of childhood poverty are persistent and detrimental, and poverty in early childhood is consistently the most harmful.[74,75] Early childhood seems to offer a window of epigenetic and immunologic patterning particularly vulnerable to the disruptive stress of poverty. A bulk of evidence demonstrates the strongest correlations between poor adult health and poverty in early childhood,[61] as do studies showing early poverty results in dysregulation of proinflammatory and glucocorticoid pathway genetic loci along with increased risk of immune-mediated chronic conditions.[76,77] Although persistent poverty during the entire life course is the strongest predictor of poor health overall, time spent impoverished in early childhood seems to most predictably alter physiologic and neuroendocrine function.[78] The existence of specific sensitive periods of health development during which adverse epigenetic and neuroendocrine changes are biologically embedded in response to nutritional or emotional strain has led to a reconceptualization of how social exposures alter life course health development.[79–83] Although it is important to understand that these trajectories are embedded early on, it is equally important to remember that they are by no means immutable.

PREVENTION OF CHILD POVERTY AND ITS ADVERSE EFFECTS ON HEALTH AND WELL-BEING

How can pediatricians intervene to reduce child poverty and mitigate its harms? Given what is known about the widespread prevalence of financial hardship and its effects on children's lives, the most challenging decision may be how to begin. There is no single right place to start to prevent the harms of poverty. Poverty's impact on multiple domains of social determinants, child health, and family well-being means there is no simple silver bullet. Solving such a multifaceted problem requires a multifaceted approach.

A Prevention Framework for Action to Reduce Child Poverty and Its Harms to Health and Well-Being

Child poverty in America behaves much like a highly prevalent chronic condition that, along with its complications for health and well-being, is driven and compounded in severity by the architecture of public policies and harmful dynamics of economic inequality and disadvantage. We propose a strategic framework for the prevention of child poverty, its consequences, and their harms from the pediatrician's perspective. Three levels of prevention of poverty are described (**Table 2**) that aim to (1) keep children out of poverty in the first place, (2) preserve the health and well-being of those children who do live in poverty, and (3) restore optimal wellness for children who have already experienced poverty-attributable harms. Each prevention level requires different tools, strategies, scale, domains, and types of intervention: high-level professional advocacy for systematic and transformative policy changes in primary poverty prevention; coordination and expansion of services for secondary poverty prevention across sectors; and clinical identification, diagnosis, and treatment of harms to health and well-being from poverty in tertiary prevention. At each level, pediatricians have important roles to play—from front-line service delivery to policy advocacy to leadership in collaboration with professionals from other fields.

Primary Child Poverty Prevention: Public Advocacy and Leadership from Pediatricians

Primary prevention of child poverty can take place through changes to the economic policies and structures that have allowed 1 in 5 American children to live in poverty and nearly half to live on the razor's edge financially. As a profession dedicated to child health and well-being, pediatricians are ideally positioned to advocate on behalf of public policies that benefit low-income children and build on the work of a broad coalition of child advocates committed to poverty reduction. Leadership at all levels is needed: clinical to neighborhood to national. At the neighborhood level, community asset development programs, such as the Promise Neighborhoods,[84] are built on cross-sector collaboration to create social and economic capital in high-risk areas. These collaborations connect community development and clinical care to form and evaluate new models of integrated economic-health promotion.[85–89] Partnerships with health care are critically important in the development and implementation of these neighborhood initiatives[90] and pediatricians are ideally suited for this role.

Pediatric advocacy around matters of public policy at the local, state, and national levels is critical to promote and preserve programs to level the playing field for low-income families. Various developing legislative efforts, from minimum wage increases and closing the wage gap[91] to expanding access to high-quality preschool,[92] are highly relevant to child health and within the purview of engaged pediatrician advocates. Access to other well-established public programs, including the Supplemental Nutrition Assistance Program; progressive tax polices like the earned income tax credit; Women, Infants, and Children (WIC); subsidized school meals; and low-income housing support, also provide lifelines for poor families. Indeed, reports by the Urban Institute and Children's Defense Fund suggest that relatively small public investments could cut child poverty dramatically, perhaps by more than half.[85,93] Expanding access to affordable health insurance coverage for children, perhaps the legislative issue most squarely in the pediatrician's wheelhouse, has new importance in light of the

Table 2
Framework for action to reduce child poverty and its harms to health and well-being

Level of Prevention and Definition	Major Aim	Central Outcome	Level of Intervention	Key Strategies	Pediatricians' Roles	Domains of Intervention	Example Interventions
Primary Prevention — Prevention of children and families from falling into poverty	Elimination of poverty and its risks to health and well-being	Reduce the rate of child poverty and the degree of income inequality	City State National	Systematic poverty-reduction policy and transformative social and political change	Vision and leadership Policy advocacy	Public policy Public discourse	Federal minimum wage increase Progressive tax reform through earned income tax credit expansion Universal high-quality early child care
Secondary Prevention — Prevention of harms for children already in poverty	Preservation of optimal health and well-being despite poverty-related risk	Reduce rates of poverty-attributable disease and disadvantage	Individual Family Community Neighborhood	Alignment, networking, and expansion of effective poverty-related services across sectors	Screening and identification Intervention and referral Improvement and innovation Cross-sector collaboration Service coordination Partnered evaluation	Clinical care Health systems Public agencies Community development organizations	Poverty-relevant clinical services (eg, Reach Out and Read) Home visitation programs Promise Neighborhoods
Tertiary Prevention — Management of harms already befallen children in poverty	Restitution toward optimal health and well-being after poverty-related harms occur	Reduce the degree of harm from identified poverty-attributable disease and disadvantage	Individual Family Community	Implementation of standardized, effective approaches to identification, diagnosis, treatment of poverty-related harms	Screening and identification Intervention and management Resource referral Improvement and innovation	Clinical care Child care and education Homes and communities	Trauma-informed care Social determinant screening in EHR Poverty-relevant clinical services (eg, medical–legal partnerships)

growing cost of insurance premiums[94] and out-of-pocket care. The economic savings and the return on investment in child health insurance coverage through lifelong productivity gains[95] argue strongly that public insurance for low-income families is wise policy. Although substantial gains in health insurance coverage for children have occurred over the last 20 years due to the implementation of the Child Health Insurance Program and Medicaid expansion, significant gaps still exist across states, especially for children in immigrant families. Leadership from pediatricians in the public discourse on programs and policies for economic stability is an immensely valuable child health intervention and must be an integral part of any unified, comprehensive strategy to reduce the harms of child poverty.

Secondary Child Poverty Prevention: Preserving Health and Well-Being for Poor Children

Preserving the health and well-being of poor individuals, families, and neighborhoods despite the risks is the central aim of secondary child poverty prevention. To prevent harm at the individual level, interventions beginning in early childhood show the greatest success. The benefits of early intervention are manifold and lasting for economic stability and health into adulthood.[96] Home visitation programs, such as the Nurse–Family Partnership and many others,[97] begin to promote the healthy development of very poor children soon after birth through improved development,[98] academic achievement,[99] parenting behavior,[100] child injury rate,[101] and all-cause mortality outcomes[102] that can last decades and reduce dependence on public assistance.[103] High-quality early childhood education, such as the Perry Preschool, has been shown many times over to significantly reduce the likelihood of children falling far behind in key areas of academic aptitude and achievement,[104] unemployment in early adulthood, imprisonment, dependence on public programs,[105] or going uninsured and underusing preventative health care well into later adulthood.[106] The broader economic ripple effects of such early intervention programs show returns to society many times over for each dollar invested.[107] Currently, these early childhood enrichment programs are not widely accessible and often exist in isolation. Head Start reaches less than half of eligible children; Early Head State reaches less than 10%.[108] Even the Maternal, Infant, and Early Childhood Home Visiting program funded by the Affordable Care Act is only funded to reach 1 to 2 percent of eligible children. Early childhood supports can be effective in the clinical setting.[109] In addition to scaling these programs, there is a need to integrate programs horizontally (across sectors) and longitudinally (across developmental time periods) to scaffold and promote children's success well beyond their early years (**Fig. 3**). This integration is essential to buffer against predictable, cumulative, and preventable risks of child poverty.[81]

A different set of tools and services support optimal health and well-being for poor older children and adolescents, including access to high-quality public schools for college or workforce readiness. Also critical are programs that can prevent children from being derailed by life-changing, poverty-related insults. For instance, early evidence suggests that supportive housing programs for unstably housed families result in greater parental self-sufficiency and less than half the incidence of child abuse and neglect.[110,111] Seeing potential health and economic benefits, health delivery systems have begun providing supportive housing programs for high-risk patients.[112] Programs that prevent high rates of unwanted teen pregnancy can also be potent in reducing the impact of poverty across generations. When long-acting reversible contraception was made available through statewide funding in Colorado in 2009, intrauterine device use increased from 5% to 19% of teens with a 30% decline in low-income teen pregnancy, 24% decline in high-risk births, 34% decline in abortion rates,

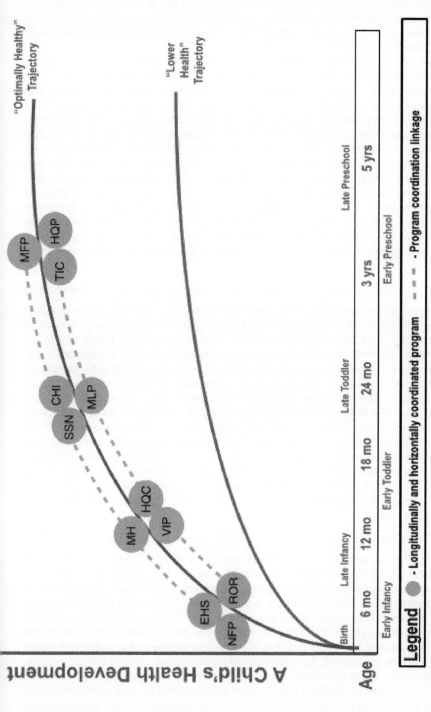

Fig. 3. Benefit of service integration for buoying the health and development of a high-risk children in poverty. CHI, community health initiative; EHS, Early Head Start; HQC, high-quality childcare; HQP, high-quality preschool; MFP, medical–financial partnership; MH, medical home; MLP, medical–legal partnership; NFP, nurse–family partnership; ROR, Reach Out and Read; SSN, social service navigation; TIC, trauma-informed care; VIP, Video Interaction Project. (*Adapted from* Halfon N. Life Course Health Development: a new approach for addressing upstream determinants of health and spending. National Institute for Health Care Management. Expert Voices (February 2009). Available at: http://www.nihcm.org/pdf/ExpertVoices_Halfon_FINAL.pdf. Accessed February 16, 2015.)

and 23% drop in need for WIC.[113] Such programs can open up worlds of opportunity for low-income women to pursue higher education and careers, increase lifelong productivity, and escape cycles of poverty. Access to higher education through financial aid and low tuition is also a key to attaining living-wage jobs and financial stability, with lifelong benefits for health and well-being.[114]

Neighborhood-level approaches to prevent poverty's health harms in poor communities match the multifactorial risks of poverty with ecological, multifaceted sets of interventions. When properly funded and implemented, wraparound community development focused on low-income children can achieve dramatic improvements in primary school readiness, high school graduation, and college entry. The Harlem Children's Zone has shepherded 95% of high school seniors in their birth-through-college pipeline on to college acceptance from a neighborhood where almost two-thirds of children are born into poverty.[115] Other neighborhood-based models have taken a less costly approach of linking existing services and resources to provide networked, wraparound supports for families.[116] Through the federally funded Promise Neighborhoods[117] and Promise Zones[118] initiatives, neighborhood-based approaches focusing on diverse areas of poverty-related community needs, from community-engaged policing to food security, are being carried out nationally.[119] These have great promise for lifelong reduction in the harms experienced by children in poverty.

Tertiary Child Poverty Prevention: Healing the Harms to Child Health and Well-Being

The pervasive harms of poverty may never be completely prevented, so these harms will need to be treated and managed through tertiary child poverty prevention to reduce their impact on poor children, families, and communities. This is definitively the purview of pediatricians. Much of pediatric practice consists of treating complications of economic hardship, whether as stubbornly hard-to-control asthma, obesity counseling undermined by cheap fast food, screening and referral of a new mother for postpartum depression, a positive serum lead test, or any number of other familiar encounters.[120,121] With more than half of pediatric patients' families reporting poverty-related social problems (housing insecurity, food insecurity, or unemployment),[122,123] standardized strategies to move clinical care toward coherently identifying and addressing socioeconomic determinants of poor child health are needed. Although most clinicians recognize poverty as a root cause of many ills they treat,[124] this work is not often thought of as treating poverty as an illness. The following are ways in which new models of pediatric care can promote both secondary and tertiary child poverty prevention.

Engineering Pediatric Care and Practice for Child Poverty Prevention

Pediatricians can and should do more to directly prevent and treat child poverty's short-term and long-term harms for several reasons. This makes sense from the perspective of health systems interested in minimizing costs of care for high-risk, socially complex poor patients[125] and it is simply better medicine in light of socioeconomic drivers of population health and disease.[126,127] Some argue that focusing on economic needs and their social consequences is the purview of social work and case management. Whereas it is true that the importance of social workers in this area cannot be overstated, the goal is not to replace social workers with physicians. Instead, core clinical processes and programs within the pediatric medical home should be reshaped to facilitate identification and treatment of adverse effects of child poverty as standard practice. This will allow social workers, who are often stretched thin with overflowing caseloads, to operate at the top of their license (rather than filling their time with rote screening and referral) and other members of the pediatric team to more effectively treat root economic causes of common ills.

The first step in this transformation of pediatric practice is to better screen for child poverty and its harms. The Institute of Medicine recommends screening patients for economic stress as part of standardized collection of information on social determinants of health via electronic health records and provides screening construct and content guidance.[128,129] With these tools, pediatric medical homes can more fully contextualize clinical information against the backdrop of patients' economic and social circumstances, opening up new avenues of diagnosis and treatment for poverty-related illnesses. With established methods to screen for symptoms of poverty and low-income, as well as structural and financing supports from policymakers and health systems, new clinical care models can be engineered to directly respond to poverty-related needs, interface with appropriate social nonmedical programs, and serve as referral hubs for community-based services to help poor families manage.

When it comes to connecting patients with services to prevent the harms of poverty (ie, secondary child poverty prevention), the paper-based community resource binder will not cut it anymore. As opposed to collecting dust on a bookshelf, integration into practice processes and workflows is a hallmark of successful community–clinic linkages. Many programs bring critical community partners into the clinic as part of routine care, such as medical–legal partnerships.[130] Others bring bundled resources in a particular domain of poverty-related need, such as Reach Out and Read's early literacy-promotion strategies that include models for parents learning to read aloud with their children and age-appropriate books families take home from their pediatrics visits.[131] Reach Out and Read has been shown to increase parental enjoyment and frequency of reading with their children,[132] promote satisfaction with pediatric providers,[133] and improve standardized language scores.[134,135] The clinic-based Video Interaction Project (VIP) to improve parenting skills through 1-to-1 sessions and feedback from a child development specialist plus parenting resources has demonstrated marked improvements in enhanced parent–child interactions and responsive parenting practices among low-income families. In addition, the VIP is associated with increased reading,[136] decreased screen time,[137] reduced parenting stress, and fewer symptoms of maternal depression.[138] These clinically-integrated programs support long-term health and well-being, especially when implemented widely.

Care coordination through the medical home to link families to services outside the health delivery system is also vital for prevention of poverty's harms. Help Me Grow exemplifies cross-sector integration in which pediatric care, early education, and family supports are coordinated through information and referral centers to link disadvantaged families with a network of programs and services.[139] Several other promising programs and organizations also provide a scaffold of coordinated poverty-related services for poor families. Notable examples are clinic-based help desks such as Health Leads[140] and community-based organizations such as LIFT[141] that provide longitudinal individualized support for families in poverty. Clinic-based help desk navigators typically offer patient screening for poverty-related social needs, referral to appropriate services in the community, and follow-up to ensure that helpful resource connections have been made. Well-implemented help desks can increase patient satisfaction[142] in the pediatric setting and increase the number of connections families make to community-based and public assistance services. A small literature on high-stakes social outcomes of help desks shows significant increases in family housing stability, child care, and employment, compared with usual care.[143] Other promising services provide web-based and call-center infrastructure to facilitate clinic-community referrals, both publicly for free (eg, the national 211 network) and as proprietary solutions,[144–146] with outcome studies underway.

New clinical care models are already reshaping the pediatric medical home to directly address poverty-related harms (ie, tertiary poverty prevention) and even improve the financial circumstances of families (ie, primary poverty prevention). As a foundation for tertiary poverty prevention, trauma-informed care practices involve raising sensitivity to the prevalence of pediatric trauma and ACEs, minimizing the risk that patients will be retraumatized,[147] and increasing family resiliency through safe, connected, and emotionally attuned care.[148] Pediatricians have also begun to reorganize processes of care to better respond to the needs of poor and low-income families and integrate poverty-related data into clinical care. Cincinnati Children's Hospital, for instance, uses geocoded asthma patients' addresses to identify and address environmental hotspots triggering neighborhood-wide flares,[149] often in poor areas. Finally, through medical–financial partnerships pediatric care delivery can directly integrate access to asset-building services and individualized financial planning with professional financial counselors familiar with the needs of low-income communities.[150] Studies of financial counseling in nonclinical settings demonstrate significantly increased income,[151] improved credit scores with reduced debt levels,[152] and higher net worth for low-income families,[153] with trials of their clinical impact underway.

How will these changes in pediatric care be paid for? It is worth noting the exceptionally strong economic argument for reducing child poverty and investing in low-income children. Early childhood intervention has been shown to return 7 to 12 dollars to society over a child's lifetime for every dollar spent.[154,155] The business case for investing in economically disadvantaged children has resonance within health care as well, especially given the growth of reimbursement models that increasingly will hold providers and health systems accountable for improving poor health outcomes that are rooted in child and family poverty. As capitation, accountable care, and shared savings reimbursement gain market share, the business case for reshaping pediatric care to address poverty only gets stronger. The advantages of retaining patients and controlling lifelong costs for payers like the Centers for Medicaid and Medicare Services and managed care plans offer opportunities in reimbursement for poverty-reduction interventions.[156] These trends will continue to advance pediatrics and pediatric care models as the foundation of lifelong health and high-value, cost-effective care.

SUMMARY

Economic adversity begets more adversity and poorer health. Therefore, interrupting the cycle of poverty has significant benefits for families today and their children tomorrow. There is much to do in reducing child poverty and many important roles for pediatricians to play in improving the health and well-being of poor families. It can be done, evidenced by efforts in the United Kingdom that cut rates of child poverty by half over the last decade.[157] Even in the United States there is remarkable success protecting another vulnerable age group, seniors, from historically high rates of poverty through health programs and social and legislative action. The same can be done for child poverty. Not only does it makes sense for the health and vitality of the nation but it is the right thing to do for children.

Although the size of the problem may be daunting, change is possible through collective action. The assertion that it is within the power and the purview of the pediatrician to address this most prevalent of child-health risk factors is borne out by a large and growing body of evidence. This evidence not only shows the physical and emotional harm wrought by living with low income in a profoundly unequal society, it also shows the mechanisms by which poverty endangers health during critical windows of development and across generations. Effective strategies at the clinic, neighborhood, community, and policy levels can prevent the harms of poverty when implemented in concert and supported by pediatric care and advocacy. With better understanding of the biomedical, behavioral, and biographic consequences of growing up poor, now, more than ever, there is opportunity to protect and prevent this nation's children from the dangers of poverty.

There is nothing new about poverty. What is new is that we now have the techniques and the resources to get rid of poverty. The real question is whether we have the will.
—*Dr Martin Luther King Jr, Remaining Awake Through a Great Revolution. Delivered at the National Cathedral in 1968.*

REFERENCES

1. DeNavas-Walt C, Proctor BD. Income and poverty in the United States: 2013. Washington, DC: United States Census Bureau; 2014. Available at: https://www.census.gov/content/dam/Census/library/publications/2014/demo/p60-249.pdf. Accessed February 16, 2015.
2. Adamson P. Measuring child poverty: New league tables of child poverty in the world's rich countries. Florence (Italy): United Nation's Children's Fund (UNICEF); 2012. Available at: http://www.unicef-irc.org/publications/pdf/rc10_eng.pdf. Accessed February 16, 2015.
3. Judge L, editor. Ending child poverty by 2020: progress made and lessons learned. London: Child Poverty Action Group; 2012.
4. Fisher GM. The development of the Orshansky poverty thresholds and their subsequent history as the official U.S. poverty measure. Washington, DC: U.S. Department of Commerce, Census Bureau; 1997. Available at: http://www.census.gov/hhes/www/povmeas/papers/orshansky.html. Accessed February 16, 2015.
5. Citro C, Michael R, editors. Measuring poverty: a new approach. Washington, DC: National Academy Press; 1995. Available at: http://www.census.gov/hhes/www/povmeas/nas.html. Accessed February 16, 2015.
6. Short K. The Supplemental Poverty Measure: 2013. Census Current Population Reports. 2014. Available at: http://www.census.gov/content/dam/Census/library/publications/2014/demo/p60-251.pdf. Accessed February 16, 2015.
7. Allen JT. Re-counting poverty. Washington, DC: Pew Research Center; 2011. Available at: http://www.pewsocialtrends.org/2011/11/30/re-counting-poverty/. Accessed February 16, 2015.
8. Renwick T. Geographic adjustments of Supplemental Poverty Measure thresholds: using the American community survey five-year data on housing costs. Washington, DC: U.S. Census Bureau; 2011.
9. Alegretto S. Basic family budgets. Washington, DC: Economic Policy Institute; 2005. Available at: http://www.epi.org/publication/bp165/. Accessed February 16, 2015.
10. Corporation for Enterprise Development. Assets & opportunity scorecard. Liquid asset poverty rate. 2015. Available at: http://scorecard.assetsandopportunity.org/2013/measure/liquid-asset-poverty-rate. Accessed February 16, 2015.
11. Fremstad S. A modern framework for measuring poverty and basic economic security. Washington, DC: Center for Economic and Policy Research; 2010.

Available at: http://www.cepr.net/documents/publications/poverty-2010-04.pdf. Accessed February 16, 2015.

12. Jiang Y, Ekono M, Skinner C. Basic facts about low-income children. New York: National Center for Children in Poverty; 2015. Available at: http://www.nccp.org/publications/pub_1100.html. Accessed February 16, 2015.

13. Agency for Healthcare Research and Quality. National healthcare disparities report. Rockville (MD): AHRQ Publication No. 14-0006 2013.

14. Kawachi I, Subramanian SV. Income inequality. Social epidemiology. 2nd edition. In: Berkman LF, Kawachi I, Glymour MM, editors. New York: Oxford University Press; 2014. p. 127–152.

15. Eckenrode J, Smith EG, McCarthy ME, et al. Income inequality and child maltreatment in the United States. Pediatrics 2014;133:454–61.

16. Pickett KE, Wilkinson RG. Child wellbeing and income inequality in rich societies: ecological cross-sectional study. BMJ 2007;335(7629):1080–6.

17. National Center for Children in Poverty. Young children at risk. New York. 2012. Available at: http://www.nccp.org/publications/pub_1073.html. Accessed February 16, 2015.

18. National Center for Children in Poverty. Poor children by parents' nativity. New York. 2011. Available at: http://www.nccp.org/publications/pub_1006.html. Accessed February 16, 2015.

19. Passel JS. A portrait of unauthorized immigrants in the United States. Pew Hispanic Center Report. 2009. Available at: http://www.pewhispanic.org/files/reports/107.pdf. Accessed February 16, 2015.

20. Cingano F. Trends in income inequality and its impact on economic growth. OECD Social, Employment, and Migration Working Papers. 2014. Available at: http://www.oecd-ilibrary.org/social-issues-migration-health/trends-in-income-inequality-and-its-impact-on-economic-growth_5jxrjncwxv6j-en. Accessed February 16, 2015.

21. Holzer HJ, Schanzenbach DW, Duncan GJ, et al. The economic costs of childhood poverty in the United States. J Child Poverty 2008;14(1):41–61.

22. Kozyrsky A, Kendall G, Jacoby P, et al. Association between socioeconomic status and the development of asthma. Am J Public Health 2010;100(3): 540–6.

23. Blackburn C, Spencer N, Read J. Is the onset of disabling conditions later childhood associated with social disadvantage in earlier childhood? BMC Pediatr 2013;13:101.

24. Saegert S, Evans G. Poverty, housing niches, and health in the United States. J Soc Issues 2003;59(3):569–89.

25. Ahnquist J, Wamala S, Lindstrom M. Social determinants of health—a question of social or economic capital? Soc Sci Med 2012;74:930–9.

26. Shonkoff JP, Phillips DA, editors. Committee on Integrating the Science of Early Childhood Development. From neurons to neighborhoods: the science of early childhood development. Washington, DC: National Academy Press; 2000.

27. Larson K, Halfon N. Family income gradients in the health and health care access of US children. Matern Child Health J 2010;14:332–42.

28. Case A, Lubostsky D, Paxson C. Economic status and health in childhood. Am Econ Rev 2002;92(5):1308–34.

29. Aizer A, Stroud L, Buka S. Maternal stress and child outcomes: evidence from siblings. Cambridge (MA): National Bureau of Economic Research; 2012. NBER Working Paper Number 81422.

30. Hanson JL, Hair N, Shen DG, et al. Family poverty affects the rate of human infant brain growth. PLoS One 2013;8:e80954.
31. Hanson JL, Chandra A, Wolfe BL, et al. Association between income and the hippocampus. PLoS One 2011;6:e18712.
32. Hart B, Risley TR. Meaningful differences in the everyday experience of young American children. Baltimore (MD): Paul H Brookes Publishing; 1995.
33. Lee VE, Burkham DT. Inequality at the starting gate: social background differences in achievement as children begin school. Washington, DC: Economic Policy Institute; 2002.
34. Fiester L. Early warning confirmed: a research update on third-grade reading. Baltimore (MD): Annie E. Casey Foundation; 2013.
35. Heuer R, Stullich S. Comparability of state and local expenditure among schools within districts: a report from the study of school-level expenditures. Washington, DC: US Department of Education; 2011.
36. Ingersoll R. The problem of under qualified teachers in American secondary schools. Educ Res 1999;28(2):26–37.
37. Muijs D, Harris A, Chapman C, et al. Improving schools in socioeconomically disadvantaged areas? A review of research evidence. Sch Effect Sch Improv 2004;15(2):149–75.
38. Palardy G. Differential school effects among low, middle, and high social class composition school: a multiple group, multilevel latent class growth curve analysis. Sch Effect Sch Improv 2008;19(1):21–49.
39. Cass J, Liss S. National Center for Education Statistics. Available at: http://nces.ed.gov/fastfacts/display.asp?id=16. Accessed February 16, 2015.
40. America's cradle to prison pipeline. Washington, DC: Children's Defense Fund; 2007.
41. Browne-Yung K, Ziersch A, Baum F. 'Faking til you make it': social capital accumulation of individuals on low-incomes living in contrasting socio-economic neighborhoods and its implications for health and well-being. Soc Sci Med 2013;85:9–17.
42. Mani A, Mullainathan S, Shafir E, et al. Poverty impedes cognitive function. Science 2013;341(6149):976–80.
43. Nobles J, Weintraub M, Adler N. Subjective socioeconomic status and health. Soc Sci Med 2013;82:58–66.
44. Browne D, Jenkins J. Health across early childhood and socioeconomic status. Soc Sci Med 2012;74:1622–9.
45. Breslau N, Wilcox HC, Storr CL, et al. Trauma exposure and post-traumatic stress disorder: a study of youths in urban America. J Urban Health 2004; 81(4):531–44.
46. Finkelhor D, Turner H, Ormrod R, et al. Children's exposure to violence: a comprehensive national survey. Washington, DC: U.S. Department of Justice; 2009.
47. Paxson C, Waldfogel J. Work, welfare, and child maltreatment. NBER Working Paper No. 7343. 1999. Available at: http://www.nber.org/papers/w7343. Accessed February 16, 2015.
48. National Center for Children in Poverty. Promoting resilience: helping young children and parents affected by substance use, domestic violence, and depression in the context of welfare reform. New York; 2000. Mailman School of Public Health at Columbia University. Available at: http://www.nccp.org/publications/pdf/download_95.pdf. Accessed February 16, 2015.

49. Beeber LS, Miles MS. Maternal mental health and parenting in poverty. Annu Rev Nurs Res 2003;21:303–31.

50. Herman-Stahl M, Kan ML, McKay T. Incarceration and the family: a review of research and promising approaches for serving fathers and families. Washington, DC: U.S. Department of Health & Human Services Assistant Secretary for Planning and Evaluation; 2008. Available at: http://aspe.hhs.gov/hsp/08/mfs-ip/incarceration&family/index.shtml. Accessed February 16, 2015.

51. Felitti VJ, Anda RF, Nordenberg D, et al. Relationship of childhood abuse and household dysfunction to many of the leading causes of death in adults: the adverse childhood experiences study. Am J Prev Med 1998;14(4):245–58.

52. Bethell CD, Newacheck P, Hawes E, et al. Adverse childhood experiences: assessing the impact on health and school engagement and the mitigating role of resilience. Health Aff 2014;33:2106–15.

53. Child and Adolescent Health Measurement Initiative. Overview of adverse child and family experiences among US children. Rockville (MD): Data Resource Center, supported by a cooperative agreement between the US Department of Health and Human Services, Health Resources and Services Administration, and Maternal and Child Health Bureau; 2013. Available at: http://www.childhealthdata.org/docs/drc/aces-data-brief_version-1-0.pdf?Status=Master. Accessed February 16, 2015.

54. Halfon N, Wise PH, Forrest CB. The changing nature of children's health development: new challenges require major policy solutions. Health Aff 2014;33:2116–24.

55. The Philadelphia urban ACE study. Institute for Safe Families; 2013. Available at: http://www.rwjf.org/content/dam/farm/reports/reports/2013/rwjf407836. Accessed February 16, 2015.

56. Committee on Psychosocial Aspects of Child and Family Health, Committee on Early Childhood, Adoption, and Dependent Care, Section on Developmental and Behavioral Pediatrics, et al. Early childhood adversity, toxic stress, and the role of the pediatrician: translating developmental science into lifelong health. Pediatrics 2012;129(1):e224.

57. Manchester J, Topoleski J. Growing disparities in life expectancy. Washington, DC: Congressional Budget Office; 2008. Available at: http://www.cbo.gov/sites/default/files/04-17-lifeexpectancy_brief.pdf. Accessed February 16, 2015.

58. Braveman P, Egerter S. Overcoming obstacles to health: report from the Robert Wood Johnson Foundation to the Commission to Build a Healthier America. Princeton (NJ): Robert Wood Johnson Foundation; 2008.

59. Adler NE, Newman K. Socioeconomic disparities in health: pathways and policies. Health Aff 2002;21(2):60–76.

60. Seeman T, Epel E, Gruenewald T, et al. Socioeconomic differentials in peripheral biology: cumulative allostatic load. Ann N Y Acad Sci 2010;1186:223–39.

61. Gruenewald TL, Karlamangla AS, Hu P, et al. History of socioeconomic advantage and allostatic load in later life. Soc Sci Med 2012;74:75–83.

62. Karlamangla AS, Friedman EM, Seeman TE, et al. Daytime trajectories of cortisol: demographic and socioeconomic differences — findings from the National Study of Daily Experiences. Psychoneuroendocrinology 2013;38:2585–97.

63. Azad MB, Lissitsyn Y, Miller GE, et al. Influence of socioeconomic status trajectories on innate immune responsiveness in children. PLoS One 2012;7:e38669.

64. Jousilahti P, Salomaa V, Rasi V, et al. Association of markers of systemic inflammation, C reactive protein, serum amyloid A, and fibrinogen with socioeconomic status. J Epidemiol Community Health 2003;57:730–3.

65. Juster RP, McEwen BS, Lupien SJ. Allostatic load biomarkers of chronic stress and impact on health and cognition. Neurosci Biobehav Rev 2010;35:2–16.

66. Janicki-Deverts D, Cohen S, Adler NE, et al. Socioeconomic status is related to urinary catecholamines in the Coronary Artery Risk Development in Young Adults (CARDIA) study. Psychosom Med 2007;69:514–20.

67. Spruill TM, Gerin W, Ogedegbe G, et al. Socioeconomic and psychological factors mediate race differences in nocturnal blood pressure dipping. Am J Hypertens 2009;22:637–42.

68. Alley DE, Seeman TE, Kim J, et al. Socioeconomic status and C-reactive protein levels in the US population: NHANES IV. Brain Behav Immun 2006;20:498–504.

69. Adler NE, Rehkopf US. Disparities in health: descriptions, causes, and mechanisms. Annu Rev Public Health 2008;29:235–52.

70. Cohen S, Janicki-Deverts D, Chen E, et al. Childhood socioeconomic status and adult health. Ann N Y Acad Sci 2010;1186:37–55.

71. Crimmins EM, Kim JK, Seeman TE. Poverty and biological risk: the earlier "aging" of the poor. J Gerontol A Biol Sci Med Sci 2009;64:286–92.

72. Cohen S, Janicki-Deverts D, Turner RB, et al. Childhood socioeconomic status, telomere length, and susceptibility to upper respiratory infection. Brain Behav Immun 2013;34:31–8.

73. Needham B, Fernandez J, Lin J, et al. Socioeconomic status and cell aging in children. Soc Sci Med 2012;74:1948.

74. Miller G, Chen E. Unfavorable socioeconomic conditions in early life presage expression of proinflammatory phenotype in adolescence. Psychosom Med 2007;69:402–9.

75. Miller GE, Chen E. The biological residue of childhood poverty. Child Dev Perspect 2013;7:67–73.

76. Miller GE, Chen E, Fok AK, et al. Low early-life social class leaves a biological residue manifested by decreased glucocorticoid and increased pro inflammatory signaling. Proc Natl Acad Sci U S A 2009;106:14716–21.

77. Ziol-Guest KM, Duncan GJ, Kalil A, et al. Early childhood poverty, immune-mediated disease processes, and adult productivity. Proc Natl Acad Sci U S A 2012;109(Suppl 2):17289–93.

78. Finch CE, Crimmins EM. Inflammatory exposure and historical changes in human lifespan. Science 2004;305(5691):1736–9.

79. Hanson MA, Gluckman PD. Developmental origins of health and disease—global public health implications. Best Pract Res Clin Obstet Gynaecol 2015;29(1):24–31.

80. Gluckman PD, Hanson MA, Buklijas T. A conceptual framework for the developmental origins of health and disease. J Dev Orig Health Dis 2010;1(1):6–18.

81. Halfon N, Larson K, Lu M, et al. Lifecourse health development: past, present, and future. Matern Child Health J 2014;18:344–65.

82. Barker DJ. The origins of the developmental origins theory. J Intern Med 2007;261:412–7.

83. Tottenham N, Sheridan MA. A review of adversity, the amygdala and the hippocampus: a consideration of developmental timing. Front Hum Neurosci 2009;3:68.

84. Promise Neighborhoods Program. US Department of Education. Available at: http://www2.ed.gov/programs/promiseneighborhoods/index.html. Accessed February 16, 2015.

85. Ending child poverty now. Washington, DC: Children's Defense Fund; 2015.

86. Rogerson B, Lindberg R, Givens M, et al. A simplified framework for incorporating health into community development initiatives. Health Aff 2014;33(11):1939–47.

87. Erickson D, Andrews N. Partnerships among community development, public health, and health care could improve the well-being of low-income people. Health Aff 2011;30(11):2056–63.

88. Mattessich PW, Rausch EJ. Cross-sector collaboration to improve community health: a view of the current landscape. Health Aff 2014;33(11):1968–74.

89. Schuchter J, Jutte DP. A framework to extend community development measurement to health and well-being. Health Aff 2014;33(11):1930–8.

90. Braunstein S, Lavizzo-Mourey R. How the health and community development sectors are combining forces to improve health and well-being. Health Aff 2011;30(11):2042–51.

91. United States Department of Labor. Minimum wage laws in the states. Available at: http://www.dol.gov/whd/minwage/america.htm. Accessed February, 2015.

92. US Department of Education. 18 states awarded new preschool development grants to increase access to high-quality preschool programs. Available at: http://www.ed.gov/news/press-releases/18-states-awarded-new-preschool-development-grants-increase-access-high-quality-preschool-programs. Accessed February 16, 2015.

93. Giannarelli L, Lippold K, Minton S, et al. Reducing child poverty in the US: costs and impacts of policies proposed by the Children's Defense Fund. Washington, DC: Urban Institute; 2015.

94. Erickson J. The middle class squeeze: a picture of stagnant incomes, rising costs, and what we can do to strengthen America's middle class. Washington, DC: Center for American Progress; 2014.

95. Brown DW, Kowalski AE, Lurie IZ. Medicaid as an investment in children: what is the long-term impact on tax receipts? Cambridge (MA): National Bureau of Economic Research Working Paper Series; 2015. Working paper number: 20835. Available at: http://www.nber.org/papers/w20835. Accessed February 16, 2015.

96. Campbell F, Conti G, Heckman JJ, et al. Early childhood investments substantially boost adult health. Science 2014;343:1478–84.

97. Help Me Grow. Available at: http://www.helpmegrownational.org. Accessed February 16, 2015.

98. Olds DL, Kitzman H, Cole R, et al. Effects of nurse home-visiting on maternal life course and child development: age six follow-up results of a randomized controlled trial. Pediatrics 2004;114(6):1550–9.

99. Olds DL, Kitzman H, Hanks C, et al. Effects of nurse home visiting on maternal and child functioning: age nine follow-up of a randomized trial. Pediatrics 2007; 120:e832–45.

100. Olds DL, Eckenrode J, Henderson CR, et al. Long term effects of home visitation on maternal life course and child abuse and neglect: fifteen year follow-up of a randomized trial. JAMA 1997;278(8):637–43.

101. Kitzman H, Olds DL, Henderson CR, et al. Effect of prenatal and infancy home visitation by nurses on pregnancy outcomes, child injuries, and repeated childbearing: a randomized controlled trial. JAMA 1997;278(8):644–52.

102. Olds DL, Kitzman H, Knudtson M, et al. Impact of home visiting by nurses on maternal and child mortality: results of a two-decade follow-up of a randomized, clinical trial. JAMA Pediatr 2014;168(9):800–6.

103. Olds DL, Kitzman H, Cole R. Enduring effects of prenatal and infancy home visiting by nurses on maternal life course and government spending. Arch Pediatr Adolesc Med 2010;164(5):419–24.

104. Berrueta-Clement JR, Schweinhart LJ, Steven Barnett W, et al. Changed lives: the effects of the Perry Preschool program on youths through age 19. Ypsilanti (MI): High/Scope Press, Monographs of the HighScope Educational Research Foundation; 1984. p. 8.

105. Schweinhart LJ, Barnes HV, Weikart DP. Significant benefits: the high/scope preschool study through age 27. Ypsilanti (MI): High/Scope Press, Monographs of the HighScope Educational Research Foundation; 1993. p. 10.

106. Muennig P, Schweinhart L, Montie J, et al. Effects of a prekindergarten educational intervention on adult health: 37-year follow-up results of a randomized controlled trial. Am J Public Health 2009;99:1431–7.

107. Karoly LA, Greenwood PW, Everingham SS, et al. Investing in our children: what we know and don't know about the costs and benefits of early childhood interventions. Santa Monica (CA): RAND Corporation; 1998. MR-898-TCWF. Available at: http://www.rand.org/pubs/monograph_reports/MR898/. Accessed August 20, 2009.

108. The state of America's children 2014. Washington, DC: Children's Defense Fund; 2014. Available at: http://www.childrensdefense.org/library/state-of-americas-children/2014-soac.pdf?utm_source=2014-SOAC-PDF&utm_medium=link&utm_campaign=2014-SOAC. Accessed February 16, 2015.

109. Mendelsohn A, Dreyer BP, Brockmeyer CA, et al. Fostering early development and school readiness in pediatric settings. In: Neuman SB, Dickinson DK, editors. Handbook of early literacy research, vol. 3. New York: Guilford Press; 2011. p. 279–94.

110. Tapper D. Keeping families together: an evaluation of the implementation and outcomes of a pilot supportive housing model for families involved in the child welfare system. New York: Metis Associates; 2010. Available at: http://www.csh.org/wp-content/uploads/2011/12/Report_KFTFindingsreport.pdf. Accessed February 16, 2015.

111. Cunningham M, Pergamit M, McDaniel M, et al. Supportive housing for high need families in the child welfare system. Washington, DC: Urban Institute; 2014.

112. Children's National Healthy Homes Initiative. Los Angeles County Department of Health Services' Housing for Health Program. Available at: http://www.nationwidechildrens.org/healthy-homes-infographic; http://dhs.lacounty.gov/wps/portal/dhs/housingforhealth. Accessed February 16, 2015.

113. Ricketts S, Klingler G, Schwalberg R. Game change in Colorado: widespread use of LARC and rapid decline in births among young, low-income women. Perspect Sex Reprod Health 2014;46(3):125–32.

114. Brunello G, Fort M, Schneeweis N, et al. The causal effects of education on health: what is the role of health behaviors? Health Econ 2015. [Epub ahead of print].

115. Harlem Children's Zone: A national model for breaking the cycle of poverty with proven success. Fact Sheet. Available at: http://hcz.org/wp-content/uploads/2014/04/FY-2013-FactSheet.pdf. Accessed February 16, 2015.

116. Halfon N, Long P, Chang DI, et al. 3.0 transition framework to guide large-scale health system reform. Health Aff 2014;33(110):2003–11.

117. US Department of Education Promise Neighborhoods. Available at: http://www2.ed.gov/programs/promiseneighborhoods/index.html. Accessed February 16, 2015.

118. US Department of Housing and Urban Development Promise Zones. Available at: http://portal.hud.gov/hudportal/HUD?src=/program_offices/comm_planning/economicdevelopment/programs/pz/overview. Accessed February 16, 2015.

119. Building Healthy Neighborhoods Initiative. California Endowment. Available at: http://www.calendow.org/communities/building-healthy-communities/. Accessed February 16, 2015.

120. Blustein J, Hanson K, Shea S. Preventable hospitalizations and socioeconomic status. Health Aff 1998;17(2):177–89.

121. Coker TR, Thomas T, Chung PJ. Does well-child care have a future in pediatrics? Pediatrics 2013;131(2):S149.

122. Fleegler EW, Lieu TA, Wise PH, et al. Families' health-related social problems and missed referral opportunities. Pediatrics 2007;119:e113.

123. Hassan A, Blood EA, Pikcilingis A, et al. Youths' health-related social problems: concerns often overlooked during the medical visit. J Adolesc Health 2013; 53(2):265–71.

124. Health Care's blind side: the overlooked connection between social needs and good health. Princeton (NJ): Robert Wood Johnson Foundation; 2011.

125. Bachrach D, Pfister H, Wallis K, et al. Addressing patients' social needs: an emerging business case for provider investment. New York: The Commonwealth Fund; 2014. Available at: http://www.commonwealthfund.org/~/media/files/publications/fund-report/2014/may/1749_bachrach_addressing_patients_social_needs_v2.pdf. Accessed February 16, 2015.

126. McGinnis JM, Williams-Russo P, Knickman JR. The case for more active policy attention to health promotion. Health Aff 2002;21(2):78–93.

127. Canadian Institute of Advanced Research, Health Canada, population and public health branch. AB/NWT 2002, quoted in Kuznetsova, D. (2012) Healthy places: councils leading on public health. London: New Local Government Network.

128. Adler NE, Stead WW. Patients in context—EHR capture of social determinants of health. N Engl J Med 2015;372:698–701.

129. Committee on the Recommended Social and Behavioral Domains and Measures for Electronic Health Records. Capturing social and behavioral domains and measures in electronic health records, phases 1 & 2. Washington, DC: National Academies Press; 2014.

130. Rosenberg T. When poverty makes you sick, a lawyer can be the cure. New York: The New York Times; 2014. Available at: http://opinionator.blogs.nytimes.com/2014/07/17/when-poverty-makes-you-sick-a-lawyer-can-be-the-cure/?_php=true&_type=blogs&_php=true&_type=blogs&_r=2&. Accessed February 16, 2015.

131. Reach Out and Read Annual Report 2013–2014. Available at: http://www.reachoutandread.org/media/40159/ror_fy14_ar_vf_web.pdf. Accessed February 16, 2015.

132. Needleman R, Fried LE, Morley DS, et al. Clinic-based intervention to promote literacy: a pilot study. Am J Dis Child 1991;145:881–4.

133. Jones VF, Franco SM, Metcalf S, et al. The value of book distribution in a clinic-based literacy intervention program. Clin Pediatr (Phila) 2000;39:535–41.

134. Theriot JA, Franco SM, Sisson BA, et al. The impact of early literacy guidance on language skills of 3-year-olds. Clin Pediatr 2003;42:165–72.

135. Mendelsohn AL, Mogliner LN, Dreyer BP, et al. The impact of a clinic-based literacy intervention on language development in inner-city preschool children. Pediatrics 2001;107(10):130–4.

136. Mendelsohn AL, Huberman HS, Berkule SB, et al. Primary care strategies for promoting parent-child interactions and school readiness in high-risk families: the Bellevue Project for early language, literacy, and education success. Arch Pediatr Adolesc Med 2011;165(1):33–41.

137. Mendelsohn AL, Dreyer BP, Brockmeyer CA, et al. Randomized controlled trial of primary care pediatric parenting programs. Arch Pediatr Adolesc Med 2011;165(1):42–8.
138. Berkule SB, Cates CB, Dreyer BP, et al. Reducing maternal depressive symptoms through promotion of parenting in pediatric primary care. Clin Pediatr 2014;53(5):460–9.
139. What is Help Me Grow? Available at: http://www.helpmegrownational.org/pages/hmg-national/what-is-hmg.pdf. Accessed February 16, 2015.
140. Available at: https://healthleadsusa.org. Accessed February 16, 2015.
141. Available at: http://www.liftcommunities.org. Accessed February 16, 2015.
142. Vasan A, Solomon B. Use colocated multidisciplinary services to address family psychosocial needs at an urban pediatric primary care clinic. Clin Pediatr (Phila) 2015;54:25–32.
143. Garg A, Toy S, Tripodis Y, et al. Addressing social determinants of health at well child care visits: a cluster RCT. Pediatrics 2015;135:e296–304.
144. Available at: https://www.healthify.us/en. Accessed February 16, 2015.
145. Available at: http://healtherx.org. Accessed February 16, 2015.
146. Available at: http://purplebinder.com. Accessed February 16, 2015.
147. Ko S, Ford J, Kassam-Adams N, et al. Creating trauma-informed systems: child welfare, education, first responders, health care, juvenile justice. Prof Psychol Res Pract 2008;39(4):396–404.
148. Greenwald R. Child trauma handbook: a guide for helping trauma-exposed children and adolescents. New York: The Haworth Maltreatment and Trauma Press; 2005.
149. Waters R. It's all in the data: Cincinnati Children's Hospital gets wonky to transform the health of its community. Jersey City (NJ): Forbes; 2013. Available at: http://www.forbes.com/sites/robwaters/2013/11/26/its-all-in-the-data-cincinnati-childrens-hospital-gets-wonky-to-transform-a-communitys-health/. Accessed February 16, 2015.
150. Schickedanz A, Bennett H, Shea S, et al. Money matters: a medical-financial partnership to reduce financial hardship and improve patient health. Oral presentation, abstract delivered at the Academic Pediatric Association Joint Region IX & X Community, Advocacy, Research, and Education Conference. Monterey, January 28, 2012. Poster presentation, Pediatric Academic Societies Annual Conference, April, 2012.
151. Delia K. Compass financial stability and savings program pilot evaluation. Waltham (MA): Institute on Assets and Social Policy; 2013.
152. Wiedrich K, Gons N, Michael Collins J, et al. Financial counseling & access for the financially vulnerable. Corporation for Enterprise Development; 2014.
153. Collins M, Murrell K. Using a financial coaching approach to help low-income families achieve economic success. Madison (WI): University of Wisconsin-Madison and PolicyLab Consulting Group; 2010.
154. Heckman JJ. Schools, skills, and synapses. Econ Inq 2008;46(3):289–324.
155. Heckman JJ, Masterov DY. The productivity argument for investing in young children. Appl Econ Perspect Policy 2007;29(3):446–93.
156. Halfon N, Conway P. The opportunities and challenges of a lifelong health system. N Engl J Med 2013;368(17):1569–71.
157. Smeeding T, Waldfogel J. Fighting childhood poverty in the US &UK: and update. Madison (WI): Institute for Research on Poverty; 2010.

Youth Violence Prevention and Safety

Opportunities for Health Care Providers

Naomi Nichele Duke, MD, MPH[a],*, Iris Wagman Borowsky, MD, PhD[b]

KEYWORDS

- Youth violence involvement • Adverse childhood experiences • Resilience
- Public health prevention • Youth health screening

KEY POINTS

- Violence involvement remains a threat to the healthy development of US youth.
- Evidence linking adverse childhood experiences to interpersonal and self-directed violence-related outcomes in adolescence and adulthood is mounting.
- Use of a resilience framework for violence prevention and intervention efforts is the key, as it focuses on building developmental assets and resources.
- Brief and validated resources are available to support screening and counseling for youth violence involvement in the office setting.
- Investment in youth, from birth to adolescence and across developmental domains including family, school, and neighborhood, is proving effective in reducing violence involvement.

INTRODUCTION

Despite declining rates of violence among youth in the last 2 decades, youth violence involvement remains a significant public health problem. Violence involvement is a leading cause of life lost and lost potential among youth ages 10 to 24 years; this is particularly disturbing because youth violence involvement is completely preventable. As advocates of prevention and health advancement, health care providers are in a unique position to help stem the problem of youth violence. This review begins with a summary of the scope of youth violence and violence-related behavior, a discussion

Disclosures: None.
[a] Division of General Pediatrics and Adolescent Health, Department of Pediatrics, University of Minnesota, 3rd Floor, #385, 717 Delaware Street Southeast, Minneapolis MN 55414, USA;
[b] Division of General Pediatrics and Adolescent Health, Department of Pediatrics, University of Minnesota, 3rd Floor, #389, 717 Delaware Street Southeast, Minneapolis MN 55414, USA
* Corresponding author.
E-mail address: duke0028@umn.edu

of adverse childhood experiences implicated in increasing risk for youth violence involvement, and an outline of additional risk and protective factors for violence. The review concludes with information on evidence-based strategies for prevention, the importance of screening for violence involvement and the delivery of prevention messaging in the office setting, and examples of online resources to support providers in intervening and advocating on behalf of youth. The article draws attention to the importance of fostering resilience as a youth violence prevention strategy.

YOUTH VIOLENCE OVERVIEW: SCOPE OF THE PROBLEM

Violence involvement, including interpersonal and self-directed violence, is a significant cause of life lost for youth and young adults in the United States. In 2012, suicide and homicide were the second and third leading causes of death among young people ages 15 to 24 years, and the third and fourth leading causes of death among youth ages 10 to 14 years, respectively.[1] In this same year, more than 4700 youth ages 10 to 24 years lost their life due to homicide in the United States, representing an average of 13 individuals each day.[2] The average daily loss of young lives due to homicide was stable from 2010 to 2012 (2010: 13.2 lives lost each day; 2011: 12.8 lives lost each day; 2012: 13.1 lives lost each day).[2] The use of firearms was particularly lethal among youth ages 10 to 24 years in 2012; homicide by firearm was the second leading cause of injury death among 15 to 24 year olds, and the third leading cause of injury death among 10 to 14 year olds.[3]

Closer scrutiny of the numbers reveals disparities in burden. Male homicide rates are 5.5 times that of female homicide rates.[2] Homicide rates for black, non-Hispanic, Hispanic, and American Indian/Alaska Native youth ages 10 to 24 years are 14, 3, and 4 times that of white, non-Hispanic youth, respectively.[2] Among youth ages 10 to 24 years, homicide is the leading cause of death for black, non-Hispanic youth, the second leading cause of death for Hispanic youth, the third leading cause of death among American Indian/Alaska Native youth, and the fourth leading cause of death for white, non-Hispanic, and Asian/Pacific Island youth.[4]

Results from the 2013 Youth Risk Behavior Survey (YRBS, grades 9–12) reveal some trends toward increasing suicide-related behavior. Among youth in grades 9 to 12, approximately 1 in 6 youth reported seriously considering suicide during the 12 months before the survey as compared with about 1 in 6.5 in 2011 and more than 1 in 7.5 in 2009.[5] In this same survey, about 1 in 7.5 youth reported having made a plan about how they would attempt suicide in the preceding 12 months, as compared with more than 1 in 8 in 2011 and about 1 in 9.5 in 2009.[5] In 2013, 8% of respondents reported at least one suicide attempt in the 12 months before taking the YRBS, compared with 7.8% in 2011 and 6.3% in 2009.[5] Across race and ethnic groups for individuals ages 10 to 24 years, suicide is the second leading cause of death for American Indian/Alaska Native, Asian/Pacific Island, and white, non-Hispanic youth; it is the third leading cause of death for black, non-Hispanic, and Hispanic youth.[4] In 2013, suicide by firearm accounted for almost 24% of all violence-related injury deaths for youth ages 10 to 24 years.[4]

Nonfatal injuries related to violence are a significant source of physical and emotional distress for young people. Almost 800,000 youths aged 10 to 24 years were treated in emergency departments for nonfatal violence-related injuries in 2013.[6] In this same year, assault (physical fighting, striking) ranked first and accounted for more than half (56%) of nonfatal violence-related injuries for youth ages 10 to 24 years, resulting in 444,350 injuries.[6] Assault (physical fighting, striking) was the sixth leading cause of nonfatal injury treated in emergency departments among 15 to

24 year olds and the ninth leading cause among 10 to 14 year olds.[7] Assault by firearm (gunshot) resulted in nonfatal injury for almost 29,000 youths aged 10 to 24 years in 2013.[6] Among youth taking the 2013 YRBS, 1 in 4 reported having been in at least one physical fight in the 12 months preceding the survey; approximately 3% reported being in a physical fight with injuries requiring medical attention from a doctor or nurse at least once during the same time period.[8] Among the 2013 YRBS respondents who reported dating or going out with someone in the 12 months before the survey, 10.3% reported being assaulted by someone they were dating or going out with (eg, intentionally hit, slammed into something, or injured with an object or weapon).[9] Within this same group, 10.4% reported being kissed, touched, or physically forced to have sexual intercourse when they did not want to by someone they were dating or going out with.[9]

Multiple behaviors contribute to youth violence involvement. Among respondents for the 2013 YRBS, almost 18% reported carrying a weapon (eg, gun, knife, or club) at least once in the month preceding the survey; 5.5% of respondents carried a gun at least once during the same time period.[8] Respondents for the 2013 YRBS reported bully victimization in multiple contexts during the year before survey administration: 14.8% via electronic methods (e-mail, chat rooms, instant messaging, Web sites, or text) and 19.6% while on school property.[8] The use of alcohol and other drugs may diminish good decisional capacity and increase chances for youth violence involvement. For example, consumption of 5 or more drinks within a couple of hours at least once during the 30 days before the 2013 YRBS administration was reported by 1 in 5 respondents; consumption of 10 or more drinks within a couple of hours at least once during the same time period was reported by almost 1 in 15 respondents.[9]

The school environment is a context in which exposure to violence as a perpetrator, victim, and witness occurs for some young people. In 2013, more than 7% of YRBS respondents reported not going to school on at least 1 day in the 30 days before the survey because of fears about safety at school or on the way to or from school; overall, there has been an increasing trend in this occurrence in the last decade (1993–2013).[10] Among 2013 YRBS participants, more than 8% reported being in a physical fight and almost 7% reported being threatened or injured with a weapon while on school property in the 12 months before the survey.[10] The Bureau of Justice estimates that, in 2012, students ages 12 to 18 years experienced 1,364,900 nonfatal victimizations at school (theft and violent crime—includes serious violent crime [rape, sexual assault, aggravated assault] and simple assault [threats, attacks without weapon or serious injury]).[11] This finding represents about 52 victimizations per 1000 youths aged 12 to 18 years at school (inside the school building, on school property, or on the way to or from school).[11] In 2011, almost 18% of 12 to 18 year olds reported gangs were present in their school during the school year; reports varied according to geographic location (urban areas: 23%; suburban areas: 16%; rural areas: 12%).[11]

Youth violence involvement is costly to our society. Beyond the great loss of human potential (life lost, physical and emotional disability; **Table 1**), impact may be seen in multiple contexts: family disruption and loss of earnings, loss of school safety and the effectiveness of the learning environment, loss of social cohesion and increased fear within communities, and declining economic development and property values in communities.[12] Impact is also evident in multiple systems, including the medical and mental health care systems (triage and treatment), law enforcement and the courts (arrest, detention), and social services.[12] Although exact dollar amounts are an underestimate of the cost of youth violence (estimated $17.5 billion in 2010),[12] estimates provide another point of reference and motivation for

Table 1
Symptoms and long-term consequences of youth violence involvement

	Symptoms, Associated Behaviors	Long-Term Consequences
Perpetration	• Low academic achievement, school truancy • Alcohol, other drug use • Unexplained injuries, bruising	• Academic failure • Alcohol, other drug use • Criminal behaviors, confinement • Violence against partners, children
Victimization	• Symptoms of depression, anxiety • Sleep disturbance (nightmares, frequent waking, extended periods of sleep) • Multiple somatic complaints (multiples sites for complaint of pain in setting of normal examination) • Unexplained injuries, bruising • Abrupt change in behaviors, temperament • School avoidance, absenteeism, falling grades	• Poor mental health: depression, anxiety, posttraumatic stress disorder • Physical disability, chronic pain • Low self-esteem • Isolation, loneliness • Poor relationship quality, low trust
Witness	• Symptoms of depression, anxiety, repeated expression of worries and fears, separation anxiety • Sleep disturbance (frequent waking, nightmares, fear of falling asleep) • Regression of developmental milestones • Multiple somatic complaints (abdominal pain, headache, generalized aches with normal examination) • Acute change in temperament, angry outbursts, aggressive behaviors, inability to settle down, withdrawal • Acting out violent scenarios	• Poor mental health: depression, anxiety • Poor relationship quality, low trust • Low self-esteem

identification and dissemination of evidence-based strategies for youth violence prevention.

CHILDHOOD EXPERIENCES AND EXPOSURES: IMPACT ON YOUTH VIOLENCE POTENTIAL

Unfortunately, children and adolescents in the United States are often exposed to crime, violence, and abuse over the course of their development, placing them at risk for negative health behavior in the short and long term. Using data from the 2011 National Survey of Children's Exposure to Violence, Finkelhor and colleagues[13] found that almost 60% (57.7%) of children and youth, ages 1 month to 17 years, had experienced or witnessed at least 1 of 5 aggregate exposures, including (1) assaults and bullying (perpetrated by an adult, juvenile sibling, peer, gang/group; with or without weapon and injury; dating violence; bias attack; Internet/cell phone harassment); (2) sexual victimization (assault or attempted rape/rape by adult stranger, known adult, peer; being flashed; harassment; Internet sex talk); (3) maltreatment by a caregiver (sexual abuse, physical abuse, psychological or emotional abuse, neglect, custodial interference or family abduction); (4) property victimization (nonsibling peer or adult: robbery, vandalism, theft); or (5) witnessing victimization (witness assault: between family members, including parents and siblings, between family member and stranger/extended family, in community; exposure to shootings, bombings, riots), in the year before survey administration. Having one type of exposure increased the chances that a youth experienced another type of exposure, in most cases by a factor of 2 to 3.[13] Just less than half of the youth (48.4%) had experienced more than 1 of 50 exposure types involving direct or witnessed victimization: 15.1% experienced 6 or more types; almost 5% experienced 10 or more types.[13] Using data from the 2009 National Survey of Children's Exposure to Violence, Hamby and colleagues[14] found that youth witness of partner violence (between parents/parent figures) was especially closely linked to all forms of child maltreatment and family violence; for example, more than a third of youth witnessing partner violence in the past year and more than half of youth witnessing partner violence in their lifetime were also victims of child maltreatment. Adverse violence-related experiences and exposures during childhood and adolescence have the potential for lasting impact on an individual's health and health behaviors.

Chronic and multiple adverse life experiences negatively impact youth's potential for healthy adaptation, good problem-solving, and the development of positive decisional capacity via change in brain physiology and function. The brain is the principal mediator and target of stress, resiliency, and vulnerability processes as it regulates behavioral and physiologic responses to experiences.[15] Alterations in the neuroplasticity of brain regions, such as the hippocampus, amygdala, and prefrontal cortex, impact stress reactivity, coping, and recovery.[15] Using a life course framework, these alterations in neuroplasticity are hypothesized to become consolidated and hardwired into neural networks as the brain continues to develop during adolescence and young adulthood. In a series of studies examining the relationship between risk exposure in childhood and health and behavioral outcomes in adulthood, researchers conducting the Adverse Childhood Experiences Study have demonstrated risk experiences to be interrelated and associated with increased likelihood of alcohol and other drug abuse, depression, and suicidality.[16,17] Using data from the population-based 1998 Minnesota Student Survey to examine the relationship between different experiences of familial physical violence and violent behaviors among adolescents, Yexley and colleagues[18] note that experience of being a direct victim of physical violence and witness of physical violence in the family are each associated with greater odds of violent adolescent behavior (suicide attempt, fighting, carrying a gun at school); however, the combination of being a witness and direct victim of violence was associated with even greater odds of violence or violence-related behavior than experience of each type of victimization by itself. Using the 2007 Minnesota Student Survey, Duke and colleagues[19] link adverse childhood experiences (physical abuse, sexual abuse, witnessing violence, household dysfunction caused by family alcohol or other drug use) with violence involvement during adolescence, including interpersonal violence (delinquency, fighting, bullying, dating violence, carrying a weapon on school property) and self-directed violence (self-injury, suicidal ideation and attempt). Findings in this study revealed that each additional type of adverse event experienced increased the risk of violence perpetration by 35% to 144%.[19] Similarly, studies with school and community samples of youth find that exposures in the family/household context, including experiences of child abuse (physical and sexual abuse), child maltreatment, and witnessing of violent victimization-perpetration among parents or adult members in the household are linked to weapon-carrying and dating violence perpetration (threatening behaviors, physical abuse) in adolescence.[20,21]

Risk Factors for Youth Violence Involvement

As alluded to earlier, the literature links multiple types of adverse experiences and exposures to negative health outcomes, including youth interpersonal and self-directed violence. Experiences are multiple, complex, and interrelated. Although understanding of the mechanisms by which adverse experiences increase risk for negative health behaviors such as violence involvement is emerging, the research documenting factors associated with risk for youth violence is broad, touching on individual, family/household, and community characteristics (**Table 2**).

Table 2
Risk and protective factors for youth violence involvement

	Individual	Family/Household	Community
Risk factors	Previous violence involvement: victimization and perpetration	Violence, criminal history	Neighborhood violence
	Antisocial beliefs, attitudes, behaviors	Conflict, household dysfunction	Media violence
	Hyperactivity, poor impulse control	Family socioeconomic disadvantage	Concentrated poverty, limited economic opportunity
	Poor socioemotional health: depression, anxiety, anger, low self-esteem, hopelessness, deficits in social cue processing and emotional regulation	Adverse childhood experience (emotional, physical, sexual abuse; witness of violence; parental substance use)	Antisocial groups and opportunities for association, gang involvement
	Academic problems, school failure	Poor monitoring, supervision	Limited opportunity for prosocial activity
	Learning disorders	Rigid, indifferent, variable disciplinary style	Neighborhood social disorganization
	Substance use	Guns in the home	Firearm, lethal weapon access
Protective factors	Socioemotional health	Parent-family connection, shared activities	Neighborhood safety
	Spirituality	Stable supervision, monitoring	Positive connection to community adults
	Strong social skills	Expectations for academic achievement, success	School connectedness
	Academic achievement	Consistent, nonviolent disciplinary practices	Neighborhood social control (informal norms and values related to behavior, adult monitoring of youth)
	Future orientation, sense of purpose	Facilitation of open lines of communication	Economic opportunity
	Self-efficacy, self-esteem	Good problem-solving skills	Opportunity for prosocial activity
	Prosocial involvement	Authoritative parenting style	—

At a national level, several studies have documented factors associated with greater risk of youth violence involvement. Using data from the National Longitudinal Study of Adolescent Health (Add Health, Wave I), Resnick and colleagues[22] found multiple factors associated with youth violence, including history of victimization or witnessing violence, individual deviant and antisocial behavior, selling drugs, perceived high risk for premature death, household access to a gun, and recent family history of suicide or suicide attempt. In follow-up, using Add Health Wave I characteristics to predict youth violence involvement in Wave II approximately 1 year later, Resnick and colleagues[23] found that for male and female youths, risk for violence perpetration was associated with a history of violence victimization and involvement, weapon-carrying at school, substance use (marijuana, alcohol), grade retention, and learning problems (self-report). In this same study, a few additional risk factors were gender-specific: previous treatment for emotional problems (male youths); feelings of emotional distress (female youths); and somatic complaints (female youths).[23] Using Add Health, Waves I and II, Borowsky and Ireland[24] identified factors predicting future fight-related injury requiring medical care. Findings parallel earlier work: for boys and girls, previous fight-related injury, fighting, and previous victimization or witness of violence predicted injury requiring medical intervention. In addition, illicit drug use among male youths and symptoms of depression among female youths forecast fight-related injury requiring medical care.[24] Also, at the national level, findings from McNulty and Bellair[25] using data from the National Educational Longitudinal Survey suggest intervention to mitigate concentrated poverty (community and family disadvantage) as a means to address race and ethnic group differences in fighting behavior.[25] Media outlet portrayal of neighborhoods with concentrated poverty as crime ridden, menacing, and dangerous may increase the risk for violence as residents become marginalized and develop a collective sense of hopelessness.[26]

Multiple regional and population-based studies advance our knowledge of factors associated with youth violence involvement. For example, among a subsample of youth participating in the Mobile Youth Survey (a community-based, multiple cohort sample of youth living in extremes of poverty), Stoddard and colleagues[27] found that increasing and accelerating trajectories for hopelessness among middle adolescents forecast violence involvement later in adolescence (eg, violence with a weapon). Using data from the 2007 Minnesota Student Survey, Duke and colleagues[28] also found a significant relationship between hopelessness and violence involvement. In this study, moderate to high levels of hopelessness, independent of low affect, among participants were associated with weapon-carrying at school, delinquency, and self-directed violence.[28] For participants in the Urban Indian Youth Health Survey conducted from 1995 to 1998 in Minneapolis, Minnesota, the strongest factors associated with violence involvement were substance use and suicidal thoughts and behaviors.[29] In a sample of rural adolescents in North Carolina, Foshee and colleagues[30] found that the odds of assignment to a violence profile that included perpetration against peers and dating partners was significantly increased by higher levels of individual anger, anxiety, and substance use (alcohol and marijuana). Within a clinic sample of youth who scored positive on a brief psychosocial screen in 8 outpatient pediatric practices in Minnesota, youth report of corporeal punishment as a disciplinary method by his or her parent(s) was significantly associated with youth report of intention to fight if pushed or hit, fighting in the last year, bullying, and violent victimization.[31] In multiple school and community samples, childhood exposure to media violence is implicated in contributing to risk of youth violence and aggressive behaviors and perpetration of physical violence in young adulthood.[32–34] In their longitudinal follow-up of children growing up in Chicago in the 1970s, Huesmann and colleagues[32] noted that television violence viewing (youth ages 6–9 years), childhood perceptions of television violence as a reflection of real life, and childhood identification with aggressive television characters who were the same sex as the child significantly predicted a composite measure of adult aggression 15 years later.

Protective Factors Against Youth Violence Involvement

Many risks associated with youth violence involvement are preventable or modifiable. Toxic stress results from frequent and extended periods of exposure to adversity in the absence of mitigating influence from protective factors.[35] The literature focusing on factors that buffer against negative exposures is growing. Common themes across developmental contexts are identified (see **Table 2**). Below is a brief summary of protective factors relevant for multiple types of youth violence involvement.

Across studies, connections on multiple levels, prosocial norms, and parental expectations for academic achievement are negatively associated with youth violence involvement. Parent-family connections, school connectedness, and connection to adults outside of the family reduce the risk of youth violence.[22,23,29] Peer and parent prosocial norms and parent disapproval of violence are negatively associated with multiple forms of violence perpetration, including shooting or stabbing and physical fighting.[29,31] Parent expectations for school achievement/school performance buffer against violence involvement[22,23]; as well, youth academic achievement (higher grade point average) is protective.[23] Additional factors found to be protective include having the ability to discuss problems with parents among male youths and religiosity, defined as valuing religious observance and personal prayer, among female youths.[23] Higher levels of individual social bonding (having prosocial values, ascribing to conventional beliefs), parental monitoring, and neighborhood social control (adult monitoring of youth) were associated with reduced risk of peer and dating violence perpetration in a sample of rural adolescents.[30] Intentions to contribute to the neighborhood were associated with lower levels of violence involvement in a sample of young, urban adolescents.[36]

Resilience and Youth Violence Prevention

Resilience is a process evidenced and defined on multiple levels: (1) functioning to meet normal developmental tasks that are unique and relevant for a particular time in life; (2) thriving when experiencing challenging circumstances and under conditions of adversity; (3) exhibiting healthy, sustained competence and adaptation in contexts of stress; and (4) recovery from trauma.[37,38] Resilience encompasses critical components reflecting dynamic individual characteristics and elements external to the individual (**Box 1**).[37–40]

Theoretic models of resilience include risk and promotive factors (assets and resources) in defining desired outcomes: assets or resources may counteract or compensate for risk exposures, moderate risk, or in some cases, risk may be defined on a continuum in which a stress may be promotive of a positive outcome (eg, the development of a coping strategy).[40] In addition, the positive or mitigating effect of assets or resources may be context-specific, such that impact may not be the same across populations differing by age, geographic location, or cultural group.[26,40] As a point of reference, assets such as academic achievement and resources such as family connectedness in resilience models, are synonymous with the concept of protective factors. For example, in their study of protective factors for youth participating in the Project on Human Development in Chicago Neighborhoods Study, Jain and colleagues[41] found that positive peers and supportive relationships with parents and other adults (called resources in resilience literature) were predictive of emotional resilience for youth exposed to community violence.

Box 1
Components contributing to the process of resilience in youth

- Having stable and positive relationships with adults (parental support, adult mentoring)
- Positive self-perception
- Belief in purpose, meaning in life
- Empathy
- Perspective-taking skills
- Problem-solving skills
- Capacity to engage others
- Strong verbal and communication skills
- Easy temperament, emotional regulation
- Use of humor
- Spirituality
- Developed competencies in societal perceived areas of value (eg, academics, arts, athletics)
- Prosocial friends
- Bonding in other domains: school, community

Given its focus on building developmental assets and resources, a resilience approach has much to offer in informing violence prevention efforts. For example, interventions that support growth in problem-solving, general social and life skills, or family-level resources, including parenting skill, monitoring, and communication, are examples of using a resilience approach[40] that are relevant to youth violence prevention. Development of interventions focused on building resources for youth in other contexts, such as school, neighborhood, and community, are also represented in emerging research defining evidence-based strategies for the prevention of youth violence involvement that use a resilience approach (**Table 3**).

YOUTH VIOLENCE PREVENTION: BACKGROUND AND OPPORTUNITIES FOR HEALTH CARE PROVIDERS

Evidence for the impact and cost-effectiveness of youth violence prevention programs is mounting. Examples of programs exhibiting impact include (1) universal school-based prevention programming—focused on information and skills development for conflict avoidance and resolution (estimated 15% reduction in youth violence); (2) family-focused interventions—building networks of social support and parents' skills development around communication, problem-solving, modeling conflict resolution, and monitoring (estimated 24%–50% reduction in youth violence); and (3) community development—increasing security, adding green space, investment in local services, and youth engagement (estimated 8% reduction in violent crime).[12,42] It is estimated that model youth violence prevention programs save $2.73 to $49.53 for every dollar spent.[42,43] This estimate compares favorably to another well-known prevention intervention, childhood immunization programs, which are estimated to save $18.40 for every dollar spent.[42] Despite promising impact for youth violence prevention strategies, there is work to do in dismantling remaining barriers to implementation. Primary barriers include difficulty in changing existing practices, such as continued focus on

Table 3
Example prevention strategies: building youth strengths and resources

Approach/Program	Focus
Wrap-around services for youth	• Team-based needs assessment • Intervention to address mental, physical, and behavioral health • Intervention to improve safety of living space • Crisis and safety planning
Mentoring	• Building positive relationships between youth and caring adults in the community • Monitoring and role modeling of problem-solving, communication, and navigation-cooperative skills
Home visitation (during pregnancy and early childhood)	• Caregiver support • Increase knowledge about child development • Skill development for child care
Early childhood education	• Special education services to youth (and families) spanning birth to kindergarten • Build strong base for learning and healthy development
Family relationship-family dynamics	• Building network for parent social support • Skill development: problem-solving; communication; conflict resolution; dealing with anger; youth monitoring
Universal school violence prevention	• Creating a healthy school environment: commitment to positive value systems, norms; design of physical space • Support for student skill development: conflict avoidance, resolution
Community: structure and policy	• Attention to security • Increasing the built environment, green space • Economic development; investment in local services and businesses; economic empowerment zoning: tax incentives to businesses in high poverty, unemployment areas • Youth engagement for greater voice, connection; volunteerism • Addressing alcohol outlet density, alcohol availability
Street outreach	• Use of trained staff to engage youth and communities about changing beliefs and norms contributing to tolerance of violence; build support for choice of nonviolent problem-solving and conflict resolution • Conflict mediation by trained staff

See also **Table 8** for links to information on program names, policies, and practices.

individual factors, which alone are unlikely to lead to population level change, and challenges in achieving integration of individual-level strategies with community-level interventions.[42]

The Office Setting: Screening and Referral

Screening for youth violence involvement in the clinical setting is recommended; screening should include individual behaviors for youth and parents as well as assessing potential exposures in other settings (eg, friends' homes) (**Tables 4–6**). Questions about risk of violence involvement should also take account of a range of violence-related behaviors and outcomes (**Table 7**) and should be part of a comprehensive health assessment. A functional mnemonic for organizing comprehensive screening and prevention counseling is HEADDSSS, which stands for *Home, Education,*

Table 4
Position papers and policy statements related to screening for youth and family violence involvement

Institution, Medical Organization	Policies and Statements Related to Violence Screening, Prevention, and Intervention
American Academy of Family Physicians	Violence Position Paper: http://www.aafp.org/about/policies/all/violence.html Intimate Partner Violence: http://www.aafp.org/afp/2011/0515/p1165.html
American Academy of Pediatrics	Role of the Pediatrician in Youth Violence Prevention: http://pediatrics.aappublications.org/content/124/1/393.full.pdf+html Intimate Partner Violence: The Role of the Pediatrician: http://pediatrics.aappublications.org/content/125/5/1094.full.pdf+html Firearm-Related Injuries Affecting the Pediatric Population: http://pediatrics.aappublications.org/content/130/5/e1416.full.pdf+html Gun Violence Policy Recommendations: http://www.aap.org/en-us/advocacy-and-policy/federal-advocacy/Documents/AAPGunViolencePreventionPolicyRecommendations_Jan2013.pdf
American College of Obstetricians and Gynecologists	Intimate Partner Violence: http://www.acog.org/-/media/Committee-Opinions/Committee-on-Health-Care-for-Underserved-Women/co518.pdf?dmc=1&ts=20150112T2118022948
Society for Adolescent Health and Medicine	Adolescent Firearm Violence: https://www.adolescenthealth.org/SAHM_Main/media/Advocacy/Positions/Aug-05-Firearms_and_Adolescents.pdf Bullying and Peer Victimization: http://www.adolescenthealth.org/SAHM_Main/media/Advocacy/Positions/Jan-05-Bullying_and_Peer_Victimization.pdf
US Department of Health and Human Services	Screening for Domestic Violence in Health Care Settings: http://aspe.hhs.gov/hsp/13/dv/pb_screeningDomestic.pdf

Activities (social, physical activity, work), Diet, Drugs, Safety (risk of abuse, unintentional and intentional injury), Sexuality, and Symptoms of depression/Suicidality. An alternate approach for comprehensive screening begins with questions about an adolescent's strengths before queries about risk potential: SSHADESS, which stands for Strengths or interests, School, Home, Activities, Drugs, Emotions, Sexuality, and Safety.[44] Brief, clinic-friendly tools for screening of behaviors related to violence involvement are available (see **Table 7**). Screening should be followed by counseling designed to highlight actions that will support healthy youth development and facilitate beliefs around nontolerance for violence (see **Table 6**).

Screening and appropriate intervention are facilitated by the development of protocols that normalize and standardize the assessment process.[45,46] Several resources are available for staff and provider training related to violence prevention and screening and intervention strategies (**Table 8**). As well, the creation of a repository of local resources and organizations available to assist and support in violence intervention is recommended (see **Table 8**). Screening in combination with office-based referral may be instrumental in reducing youth violence involvement. In their study of 8 outpatient pediatric and community practices, Borowsky and colleagues[47] found

Table 5
Snapshot: youth violence-related behaviors and tools for use in clinical setting

Bullying	**Definition** • Repetitive, aggressive behavior to intimidate, harass, cause physical harm **Key points** • Involves 3 groups of youth: bullies, victims, bystanders • 3 forms: direct (verbal, physical aggression); indirect (covert, relational–social isolation, rumors); technology-based (Cyber bullying) **Example questions** • Have you ever been threatened, made fun of, or isolated from activities, or through any form of electronic communication? • Have you ever threatened, made fun of, or kept someone from activities, or through any form of electronic communication? **Online resources** • Information on effective interventions for building respect, resilience, relationships; youth voice as key component: Stop Bullying Now: http://stopbullyingnow.com/ • Federal Web site providing access to state laws, policies; resources for youth, parents, educators, community members: Stop Bullying: http://www.stopbullying.gov/
Dating/relationship violence	**Definition** • In context of close, intimate relationship, behavior to intimidate, control, cause physical harm **Key points** • Multiple levels of harm: physical (shoving, hitting, punching, beating); sexual (unwanted touching, nonconsensual sex); psychological (verbal threats, isolating, name-calling) • Psychological, nonphysical threat may result in more severe forms of violence over time **Example questions** • Does the person you are seeing (individuals you hang out with) make you feel stupid, make you feel afraid, try to control you, or verbally or physically hurt you?[a] • Does the person you are seeing (individuals you hang out with) put pressure on you to do things that you do not want to?[a] **Online resources** • Practice-focused tools for creating context to discuss healthy relationships, relationship abuse with adolescents: Hanging Out or Hooking Up: Clinical Guidelines on Responding to Adolescent Relationship Abuse: https://www.futureswithoutviolence.org/userfiles/file/HealthCare/Adolescent%20Health%20Guide.pdf • Peer-led discussions on identifying healthy relationships, abuse: Love is Respect: http://www.loveisrespect.org/ • Building youth, community capacity to end dating violence: Break the Cycle: http://www.breakthecycle.org/

Physical fighting	Definition • Interpersonal aggression between 2 or more youth to cause immediate physical injury or harm Key points • Example, youth-identified causes: perceptions of disrespect by another; to save a reputation; to resolve an on-going conflict, disagreement • Severity of consequences bolstered by substance use and weapon carrying Example questions • Have you been in any fights during the past year? • If yes, were weapons used? • If yes, what injuries did you and others involved have? Online resources • Practical tips directed at parents to assist their child in coping with conflict: Everybody Gets Mad: Helping Your Child Cope with Conflict: http://www.healthychildren.org/English/healthy-living/emotional-wellness/Pages/Everybody-Gets-Mad-Helping-Your-Child-Cope-with-Conflict.aspx
Weapon carrying	Definition • Physical possession of a gun, knife, club, other object to intimidate, cause physical harm Key points • Important to recognize youth misperception of enhanced safety provided by weapon carrying • Perceptions of threat associated with the school environment may be motivation to initiate weapon carrying Example questions • Do you carry a weapon for any reason (even for self-defense)? • If yes, what kind of weapon do you carry? • Do you have access to any weapons? Online resources • Practical tips directed at parents to assist in opening lines of communication with their child; includes tips on keeping child safe (weapons, what to do about fighting): Talking with Your Teen: Tips for Parents: http://www.healthychildren.org/English/family-life/family-dynamics/communication-discipline/Pages/Talking-With-Your-Teen-Tips-For-Parents.aspx

[a] In early to middle adolescence, dating may start out in group form.

Table 6
Screening and counseling related to youth violence involvement

Screening for Youth Violence Involvement	Counseling Related to Youth Violence Involvement
Youth	*Youth*
Make screening a routine	Focal points for anticipatory guidance
• Identification of one type of violence or violence-related behavior should prompt screening and assessment for other forms of violence involvement	• Send clear messages that violence is not a desired method for problem-solving and conflict resolution
• Include separate questions for different types of violence and violence-related behaviors: bullying, dating violence, weapon carrying (access) and related injury, physical fighting and related injury	• Encourage and support youth development of strategies for good communication, conflict management, and brave bystander behavior
• Have a written questionnaire to facilitate screening and counseling	• Counsel youth to report all violence (witness, victimization) to a safe adult
• Include witnessing violence as part of screen—address potential related feelings of stress and fear about becoming a target of violence	• Explore youth perceptions of safety, and how to be safe if ever threatened
Parent	*Parent*
Make screening a routine	Focal points for anticipatory guidance
• Ask parents about intimate partner violence and other experiences with violence during health supervision visits for youth	• Counsel on the importance of modeling behavior
• Check in on communication and disciplinary style	• Counsel on communicating standard of nonviolent means of conflict resolution with child
• Screen for weapons in the home	• Encourage consistency in discipline
• Check in on other forms of violence exposure, including media content	• Encourage taking opportunities to talk with child about violence exposures, including in entertainment media
	• Address potential sources of injury to child (eg, weapon access inside and outside of home)
	• Counsel on importance of knowing child's friends and friends' parents (including dating partners, if applicable)

Table 7
Short, validated, clinically accessible screening tools on topics related to youth violence

Screen Name	Screen Characteristics	Screen Link
CRAFFT	• 3 "prescreening" items; 6 screen items • Screen for alcohol and other drug use • Translated into multiple languages; clinician (structured as brief interview) and self-administered versions	http://www.ceasar-boston.org/CRAFFT/
Patient Health Questionnaire-9 Item, modified for teens	• 13 items • Screen for major depression and suicidality • Available in English and Spanish	http://www.lfmp.com/Portals/8/PHQ-9%20(Depression%20Screener%20for%20Adolescents%2012-18).pdf http://www.ncfhp.org/Data/Sites/1/phq-9-spanish.pdf
Pediatric Symptom Checklist-17	• 17 items • 3 psychosocial problem subscales (internalizing, attention, externalizing) • Available in English, Spanish, Chinese; youth[a] and parent versions	http://www.massgeneral.org/psychiatry/services/psc_home.aspx
Rapid Assessment for Adolescent Preventive Services	• 21 items • General health risk assessment survey	https://www.raaps.org/ Accessible for clinical use with registration

[a] Validation as a self-report is pending.

that psychosocial screening and the availability of a telephone-based parenting education program was associated with decreases in violence and violence-related behaviors/outcomes, including physical fighting and fight-related injury, bullying involvement, youth aggression, and delinquent behavior.

The Office Setting: Messages and Resources to Foster Resilience in Youth

Using a strength-based approach to engage youth and families is helpful for fostering resilience. Screening, although necessary to gather information on the absence or presence of problem behaviors, should be provided in such a way to elicit current assets and potential intervention points in which to promote skills and resource building for youth and families (eg, trial dialogue for dealing with conflict; referral for mentoring program) (**Table 9**). The provision of practical tips that support positive coping and wellness for youth also contributes to the process of resilience: (1) Parents: maintaining routine, encouraging outlets for expression and connection, encouraging time away from media and electronic devices; (2) Youth: connection with others, taking time for self, centering and use of deep breathing, finding outlets for free expression. Resources are available for information and practice for youth and families, and practice and office-organizational change for health care providers (see **Table 9**).

Table 8
Online resources for general screening and anticipatory guidance, evidence-based strategies for youth violence prevention

Resource Name	Resource Components	Resource Link
Connected Kids: Safe, Strong, Secure (American Academy of Pediatrics)	• Provider focus on strength-based approach to anticipatory guidance • Reviews counseling schedule, with example questions for parents and youth according to early, middle, and late adolescence (and across age spectrum) • Focus on assisting parents in raising resilient children	Connected Kids Materials: https://www2.aap.org/connectedkids/material.htm
Massachusetts Medical Society Violence Prevention Project	• Clinical suggestions for violence screening, evaluation, anticipatory guidance, and documentation • Tools and tips for parents: praise; time out; media violence; bully prevention; dating violence; street violence; coping after witness of violence	Recognizing and Preventing Youth Violence: A Guide for Physicians and Other Health Care Professionals[a] Intimate Partner Violence: The Clinician's Guide to Identification, Assessment, Intervention, and Prevention[a] http://www.massmed.org/violence/
Striving to Reduce Youth Violence Everywhere (STRYVE) (Centers for Disease Control and Prevention)	• Database with access to names and descriptions of strategies that reflect the best available evidence in preventing youth violence[b] • Online training of key concepts and strategies for violence prevention • Platform to connect online with others working to prevent youth violence and other public health issues	STRYVE—Home: http://vetoviolence.cdc.gov/apps/stryve/

VetoViolence (Centers for Disease Control and Prevention)	• Violence prevention basics: primary prevention, public health approach, socioecological model • Example tools and trainings: Principles of Prevention; Understanding Evidence	VetoViolence: http://vetoviolence.cdc.gov/
Youth Topics—Find Youth Info (Preventing Youth Violence)[c] (in Partnership with the National Forum on Youth Violence Prevention)	• Highlights Forum Communities charged with developing and implementing youth violence prevention strategic plans[d] • Mapping feature to assist in locating federally supported youth programs in one's community (goal to promote collaboration, avoid duplication)[e] • Strategic planning tool kit for communities	Preventing Youth Violence: http://findyouthinfo.gov/youth-topics

[a] Overview information, tips, and tools are relevant for any clinical practice; information regarding laws and crisis phone numbers are unique to Massachusetts.
[b] Can select on characteristics: age; demographics (geography, race, and ethnicity); focus area (eg, bullying); setting (eg, community, school); specific populations (eg, foster care; pregnant; incarcerated).
[c] Additional topics: teen dating violence; bullying.
[d] Strategic plans available for: Boston, Camden, Chicago, Detroit, Memphis, Minneapolis, New Orleans, Philadelphia, Salinas, San Jose.
[e] Can filter by topic (eg, bullying, violence and victimization, mentoring, positive youth development); agency distance.

Table 9 Resources for resilience	
Building Resilience in Children (Ginsburg, Kenneth; American Academy of Pediatrics)	Target audience • Parents, caregivers Key points • Identifies 7 C's of resilience: competence, confidence, connection, character, contribution, coping, control • Guide to help parents help youth recognize their value and tap into their inner resources Link • http://www.healthychildren.org/English/healthy-living/emotional-wellness/Building-Resilience/Pages/Building-Resilience-in-Children.aspx
Little Children, Big Challenges (Sesame Street Workshop)	Target audience • Young children • Parents, caregivers • Teachers Key points • Focus on helping children to build self-confidence, problem-solving skills, skills to deal with day-to-day challenges and more significant transitions • Tool kit: videos, songs, tips and guides, activities for youth, links to related workshop content (bully prevention; parental incarceration; parental divorce; self-confidence) Link • http://www.sesamestreet.org/parents/topicsandactivities/toolkits/challenges#
Resilience for Teens: Got Bounce? (American Psychological Association)	Target audience • Adolescents Key points • Provides 10 tips for building resilience • Frames resilience as a journey, developing skills to be applied throughout life Link • http://www.apa.org/helpcenter/bounce.aspx
The Resilience Project (American Academy of Pediatrics)	Target audience • Clinical providers • Clinical practice staff Key points • Situates medical home as place to identify issues related to violence, connect youth and families to resources that promote healing, thriving • Provides strategies for modifying practice operations to better identify and intervene where youth have been exposed to, victimized by violence • Training tool kit: clinical vignettes, framing questions, identifying potential actions to take if violence exposure identified, discussion questions, resources Link • http://www.aap.org/en-us/advocacy-and-policy/aap-health-initiatives/Medical-Home-for-Children-and-Adolescents-Exposed-to-Violence/Pages/Medical-Home-for-Children-and-Adolescents-Exposed-to-Violence.aspx

Advocacy and Collaboration Beyond the Office

Opportunities exist for providers to embrace a role for violence prevention outside of the medical practice setting. Seeking out and working in conjunction with organizations that focus on youth violence prevention and healthy youth development will facilitate building a referral base and will help support the success of community partners. Connection and work with school personnel (school nurse, psychologist, social worker, and administration) will facilitate communication and coordination of care as well as provide opportunities for collaboration (provision of information, speaking engagements, attendance at sponsored events focused on health promotion). In addition, resources are available to identify potential collaborators in other contexts, including research and policy development; these resources also include access to sample strategic plans and tool kits to help get energized and organized (see **Table 8**).

SUMMARY

Youth violence involvement is completely preventable. The evidence base for successful prevention strategies is growing. Health care providers have a critical role to play in identifying youth at risk for violence involvement. Use of a resilience framework to guide prevention efforts and clinical activities places the development of youth assets and resources at the center of care, effectively helping youth reach their full potential.

REFERENCES

1. National Center for Injury Prevention and Control, Causes of death by age group. Available at: www.cdc.gov/injury/wisqars/pdf/leading_causes_of_death_by_age_group_2012-a.pdf. Accessed January 8, 2015.
2. Centers for Disease Control and Prevention, WISQARS, fatal injury reports, national and regional, 1999–2013. Available at: http://webappa.cdc.gov/sasweb/ncipc/mortrate10_us.html. Accessed January 8, 2015.
3. National Center for Injury Prevention and Control, Causes of injury death: highlighting violence. Available at: www.cdc.gov/injury/wisqars/pdf/leading_causes_of_injury_death_highlighting_violence_2012-a.pdf. Accessed January 8, 2015.
4. Centers for Disease Control and Prevention, WISQARS, leading causes of death reports, national and regional, 1999–2013. Available at: http://webappa.cdc.gov/sasweb/ncipc/leadcaus10_us.html. Accessed January 8, 2015.
5. National Center for HIV/AIDS, Viral Hepatitis, STD, and TB Prevention, Division of Adolescent and School Health, Youth risk behavior surveillance system: trends in the prevalence of suicide-related behavior, National YRBS: 1991–2013. Available at: http://www.cdc.gov/healthyyouth/yrbs/pdf/trends/us_suicide_trend_yrbs.pdf. Accessed January 8, 2015.
6. Centers for Disease Control and Prevention, WISQARS, leading causes of nonfatal injury reports, 2001–2013. Available at: http://webappa.cdc.gov/sasweb/ncipc/nfilead2001.html. Accessed January 8, 2015.
7. National Center for Injury Prevention and Control, Causes of nonfatal injuries treated in hospital emergency departments. Available at: www.cdc.gov/injury/wisqars/pdf/leading_causes_of_nonfatal_injury_2013-a.pdf. Accessed January 8, 2015.
8. National Center for HIV/AIDS, Viral Hepatitis, STD, and TB Prevention, Division of Adolescent and School Health, Youth risk behavior surveillance system: trends in the prevalence of behaviors that contribute to violence, National

YRBS: 1991–2013. Available at: http://www.cdc.gov/healthyyouth/yrbs/pdf/trends/us_violence_trend_yrbs.pdf. Accessed January 8, 2015.

9. Kahn L, Kinchen S, Shanklin SL, et al. Youth risk behavior surveillance—United States, 2013. MMWR Surveill Summ 2014;63(4):1–168.

10. National Center for HIV/AIDS, Viral Hepatitis, STD, and TB Prevention, Division of Adolescent and School Health, Youth risk behavior surveillance system: trends in the prevalence of behaviors that contribute to violence on school property, National YRBS: 1991–2013. Available at: http://www.cdc.gov/healthyyouth/yrbs/pdf/trends/us_violenceschool_trend_yrbs.pdf. Accessed January 8, 2015.

11. Bureau of Justice, Indicators of school crime and safety 2013. Available at: http://www.bjs.gov/content/pub/pdf/iscs13.pdf. Accessed January 8, 2015.

12. David-Ferdon C, Simon TR. Preventing youth violence: Opportunities for action. Atlanta Georgia: National Center for Injury Prevention and Control, Centers for Disease Control and Prevention, 2014. Available at: http://www.cdc.gov/violenceprevention/youthviolence/pdf/opportunities-for-action.pdf. Accessed January 8, 2015.

13. Finkelhor D, Turner HA, Shattuck A, et al. Violence, crime, and abuse exposure in a national sample of children and youth: an update. JAMA Pediatr 2013;167(7):614–21.

14. Hamby S, Finkelhor D, Turner H, et al. The overlap of witnessing partner violence with child maltreatment and other victimizations in a nationally representative survey of youth. Child Abuse Negl 2010;34:734–41.

15. McEwen BS, Gianaros PJ. Central role of the brain in stress and adaptation: links to socioeconomic status, health, and disease. Ann N Y Acad Sci 2010;1186:190–222.

16. Chapman DP, Dube SR, Anda RF. Adverse childhood events as risk factors for negative mental health outcomes. Psychiatr Ann 2007;37:359–64.

17. Felitti VJ, Anda RF. The relationship of adverse childhood experiences to adult medical disease, psychiatric disorders, and sexual behavior: implications for healthcare. In: Lanius RA, Vermetten E, Pain C, editors. The impact of early life trauma on health and disease: the hidden epidemic. New York: Cambridge University Press; 2010. p. 77–87.

18. Yexley M, Borowsky I, Ireland M. Correlation between different experiences of intrafamilial physical violence and violent adolescent behavior. J Interpers Violence 2002;17(7):707–20.

19. Duke NN, Pettingell SL, McMorris BJ, et al. Adolescent violence perpetration: associations with multiple types of adverse child experiences. Pediatrics 2010;125:e778–86.

20. Wekerle C, Wolfe DA. Dating violence in mid-adolescence: theory, significance, and emerging prevention initiatives. Clin Psychol Rev 1999;19(4):435–56.

21. Wolfe DA, Scott K, Wekerle C, et al. Child maltreatment: risk of adjustment problems and dating violence in adolescence. J Am Acad Child Adolesc Psychiatry 2001;40(3):282–9.

22. Resnick MD, Bearman PS, Blum RW, et al. Protecting adolescents from harm: findings from the National Longitudinal Study of Adolescent Health. JAMA 1997;278:823–32.

23. Resnick MD, Ireland M, Borowsky IW. Youth violence perpetration: what protects? What predicts? Findings from the National Longitudinal Study of Adolescent Health. J Adolesc Health 2004;35:424.e1–10.

24. Borowsky IW, Ireland M. Predictors of future fight-related injury among adolescents. Pediatrics 2004;113:530–6.

25. McNulty TL, Bellair PE. Explaining racial and ethnic difference in adolescent violence: structural disadvantage, family well-being, and social capital. Justice Q 2003;20(1):1–31.
26. Aisenberg E, Herrenkohl T. Community violence in context: risk and resilience in children and families. J Interpers Violence 2008;23(3):296–315.
27. Stoddard SA, Henly SJ, Sieving RE, et al. Social connections, trajectories of hopelessness, and serious violence in impoverished urban youth. J Youth Adolesc 2011;40:278–95.
28. Duke NN, Borowsky IW, Pettingell SL, et al. Examining youth hopelessness and an independent risk correlate for adolescent delinquency and violence. Matern Child Health J 2011;15:87–97.
29. Bearinger LH, Pettingell S, Resnick MD, et al. Violence perpetration among urban American Indian youth: can protection offset risk? Arch Pediatr Adolesc Med 2005;159:270–7.
30. Foshee VA, Reyes HL, Ennett ST, et al. Risk and protective factors distinguishing profiles of adolescent peer and dating violence perpetration. J Adolesc Health 2011;48:344–50.
31. Ohene S, Ireland M, McNeely, et al. Parental expectations, physical punishment, and violence among adolescents who score positive on a psychosocial screening test in primary care. Pediatrics 2006;117:441–7.
32. Huesmann LR, Moise-Titus J, Podolski CL, et al. Longitudinal relations between children's exposure to TV violence and their aggressive and violent behavior in young adulthood: 1977–1992. Dev Psychol 2003;39(2):201–21.
33. Boxer P, Huesmann LR, Bushman BJ, et al. The role of violent media preference in cumulative developmental risk for violence and general aggression. J Youth Adolesc 2009;38(3):417–28.
34. Gentile DA, Bushman BJ. Reassessing media violence effects using a risk and resilience approach to understanding aggression. Psychol Pop Media Cult 2012;1(3):138–51.
35. Shonkoff JP. Building a new biodevelopmental framework to guide the future of early childhood policy. Child Dev 2010;81(1):357–67.
36. Widome R, Sieving RE, Harpin SA, et al. Measuring neighborhood connection and the association with violence in young adolescents. J Adolesc Health 2008;43:482–9.
37. Masten AS, Best KM, Garmezy N. Resilience and development: contributions from the study of children who overcame adversity. Dev Psychopathol 1990;2:425–44.
38. Resnick MD. Protective factors, resiliency, and healthy youth development. Adolesc Med 2000;11:157–64.
39. Masten AS. Regulatory processes, risk, and resilience in adolescent development. Ann N Y Acad Sci 2004;1021:310–9.
40. Fergus S, Zimmerman MA. Adolescent resilience: a framework for understanding healthy development in the face of risk. Annu Rev Public Health 2005;26:399–419.
41. Jain S, Buka SL, Subramanian SV, et al. Protective factors for youth exposed to violence: role of developmental assets in building emotional resilience. Youth Violence Juv Justice 2012;10(1):107–29.
42. Gorman-Smith D. Centers for Disease Control and Prevention Public Health Grand Rounds Presentation Preventing Youth Violence 2014: Helping communities use the evidence for youth violence prevention. Available at: http://www.cdc.gov/cdcgrandrounds/pdf/gr-youth-violence-feb18.pdf. Accessed January 8, 2015.

43. Washington State Institute for Public Policy, Benefit-Cost Results. Available at: http://www.wsipp.wa.gov/BenefitCost. Accessed January 8, 2015.
44. Ginsburg KR. Viewing our patients through a positive lens. Contemp Pediatr 2007;24:65–75.
45. Borowsky IW, Ireland M. National survey of pediatricians' violence prevention counseling. Arch Pediatr Adolesc Med 1999;153:1170–6.
46. Borowsky IW, Ireland M. Parental screening for intimate partner violence by pediatricians and family physicians. Pediatrics 2002;110:509–16.
47. Borowsky IW, Mozayeny S, Stuenkel K, et al. Effect of a primary-care based intervention on violent behavior and injury in children. Pediatrics 2004;114:e392–9.

Systematic Review to Inform Dual Tobacco Use Prevention

William Douglas Evans, PhD, Kimberly A. Horn, EdD*,
Tiffany Gray, MPH

KEYWORDS

- Adolescent tobacco use • Dual tobacco use • Tobacco prevention
- Health communications • Systematic review

KEY POINTS

- Dual tobacco use is increasing among youth, but there are few evidence-based, published interventions to combat it.
- Health communication strategies are potential areas for dual use prevention, given success of campaigns to prevent youth smoking and encourage cessation.
- The emergence of alternative products such as electronic cigarettes adds new complexities to dual use that calls for innovative research and intervention strategies.

INTRODUCTION

Dual tobacco use, the concurrent use of smoked and smokeless tobacco, is a growing US phenomenon. Approximately 15% of US adult tobacco users concurrently use some form of smoked and smokeless tobacco.[1] Dual tobacco users represent a unique high-risk population.[1] Compared with those who use cigarettes only, dual users tend to be from low socioeconomic status environments, more heavily addicted to nicotine, have extensive difficulties quitting tobacco and sustaining cessation, and may experience compounding risks of chronic diseases and certain cancers.[1–5]

With an expanding number of tobacco products now available and heavily marketed, dual tobacco use is on the increase among youth. This phenomenon may signal a new pathway to nicotine addiction among youth.[6] A recent National Youth Tobacco Survey found that 12.6% of youth ages 14 to 19 currently use 2 or more types of tobacco.[7,8] The addictive power of cigarettes is generally well accepted in the United

Disclosures: None.
The Milken Institute School of Public Health, The George Washington University, Department of Prevention and Community Health, 905 New Hampshire Avenue, Northwest, Washington, DC 20052, USA
* Corresponding author.
E-mail address: khorn1@email.gwu.edu

States. Youth, however, even when they acknowledge the dangers of cigarette smoking, perceive that other tobacco products are less harmful. Currently, the field lacks literature that illuminates the short- and long-term effects of dual use on youth, but prevention is critical. Recent evidence shows how industry marketing is one of the most significant influences of dual tobacco uptake.[9] Misperceptions are conveyed through advertisements that encourage cigarette smokers to switch to smokeless tobacco products rather than quitting, to use them in environments in which smoking is prohibited, or to use them as social alternatives.[10] Tobacco companies spend billions of dollars annually to portray tobacco use as attractive, accepted, and culturally engrained.

While we await the studies of immediate and long-term consequences on youth, experts recommend that widespread public education and aggressive product regulations are needed to prevent escalation of dual tobacco use among youth.

More specifically, a recent report by The Community Preventive Services Task Force recommends mass-reach health communication interventions as evidence-based approaches to reducing tobacco use among youth.[11] Unfortunately, we have limited knowledge of prevention efforts focused on dual tobacco use, particularly through mass health communication approaches as a part of comprehensive tobacco control initiatives. According to the Centers for Disease Control and Prevention mass-reach health communication refers to the numerous channels by which targeted public health information reaches large numbers of people.[11] Although there are many systematic reviews of mass health communication interventions for distinct tobacco products, especially cigarette smoking, there are no such published systematic literature reviews focusing on dual tobacco use. This type of review is needed to inform the understanding, design, and implementation of dual tobacco use prevention for youth.

To address this gap, this systematic review focused on the synthesis of empirical results in the context of dual tobacco use rather than particular theories or frameworks. We did not conduct a meta-analysis of extant data, rather the primary goal was to determine what portion of the existing literature had the prevention of dual use as the sole object of study. As a secondary goal, we assessed, within that body of knowledge, the extent to which studies informed population level approaches using any type of mass health communication strategy. The expected outcomes of these systematic reviews were: (1) a compilation of literature on mass health communication approaches addressing dual use tobacco prevention, (2) a methodology for identifying and categorizing such literature, and (3) recommendations for dual tobacco use prevention as gleaned from the literature review, including future development of a research agenda to build the evidence base for dual use prevention among youth.

MATERIALS AND METHODS
Search Protocol

From May to July 2013, we conducted a systematic search of literature using all relevant, major online research literature databases (specified in later discussion), following widely accepted methods for systematic review.[12] Dual tobacco use literature was operationalized as any manuscript in the published health, social science, and business literature addressing strategies to prevent or control the concurrent use of any smoked and smokeless form of tobacco. This definition included noncombustible products such as e-cigarettes. The intent of our search was to identify all articles that reported or advised on the development, delivery, or evaluation of dual use tobacco prevention or intervention, specifically. Key search terms included *smoking* (including both traditional and new products) and *smokeless* (based on a designated list of products) shown in **Table 2**, in combination with the following terms: *health promotion, counter marketing, counter advertising, social marketing, health communication, health marketing campaign, diffusion of information, diffusion of innovation,* and *advertising*. To that end, we searched the following health, social science, and business databases: PubMed, PsycINFO, Web of Science (includes Science Citation Index Expanded, Social Sciences Citation Index, and Arts & Humanities Citation Index), Communication & Mass Media Complete, Academic Search Premier, Business Source Premier, CINAHL, Health Source: Nursing/Academic Edition, and Health Source: Consumer Edition.

As a result of this literature search, we identified 46 possible references. The 2 lead authors of this report then independently reviewed all available abstracts and compared their reviews.

Inclusion/Exclusion Criteria

A set of formalized decision rules were followed consistent with the PRISMA (Preferred Reporting Items for Systematic Reviews and Meta-Analyses) guidelines (**Fig. 1**) in the subsequent assessment of articles for inclusion in the review. This procedure identified studies in which objectives were specifically related to or informed dual tobacco use prevention outcomes. Based on preset terms, we eliminated all articles that (1) did not represent original research (eg, review papers), (2) did not address prevention or intervention with dual tobacco use, (3) represented tobacco industry product market research, or (4) were not otherwise focused on dual use prevention or intervention outcomes. This screening process yielded 8 articles deemed specific to dual tobacco use health communications prevention or intervention and relevant for study inclusion. In this process, we eliminated the remaining articles because they did not meet the criteria previously noted.

Coding Form

A coding form was developed to capture descriptive information on dual use prevention or intervention health communications initiatives. Based on authors' previous systematic reviews of health communications and design of public health branding studies, several coding domains were identified. Major domains included: (1) Health Communication Intervention Development; (2) Marketing Execution; (3) Evaluation and Outcomes Reporting; and (4) Study Quality. Within each domain, specific variables of interest were further specified. An open-ended "other, please specify" response was included for many variables to ensure novel, but significant, options were not ignored.

Health Communication Intervention Development

Variables in this domain captured information on research and activities that led to the development of health communication interventions aimed at preventing and reducing dual tobacco use. Specific variables of interest identified included (1) use of scientific theory, (2) formative research, and (3) persuasive elements. We assessed and noted whether authors specified the use of scientific theory in the development of the intervention and the type of theory that was reported. Responses included psychological theory, communication theory, marketing theory, or other. We also coded whether development of dual use interventions were supported by formative research, including the type of research conducted (ie, focus groups). This variable is pertinent, as public health intervention efforts are strengthened through input from the target population during the development process.

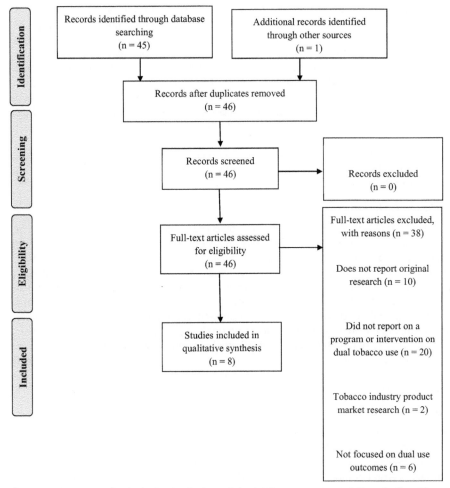

Fig. 1. Decision tree for inclusion/exclusion of dual tobacco use prevention studies. (*From* Moher D, Liberati A, Tetzlaff J, et al. Preferred reporting items for systematic reviews and meta-analyses: the PRISMA statement. Ann Intern Med 2009;151(4):264–9; with permission.)

Marketing Execution

Domain variables sought to capture reported information on the mechanisms used to promote or disseminate population level messages aimed at dual tobacco use prevention and control. Variables included (1) evidence of a social marketing or communication campaign, (2) marketing channels, and (3) marketing techniques.

We coded whether study authors described the channels used to promote interventions and identified which channels were described. Potential channels included paid mass media, unpaid mass media, earned media (ie, generating news coverage), community outreach, community mobilization, mobile phones, and social media. A broad range of strategies can be used to increase the impact and uptake of the branded health behavior. For example, audience segmentation is a common strategy used to increase the homogeneity of the group the media campaign is targeted toward. Therefore, we reported on whether authors included this information.

Evaluation and Outcomes Reporting

We assessed the completeness with which the study sample was described by indicating whether the following variables were reported: (1) sample size, (2) sample characteristics (eg, socio-demographics), and (3) response (or follow-up) rate. Each study was categorized as experimental, quasi-experimental, or observational. Also noted were the type of statistics used and reported in the evaluation of studies. These statistics include descriptive statistics, multivariate statistics (eg, analysis of variance, regression), multilevel and path models (eg, Structural Equation Models), or other statistics.

We recorded whether hypotheses were clearly stated and, if so, whether they related to awareness of dual use intervention efforts, prebehavioral/intermediate outcomes (eg, tobacco-related attitudes, beliefs, and intentions), behavioral outcomes, or specific health-related effects on morbidity and mortality. Following the manner in which research objectives were assessed, we coded for indication of the types of outcomes and whether they reported dual use awareness, behavioral outcomes, and positive or negative health impacts. A dichotomous variable indicated whether P values, standard errors, or confidence intervals were reported in the study.

Study Quality

Finally, to get an initial assessment of the quality of dual use studies reviewed, a quality scale was developed similar to those of recent systematic reviews of health communication research.[12] Several key factors should be included in a well-reported health communications study. The quality scale includes elements from each of the 4 domains described above and resulted in a scale with a range of 0 to 11 points (with 0 being the least desirable and 11 being the most desirable) with one point given for each of the following:

- The theory of change used in the intervention is clearly described.
- Role/input of formative research is reported.
- Key elements of the intervention are discussed.
- Channels used in marketing execution are described.
- Marketing techniques to increase behavior adoption are reported.
- Sample size and sample characteristics are described.
- A response or completion rate is reported.
- Explicit measures of intervention effectiveness are described.
- Hypotheses/research questions are clearly stated and match outcome measures.
- Reported outcomes include sufficient statistics.
- Measure of precision of the estimate is provided.

For this study, all studies that included all or almost all of the above elements (8–11) points) are exemplary in describing the thinking, implementation, and evaluation of the effort; studies that include most of the above elements (5–7 points) is good, and studies that include only a few of the above elements (0–4 points) are less than adequate in describing the effort.

RESULTS
Summary of Reviewed Articles

Table 1 summarizes the 8 articles (of 46) that met inclusion criteria for review. Four of the interventions were developed in the United States. Two additional interventions were in India (Delhi, Chennai, including a National study), one in Sweden (Vasterbotten

Table 1
Overview of studies included in this review

Citation	Public Health Intervention	Research Design	Location
Doi & DiLorenzo,[17] 1993	School-based, peer led curriculum; prevention	Experimental	Missouri
Lee et al,[6] 2014	Korean Youth Risk Behavior Survey; dual use assessment	Observational	Korea
McClave-Regan & Berkowitz,[26] 2011	ConsumerStyles survey (mail-in); dual use assessment	Observational	United States
Murukutla et al,[27] 2012	National television and radio mass media campaign; control	Observational	India
Norberg et al,[28] 2011	Vasterbotten Intervention; evaluation; control	Observational	Sweden
Popova et al,[29] 2014	Pre-Post survey; message testing; prevention	Experimental	United States
Regan et al,[19] 2012	ConsumerStyles survey (mail-in); dual use assessment	Observational	United States
Stigler et al,[18] 2007	Project MYTRI; School-based, multiple component intervention	Experimental	India

County), and one in Korea. Interventions were specifically developed to assess, prevent, or control dual use. Broadly, the interventions involved the use of school-based/peer-led curriculums, school-based and consumer surveys, and national television and radio campaigns. Because characteristics of these articles are generally a function of the underlying intervention, where relevant, we report below the statistics on the interventions rather than the individual articles, as recommended by previous systematic reviews.[13]

Types of Tobacco

Table 2 provides an overview of the types of tobacco (smoked and smokeless) represented in this review. Cigarettes and cigars were the most reported forms of smoked tobacco, whereas chewing tobacco, dipping tobacco, snuff, and dissolvable tobacco (including snus), were among the most reported types of smokeless tobacco in the 8 included articles.

Communication Intervention or Campaign Development

We coded for the clarity and comprehensive description of the research activities used to develop communication interventions and social marketing campaigns. We found that 3 of the studies provided enough detail to identify the main scientific theory or theories used. Three articles examined cited communication theories, and psychological theories were cited by 2 articles. Three of the studies examined reported the use of formative research in social marketing development. Interestingly, they all reported observational methods rather than traditional focus groups or in-depth interviews used in many interventions and campaigns.

Marketing Execution

Marketing execution variables describe the methods used to promote and disseminate the intervention. Community outreach was the most common channel reported (25%) whereas paid (ie, commercially placed advertising) and unpaid media were only reported in 12.5% of the interventions. Of the marketing tactics used, message

Table 2
Types of tobacco (smoked and smokeless) products

Types of Tobacco Products	Description	Category	Frequency	%
Cigars (including, blunts, cigarillos, little cigars)	Tightly rolled bundle of dried and fermented tobacco	Smoked	2[a]	25.0
Cigarettes (including kreteks, roll-your-own)	Roll of finely cut tobacco	Smoked	6[a]	75.0
Chewing tobacco	Loose leaf, pellets, plug, twist creamy snuff	Smokeless	2[a]	25.0
Dipping tobacco	Long cut, mid cut, fine cut, snuff, pouches	Smokeless	1[a]	12.5
Dissolvable tobacco (including snus)	Moist powder tobacco consumed by placing it under the upper lip for extended periods of time and does not require spitting	Smokeless	3	37.5
Snuff	Fine ground tobacco, intended for consumption by being inhaled or sniffed into the nose	Smokeless	1	12.5
Gutka	Crushed mixture of betel nuts and tobacco	Smokeless	—	—
Dokha	Finely shredded tobacco mixed with leaves, bark and herb	Smoked	—	—
Shisha or Hookah tobacco	Flavored tobacco smoked in a water pipe	Smoked	—	—

[a] Several articles addressed multiple topics.

tailoring was reported in only 12.5% of interventions, whereas audience segmentation and other techniques were not reported.

Evaluation and Outcome Reporting

All 8 articles included in this review reported information on the outcome or evaluation of the intervention. The types of outcome and evaluation information from these efforts are summarized in **Table 4**. Three of the included interventions were based on experimental designs, and 5 were based on observational designs. We found that 6 of the interventions reported outcomes indicating dual awareness and behavioral outcomes, and 3 interventions indicated prebehavioral/intermediate outcomes (eg, tobacco-related attitudes, beliefs, and intentions). We also found that all interventions provided information on the study sample, and 7 interventions provided information on sample characteristics and reported response/follow-up rates.

Quality Scale

A quality scale was constructed for this review with a range of 0 to 11 points. We analyzed quality at the campaign level (not individual studies within campaigns). Observed values ranged from 5 to 9, with a mean value of 6.8 and a standard deviation of 1.41. None of the campaigns scored 10 or 11 points, a score considered to be exemplary reporting in previous studies using this scale.[14]

We noted a wide range of quality of research and results reporting. However, most studies reviewed did have the most coded reporting procedures (7 of the 8 articles had 6 or more elements) and would thus qualify as "good" based on our subjective assessment (see Methods section).

DISCUSSION
Achieving Consensus on Dual Use Definitions

The relative newness of the research on dual tobacco use dictated the need to establish an operational definition for our review inclusion criteria, including a scheme for characterizing dual use tobacco control as a distinct strategy. At the outset, we broadly defined dual tobacco use as the concurrent use of smoked and smokeless tobacco. Klesges and colleagues[15] estimate that the varying definitions of dual use may impair prevalence estimates 50-fold (0.5%–25.3%). Because of lack of consensus on the definition of dual tobacco use, and to be exhaustive, we considered not only categories of smoked and smokeless tobacco but specific types of tobacco within the categories: cigarettes, cigars, dokha, hookah tobacco, chewing tobacco, dipping tobacco, and dissolvable tobacco.[15] See **Table 1** for definitions of each type of tobacco considered in our study. One of our objectives was to assess the extent to which studies reported on specific types of tobacco. Consistent with other studies, the preponderance of literature we reviewed reported general categories of users (eg, cigarettes only, cigarettes and other tobacco products, and other tobacco products only).[16] Although these general categories assist in identifying dual use prevalence or incidence, they don't necessarily maximize information to tailor or message strategies for specific types of dual users. Increased specificity in types of tobacco use reported is important because dual users of cigarettes and hookah tobacco, for example, may be demographically unique compared with dual users of cigarettes and chewing tobacco. In addition to age, gender, race/ethnicity, and socioeconomic status, it is also likely that there are differences in dual tobacco use patterns, all of which potentially have implications for the design, implementation, and communication of effective tobacco control strategies.[16]

As part of the primary goal, we sought to develop a scheme for characterizing extant dual use tobacco control interventions or campaigns. For example, Doi and DiLorenzo[17] and Stigler and colleagues[18] both used school-based health education and tobacco use risk communication strategies. These interventions were evaluated using experimental, school-based designs to assess the effects of an in-school curriculum on dual tobacco use outcomes. However, the 8 studies reviewed in depth covered a wide range of intervention approaches, such as communications, and were generally based on evaluation through existing surveys of the general population, such as ConsumerStyles.[19]

Characterizing dual use health communications interventions is an important aim to pursue as the field moves forward, but the small number of studies meeting our inclusion criteria and their diversity in terms of populations addressed, media channels and settings used, and specific messages delivered, leave this as a future research question. Given that we identified 43 studies that addressed dual use in some way, as more interventions are developed, we anticipate that proven health communication and social marketing approaches will become more prevalent. Future studies should aim to apply evidence-based approaches, such as the use of health branding, to create a positive identity for avoidance of dual use.[14] For example, future branded dual use campaigns could use social role modeling (eg, appealing members of the target audiences' perceived peer group or celebrities) to depict the benefits of alternative, healthier lifestyles to reach high-risk populations such as low socioeconomic status young adult men.[19]

Applying Proven Tobacco Control Health Communication Strategies to Dual Use

A secondary aim was to review existing literature on dual use tobacco control to determine the extent to which generally accepted tobacco control strategies have been applied or evaluated in the context of dual use. **Table 2** shows the various types of tobacco control strategies, in the context of health communication and social marketing interventions and campaigns. As shown in **Table 3**, we assessed the key domains of health communication and social marketing in the categories of theory, use of formative research, marketing "Ps", (place, price, product, and promotion) marketing channels, and marketing techniques.

Use of Sound Research Design and Evidence of Impact on Behavioral Outcomes

Most of the studies we reviewed included clearly described research designs, with 5 being observational studies and 3 experimental studies in school-based settings. Methods, measures, and outcomes were also clearly described, as represented in the coding shown in **Table 4**. On our quality rating scale, the articles that qualified for review scored in the middle range and on average qualified as good reporting. The scores were generally somewhat lower than they might have been because of incomplete reporting of intervention development and formative research, specific communication and social marketing components, and implementation. Future

Table 3
Health communication/social marketing intervention or campaign development (n = 8)

Variables	Frequency	%
Scientific theory		
Communication	1	12.5
Marketing	—	—
Psychology	2	25
Other	—	—
Formative research		
Focus groups	1	12.5
Interviews	—	—
Other	3	37.5
Marketing "P's"		
Product	2	25.0
Price	—	—
Place	2	25.0
Promotion	3	37.5
Marketing channels		
Paid mass media	1	12.5
Unpaid mass media	1	12.5
Earned media	—	—
Community outreach	2	25.0
Coalition building	—	—
Mobile phones	—	—
Social media (not mobile)	—	—
Other	2	25.0
Other marketing techniques		
Audience segmentation	1	12.5
Message tailoring	1	12.5
Other	—	—

Table 4 Study design and outcomes (n = 8)		
Variables	**Frequency**	**%**
Research design		
Experiment	3	37.5
Quasi-experiment	—	—
Observational study	5	62.5
Sample size reported	8	100
Sample characteristics described	7	87.5
Response/follow-up rate reported	7	87.5
Statistics reported		
Descriptive	8	100
Multivariate analysis (ANOVA/Regression)	6	75.0
Multi-level models	—	—
Path analysis	2	25.0
None reported	—	—
Objectives clearly stated		
Product/behavior awareness or reactions	4	50.0
Prebehavioral outcomes	3	37.5
Behavioral outcomes	6	75.0
Health impacts (morbidity/mortality)	—	—
Effects reported		
Product/behavior awareness or reactions	3	37.5
Pre-behavioral outcomes	6	75.0
Behavioral outcomes	5	62.5
Estimate of precision reported	8	100

research should include more experimental designs and strong quasi-experimental designs for population-level dual use prevention. Studies should address the mechanisms of behavior change. Although the programs we reviewed were generally successful, it is unclear from this review what behavioral mediators, such as changes in social norms about dual use, were responsible.

Recommendations for Future Research Agenda

Dual tobacco use is a growing problem, in part, because of the surge in use of new tobacco products, including e-cigarettes and new forms of smokeless tobacco.[20] Although not voluminous compared with tobacco control literature as a whole, there is a body of research that addresses dual use in various forms, and this research has been done worldwide. However, there has been little intervention development, and little to no focus on mass health communications. Given these facts, more intervention research is needed in the field, specifically, development and testing of tobacco control messages and social marketing campaigns using proven principles from mass health communications strategies (eg, Legacy's truth, Centers for Disease Control's TIPS).[21,22] In particular, little research, including the articles screened in this review, focused on the types of dual use by specific high-risk audiences. More studies should examine and measure unique patterns of dual use. Based on different categories of dual use—cigarettes and snus, for example—specific target populations may be specified. Additionally, given the increased prevalence of alternative tobacco products among youth, such as e-cigarettes and other noncombustible delivery methods, intervention studies should examine reductions in dual use including these products.[23,24] Based on specific target groups, health communication researchers can develop and test messages and evaluate their effectiveness in tightly controlled trials. This is the next logical step in dual tobacco use health communications research.

Limitations

One of the major challenges associated with isolating the effects of dual tobacco use interventions is a lack of consensus on a definition. Most of the original 46 studies we reviewed did not include enough information about the types of tobacco addressed in the studies, which led our initial screening being pared down to the 8 articles we reviewed. As this field advances, researchers should report on dual tobacco use with commonly accepted taxonomy or set of terms that would facilitate future research and citation of relevant articles.

There are additional limitations to this study, as is often the case with systematic reviews. One barrier is the relative newness of the field of dual tobacco use interventions research and the manner in which findings are published in the literature.[14,18] This issue has arisen in other systematic reviews of health communication because of variable use of keywords and descriptors for interventions.[25] Because dual use tobacco control is an emerging strategy, there are few well-recognized keywords that can be used to identify literature on the topic. This problem faces the larger field of public health campaigns, as reflected in recent research. This finding is not surprising given that widespread strategic use of dual use strategies is a fairly recent phenomenon. It may be that some dual tobacco use health communications or other interventions methods do not describe themselves as such. Our search protocol would have missed these articles, as it was designed to capture studies with dual tobacco use–related key words, and to exclude single-product tobacco control interventions. As dual use interventions become more widespread, we expect that use of specific taxonomies will become more widespread in the public health literature. Finally, it is possible that some interventions in the published literature did address smoking and smokeless use, but chose to report on data from one or the other tobacco use rather than on dual tobacco use. Our review may not have captured such studies if they did not explicitly mention dual tobacco use or any of the other keywords described in the methods section. It is also important to note that our search terms may not have captured tobacco prevention or control efforts inclusive of alternative products, such as electronic cigarette use. Future systematic reviews should be updated to include these terms specifically.

SUMMARY

Dual tobacco use is undeniably a health threat, and although there is extant research on the behavior, more careful segmentation and definition of dual tobacco use is needed. Categories of conjoint use of smoking and smokeless products need to be developed in light of the proliferation of new products. Moreover, differences in the segments of users who combine various products need to be identified and studied. This study operationally defined the domains of dual use tobacco and provides a potential scheme for characterizing dual use tobacco control as a distinct strategy or combination of health communication strategies.

As a next step, targeted and tailored health communication interventions need to be designed, evaluated in tightly controlled efficacy studies with consistent measurement, and then implemented and evaluated in effectiveness trials. Evidence suggests a new generation of dual tobacco users will emerge into adulthood if these types of interventions are not developed and implemented with those populations most at risk for dual use, beginning in youth.

REFERENCES

1. Tomar SL, Alpert HR, Connolly GN. Patterns of dual use of cigarettes and smokeless tobacco among US males: findings from national surveys. Tob Control 2010; 19(2):104–9.
2. Hatsukami DK, Lemmonds C, Tomar SL. Smokeless tobacco use: harm reduction or induction approach? Prev Med 2010;38(3):309–17.
3. Teo KK, Ounpuu S, Hawken S, et al. Tobacco use and risk of myocardial infarction in 52 countries in the INTERHEART study: a case-control study. Lancet 2006; 368(9536):647–58.
4. Tomar SL, Fox BJ, Severson HH. Is smokeless tobacco use an appropriate public health strategy for reducing societal harm from cigarette smoking? Int J Environ Res Public Health 2009;6(1):10–24.
5. US Department of Health and Human Services (USDHHS). How tobacco smoke causes disease [Electronic Resource]: the biology and behavioral basis for smoking-attributable disease: a report of the surgeon general [e-book]. Rockville (MD): U.S. Dept. of Health and Human Services, Public Health Service, Office of the Surgeon General; 2010 [Washington, D.C.]: for sale by the Supt. Of Docs., U.S., G.P.O. Available at: http://www.ncbi.nlm.nih.gov/books/NBK53017/. Accessed January 30, 2015.
6. Lee S, Grana RA, Glantz SA. Electronic cigarette use among Korean adolescents: a cross-sectional study of market penetration, dual use, and relationship to quit attempts and former smoking. J Adolesc Health 2014;54(6):684–90.
7. Arrazola R, Neff L, Kennedy S, et al. Tobacco use among middle and high school students-United States, 2013 [serial online]. MMWR Morb Mortal Wkly Rep 2014; 63(45):1021–6. Available at: http://www.cdc.gov/mmwr/preview/mmwrhtml/mm6345a2.htm?hc_location=ufi. Accessed January 30, 2015.
8. Arrazola R, Kuiper N, Dube S. Patterns of current use of tobacco products among U.S. high school students for 2000–2012-Findings from the National Youth Tobacco Survey. J Adolesc Health 2014;54(1):54–60. Available at: http://www.sciencedirect.com/science/article/pii/S1054139X13004291. Accessed January 30, 2015.
9. Tobacco Fact Sheet. Electronic Cigarettes (E-Cigarettes). Legacy Foundation. Available at: http://www.legacyforhealth.org/content/download/582/6926/file/LEG-FactSheet-eCigarettes-JUNE2013.pdf. Accessed January 30, 2015.
10. Bombard J, Pederson L, Nelson D, et al. Are smokers only using cigarettes? Exploring current polytobacco use among an adult population. Addict Behav 2007;32(10):2411–9. Available at: http://www.sciencedirect.com/science/article/pii/S0306460307000883. Accessed January 30, 2015.
11. Centers for Disease Control and Prevention. Best Practices for Comprehensive Tobacco Control Programs-2014 [e-book]. Atlanta (GA): U.S. Dept. of Health and Human Services, Centers for Disease Control and Prevention, National Center for Chronic Disease Prevention and Health Promotion, Office on Smoking and Health; 2014. Available at: http://www.cdc.gov/tobacco/stateandcommunity/best_practices/. Accessed January 30, 2015.

12. McLeroy KR, Northridge ME, Balcazar H, et al. Reporting guidelines and the American Journal of Public Health's adoption of preferred reporting items for systematic reviews and meta-analyses. Am J Public Health 2012;102(5):780–4.

13. Snyder LB, Hamilton MA, Huedo-Medina T. Does evaluation design impact communication campaign effect size? A meta-analysis. Commun Methods Meas 2009;3(1–2):84–104.

14. Evans W, Blitstein J, Hersey J, et al. Systematic review of public health branding [serial online]. J Health Commun 2008;13(8):721–41. Available at: http://www.tandfonline.com/doi/full/10.1080/10810730802487364. Accessed January 30, 2015.

15. Klesges RC, Sherrill-Mittleman D, Ebbert JO, et al. Tobacco use harm reduction, elimination, and escalation in a large military cohort. Am J Public Health 2010; 100(12):2487–92.

16. Rath JM, Villanti AC, Abrams DB, et al. Patterns of tobacco use and dual use in US young adults: the missing link between youth prevention and adult cessation. J Environ Public Health 2012;2012:679134.

17. Doi S, DiLorenzo T. An evaluation of a tobacco use education-prevention program: a pilot study [serial online]. J Subst Abuse 1993;5(1):73–8. Available at: http://www.sciencedirect.com/science/article/pii/089932899390124T. Accessed January 30, 2015.

18. Stigler M, Perry C, Arora M, et al. Intermediate outcomes from Project MYTRI: mobilizing youth for tobacco-related initiatives in India [serial online]. Cancer Epidemiol Biomarkers Prev 2007;16(6):1050–6. Available at: http://cebp.aacrjournals.org/content/16/6/1050.full.html. Accessed January 30, 2015.

19. Regan A, Dube S, Arrazola R. Smokeless and flavored tobacco products in the U.S.: 2009 styles survey results [serial online]. Am J Prev Med 2012;42(1):29–36. Available at: http://www.sciencedirect.com/science/article/pii/S074937971100729X. Accessed January 30, 2015.

20. Evans WD. How social marketing works in health care. BMJ 2006;33:299.

21. New smokeless tobacco products. American Lung Association. Available at: http://www.lung.org/stop-smoking/tobacco-control-advocacy/reports-resources/tobacco-policy-trend-reports/new-smokeless-tobacco-products.pdf. Accessed January 30, 2015.

22. Farrelly M, Davis K, Duke J, et al. Sustaining "truth": changes in youth tobacco attitudes and smoking intentions after 3 years of a national antismoking campaign [serial online]. Health Educ Res 2009;24(1):42–8. Available at: http://her.oxfordjournals.org/content/24/1/42.long. Accessed January 30, 2015.

23. McAfee T, Davis K, Alexander R, et al. Effect of the first federally funded US antismoking national media campaign [serial online]. Lancet 2013;382(9909):2003–11. Available at: http://www.sciencedirect.com/science/article/pii/S0140673613616864. Accessed January 30, 2015.

24. King B, Alam S, Promoff G, et al. Awareness and ever-use of electronic cigarettes among U.S. adults, 2010–2011 [serial online]. Nicotine Tob Res 2013;15(19): 1623–7. Available at: http://c.ymcdn.com/sites/www.naquitline.org/resource/resmgr/news/feb28ntt013.pdf. Accessed January 30, 2015.

25. McDermott L, Stead M, Hastings G. What is and what is not social marketing: the challenge of reviewing the evidence [serial online]. J Market Manag 2005; 21(5–6):545–53. Available at: http://www.tandfonline.com/doi/abs/10.1362/0267257054307408. Accessed January 30, 2015.

26. McClave-Regan A, Berkowitz J. Smokers who are also using smokeless tobacco products in the US: a national assessment of characteristics, behaviours

and beliefs of 'dual users' [serial online]. Tob Control 2011;20:239. Available at: http://tobaccocontrol.bmj.com/content/early/2010/12/19/tc.2010.039115.short. Accessed January 30, 2015.

27. Murukutla N, Turk T, Wakefield M, et al. Results of a national mass media campaign in India to warn against the dangers of smokeless tobacco consumption [serial online]. Tob Control 2012;21(1):12–7. Available at: http://tobaccocontrol.bmj.com/content/early/2011/04/20/tc.2010.039438.short. Accessed January 30, 2015.

28. Norberg M, Lundqvist G, Nilsson M, et al. Changing patterns of tobacco use in a middle-aged population – the role of snus, gender, age, and education. Glob Health Action 2011;4. http://dx.doi.org/10.3402/gha.v4i0.5613.

29. Popova L, Neilands T, Ling P. Testing messages to reduce smokers' openness to using novel smokeless tobacco products [serial online]. Tob Control 2014;23(4): 313–21. Available at: http://tobaccocontrol.bmj.com/content/early/2013/03/05/tobaccocontrol-2012-050723.short. Accessed January 30, 2015.

Developmental Exposure to Environmental Toxicants

Alison J. Falck, MD*, Sandra Mooney, PhD, Shiv S. Kapoor, MD,
Kimberly M.R. White, MS, Cynthia Bearer, MD, PhD,
Dina El Metwally, MD, PhD

KEYWORDS

- Toxicant • Environmental exposure • Fetus • Child

KEY POINTS

- Susceptibility to environmental toxicants depends on a child's developmental stage and interactions within the physical, biological, and social environment.
- Critical stages of growth and cellular differentiation that occur in fetuses, newborns, infants, and children represent periods of greatest vulnerability to the adverse effects of environmental toxicants.
- The floor inside the home represents an important microenvironment for young children, because their breathing zones are lower than those of adults, and many chemicals are concentrated near the floor. Ingestion, inhalation, and dermal absorption can occur.
- Toxicants are widely dispersed in the environment. It is important for pediatricians to understand the potential routes of exposure, toxic effects, and strategies for prevention of exposure in order to provide anticipatory guidance to children and their families.

OVERVIEW AND DEVELOPMENTAL ASPECTS
Introduction

Toxicants are ubiquitous in the human environment, and children are often inadvertently exposed. Infants and children are a uniquely vulnerable population, especially during early stages of growth and development. Exposure to environmental toxicants is affected by children's physical, biological, and social environment. Children and adults experience the physical environment differently. The physical environment can be more hazardous for children, especially those who are preambulatory and lack control of their surroundings. The physical environment changes as

Disclosures: None.
Department of Pediatrics, Division of Neonatology, University of Maryland School of Medicine, 110 South Paca Street, 8th Floor, Baltimore, MD 21201, USA
* Corresponding author.
E-mail address: afalck@peds.umaryland.edu

Pediatr Clin N Am 62 (2015) 1173–1197
http://dx.doi.org/10.1016/j.pcl.2015.05.005
0031-3955/15/$ – see front matter © 2015 Elsevier Inc. All rights reserved.

pediatric.theclinics.com

children gain independence and spend time away from the home.[1] The biological environment is determined by genotypic and metabolic responses to interactions with the physical environment. Routes of absorption, metabolism, distribution, and health effects vary, and are influenced by the developmental stage in which exposure occurs.[1,2] A toxicokinetic diagram illustrates how environmental toxins interact with the biological environment (**Fig. 1**). The social environment is determined by lifestyle preferences and societal regulations and policies that influence the physical environment.[3]

The Epigenome

The epigenome refers to biochemical interactions that regulate expression of the genome without modification of DNA sequence. The epigenome is heritable, and highly vulnerable to toxicants during periods of rapid growth, such as fetal embryogenesis.[4] DNA methylation is a well-described epigenetic mechanism that affects DNA expression. When the promoter region of DNA is methylated, it remains tightly coiled, affecting DNA transcription. Impaired DNA methylation in children is associated with exposure to toxicants, such as lead and polycyclic aromatic hydrocarbons (PAHs) found in cigarette smoke and motor vehicle exhaust.[4,5]

Preconception

Even before conception, environmental toxins can influence future offspring. Oogonia differentiate during fetal life and therefore become vulnerable to toxicants during fetal development. Spermatogenesis begins at puberty; thus sperm become susceptible after puberty, in the periconceptual period. Because sperm lack DNA repair mechanisms and differentiate rapidly, they are highly vulnerable to toxins.[1,6] Impaired

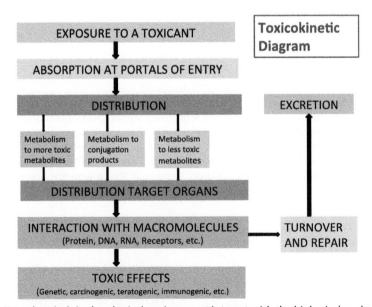

Fig. 1. How chemicals in the physical environment interact with the biological environment. Absorption, distribution, metabolism, interaction with target organs, and toxic effects vary with developmental stage. Genetic polymorphism affects metabolism and excretion of toxic metabolites.

fertility is a known consequence of environmental exposures. Examples of toxicants known to affect fertility include cigarette smoke and diethylstilbestrol (DES).[1,6,7] DES is an EDS that was prescribed to pregnant women until the 1970s to prevent miscarriage. Daughters of women exposed to DES developed vaginal clear cell carcinoma and infertility. Transgenerational effects include premature birth of DES grandchildren and hypospadias in DES grandsons.[7,8] Some environmental exposures occurring long before conception can affect future pregnancy. Certain toxins bioaccumulate before conception, and mobilize because of physiologic changes during pregnancy that promote elimination. Polychlorinated biphenyls (PCBs) are lipid-soluble organohalogens used to manufacture electrical equipment before their ban in the 1970s. PCBs are highly stable in the environment, and are stored in adipose tissue. Lead is a heavy metal that bioaccumulates in bone, and is mobilized during pregnancy because of high calcium turnover. Both PCBs and lead are known fetal neurotoxicants.[1]

The Fetus

Maternal exposures occurring during pregnancy can result in congenital malformations and fetal loss. The fetus is highly susceptible within critical stages of development, such as fetal organogenesis (weeks 3–8 of gestation).[9] Exposure to neurotoxins during neuronal differentiation, proliferation, migration, and myelination can lead to permanent neuronal loss, and affects future neurocognitive function.[2,9] For example, exposure to ionizing radiation at less than 18 weeks' gestation is correlated with microcephaly and neurocognitive delay.[2,10] Certain properties permit chemicals to cross the placental barrier and reach the fetus, such as low molecular weight, lipid solubility, and ability to use placental active transport mechanisms. Carbon monoxide is an example of a low-molecular-weight compound that is found in cigarette smoke, and is transported across the placenta via passive diffusion. Lipophilic compounds, such as ethanol, PAHs, and PCBs, also cross the placenta and can bioaccumulate in the fetus. Fetal exposures can be measured at birth via cord blood and meconium sampling.[3]

Newborns

Breast milk and formula represent important sources of exposure in newborns. Lipid-soluble toxicants, such as dioxin, PCBs, and organochlorine pesticides, are stored in maternal adipose and concentrated in breast milk.[1,11,12] Newborns fed formula may be exposed to toxins in the water supply, such as lead, arsenic, and nitrates. Nitrates are found in fertilizer and pesticides, and can contaminate soil and groundwater. Cases of methemoglobinemia have been reported in infants following exposure to nitrates from drinking water. Infants less than 3 months old are at greater risk for methemoglobinemia than older children.[13] Newborn skin is highly permeable, has a large surface/volume ratio, and is an important site of absorption of lipophilic compounds.[2] Organs in which rapid cell division continues remain highly susceptible to toxicants. Neuronal cell division is complete by 6 months, but migration, differentiation, and myelination continue into adolescence.[14] A newborn's body fat composition affects distribution of lipid-soluble toxicants. Mean body fat increases with advancing gestational age, and female infants tend to have a greater percentage body fat.[15] Infants with lower body fat levels have limited distribution of lipophilic compounds, whereas large-for-gestational-age infants with greater fat stores are more likely to sequester lipid-soluble toxicants.[16] Hepatic enzymes that metabolize toxicants are developmentally regulated, and are subject to genetic polymorphisms at all developmental stages.[17,18] At birth, glomerular filtration is a fraction of adult values, and slowly increases over the first year of life.[19]

Infants and Toddlers

Increasing ability to interact with the physical environment influences exposures during this stage. Behaviors such as oral exploration and introduction of solid foods also contribute. Processed baby foods may contain additives such as coloring, flavoring, or preservatives; safe levels of these additives are typically based on lifetime exposure in adults. Baby foods may also be contaminated by toxicants such as bisphenol-A (BPA; a plasticizer) or pesticide residue. The Food Quality Protection Act (FQPA) of 1996 provides age-appropriate safety standards for pesticide exposure based on children's dietary patterns. The FQPA requires the US Environmental Protection Agency (EPA) to account for other sources, such as drinking water and residential application, and for cumulative effects of pesticides with common mechanisms of action. The EPA uses a 10-fold margin of safety when setting standards when there are limited data available for children.[20] Infants have higher respiratory rate, resting metabolic rate, and greater oxygen consumption than older children and adults. This higher rate correlates with a proportionally higher inhaled toxicant exposure into smaller airways and lung surface area. During infancy, the ratio of skin surface area to body weight is twice that of adults. Therefore, the skin remains an important site of absorption.[2] The floor inside the home is an important microenvironment for infants and toddlers.[3] Surface contaminants, such as pesticides and volatile organic compounds (VOCs), are concentrated near the ground; oral, respiratory, or percutaneous exposures can occur while crawling or playing on the floor.[21–24] Formaldehyde is a VOC that is a known carcinogen. Formaldehyde levels are much greater indoors than outdoors, and are significantly higher following installation of new synthetic carpet or pressed wood cabinets.[1,22,23] PAHs are another carcinogenic VOC, found in cigarette smoke and concentrated in house dust.

Preschool and School-Aged Children

During this stage, food remains an important source of exposure. Children require more calories for growth than adults, increasing quantitative risk.[3,11] Qualitative differences in diet are also seen, with greater consumption of foods that may be contaminated with pesticides (fruits, vegetables, meat, and dairy).[11,25] In 2014, the Environmental Working Group published lists of fruits and vegetables most likely to contain pesticide residue, termed the Dirty Dozen. The so-called Clean Fifteen are least likely to contain pesticide residue.[25] Children have higher minute ventilation than adults, and are more vulnerable to inhaled air pollutants.[1] Breathing zones affect exposure to inhaled toxicants in young children. For adults, the typical breathing zone is approximately 120 to 180 cm (4–6 feet) above the floor. For children, the breathing zone depends on height and mobility. Certain toxicants are found in highest concentration in lower breathing zones, such as heavier particles in cigarette smoke, mercury vapor from latex paint, or radon.[1,26] Radon is of particular concern, because levels can accumulate substantially indoors and children are especially susceptible to the toxic effects. Exposure to radon is the second leading cause of lung cancer in the United States, associated with 15,000 to 20,000 deaths annually.[27,28] The physical environment changes substantially as children reach school age and spend more time away from home. School becomes an important source of environmental toxicant exposure (**Table 1**). The increasing incidence of childhood asthma is associated

Table 1
Indoor and outdoor sources of exposure

Toxicant	Indoor Source	Outdoor Source
Carbon monoxide	Malfunctioning fuel-burning appliances or home heating systems	Near high-traffic areas; auto emissions
Tobacco smoke	Smoking in child care areas Improperly vented smoking areas	Doorway near outside smoking area
Molds, biologic pollutants	Leaks, flooding	River or sewer overflows
Lead, heavy metals	Dust or paint chips Paint on furniture or toys, art supplies	Leaded soil or paint Soil contamination
Pesticides, disinfectants	Improper storage, labeling, handling; outdoor products used indoors	Improper storage, labeling, handling; infested playgrounds areas
Mercury	Ingestion of fish Broken fluorescent light bulbs	Industrial use
Asbestos	Building materials, insulation	Disasters

The physical environment changes as children mature and spend more time away from home. School and day care become sources of indoor and outdoor environmental toxicant exposure.
Adapted from American Academy of Pediatrics Council on Environmental Health, Etzel RA, editors. Pediatric environmental health. 3rd edition. Elk Grove Village (IL): American Academy of Pediatrics; 2012.

with indoor and outdoor air pollutants such as secondhand smoke and motor vehicle exhaust.[3]

Adolescents

During adolescence, freedom from parental authority begins, with the opportunity for greater control of the physical environment. However, abstract thinking and reasoning skills remain immature, leading to risk-taking behaviors such as substance abuse.[11,29] Occupational exposures may also begin during adolescence. Common routes of exposure in adolescence include dermal absorption and inhalation. Toxicants absorbed through the skin include pesticides, nicotine, solvents, and ultraviolet radiation. Those absorbed via the respiratory tract include cigarette smoke, VOCs, and particulate matter.[3,17] Although genetic polymorphisms exist, the capacity of the liver to metabolize toxicants is typically greater in adolescents than in adults. Thus, chemicals that are biologically activated to cytotoxic or carcinogenic metabolites may pose a greater risk.[17] Puberty represents period of cell growth and differentiation associated with increased susceptibility to environmental toxicants. The reproductive system is vulnerable, which could explain the increased incidence of scrotal cancer in adolescent chimney sweeps in the 1800s, after exposure to soot.[30] Toxicants such as endocrine disruptors can mimic hormones and may affect reproductive organ differentiation and onset of puberty.[29]

SPECIFIC ENVIRONMENTAL EXPOSURES
Environmental Tobacco Smoke

According to the 2009 World Health Organization (WHO) Report on the Global Tobacco Epidemic, tobacco use is the single most preventable cause of death worldwide. In 2011, 6 million deaths were secondary to tobacco; an increase to 8 million is predicted by 2030.[31] Environmental tobacco smoke (ETS) contains more than 250 harmful chemicals, including nicotine, carbon monoxide, formaldehyde, vinyl chloride, PACs, benzene, and arsenic. There is no safe level of exposure for fetuses, newborns, or growing children.[32]

Sources of exposure

ETS consists of sidestream smoke from the end of a burning cigarette, and mainstream smoke (or secondhand smoke) exhaled from the smoker's lungs.[24] Active maternal smoking and exposure to secondhand smoke during pregnancy can adversely affect fetal health.[31,32] Because smoking in public and the workplace has been restricted, the most common source of ETS exposure is in the home.[33]

Toxic effects

Active smoking is associated with infertility and early onset of menopause. This is hypothesized to be secondary to the impact of cigarette smoke on hormonal balance, follicular growth, oocyte maturation, implantation, and placentation.[34] Studies have documented the adverse effects of ETS on successful pregnancy following in vitro fertilization.[34] Male fertility is also affected; smoking has been linked to altered sperm morphology, motility, and concentration.[33] Cotinine is a metabolite of nicotine with a long half-life that is the biological marker used to measure exposure.[35] Cotinine levels in cord blood are increased in infants of mothers who smoke or are exposed to ETS.[32] Intrauterine growth restriction (IUGR) is a known outcome of in utero exposure to ETS, with a direct dose-response relationship between exposure and degree of IUGR.[32,36] Other known sequelae of maternal smoking during pregnancy include increased risk of spontaneous abortion, preterm delivery and low birth weight, perinatal depression, congenital anomalies such as cleft lip and palate, and impaired lung function that persists into childhood.[31-33] Toxic effects of secondhand smoke continue into infancy, and include upper and lower respiratory infections, reduced somatic growth, neurocognitive deficits, sudden infant death syndrome, and higher infant mortality. In childhood, secondhand smoke is linked to childhood asthma, allergies, reduced lung function, recurrent otitis media, and attention-deficit/hyperactivity disorder (ADHD).[31-33,37,38] Evidence suggests a relationship between prenatal and postnatal exposure to ETS and the development of childhood cancers such as brain tumors, leukemia, and lymphoma. Further research is warranted to further investigate this association.[31-33] Cigarette smoking and nicotine addiction often begin during adolescence.[39] Effects of smoking include abnormal pulmonary function, altered lipid profile, and impaired exercise tolerance. Teenage smokers are more likely to abuse alcohol and other drugs. Smoking in adolescence increases the risk of lung cancer in adulthood; those who smoke a pack or more of cigarettes per day live about 7 years less than nonsmokers.[40] **Table 2** summarizes toxic effects of ETS at various stages of development.

Prevention strategies

Parental smoking is a known risk factor for initiation and sustained cigarette smoking in children and adolescents.[39,41] Pediatricians should provide anticipatory guidance to parents and children that is specific to the child's developmental stage, and focused on parental smoking cessation. The WHO M-POWER campaign outlines 6 strategies to address the adverse health effects of ETS: (1) monitor tobacco use and prevention policies; (2) protect people from tobacco smoke; (3) offer help to quit tobacco use; (4) warn about the dangers of tobacco; (5) enforce bans on tobacco advertising, promotion, and sponsorship; and (6) raise taxes on tobacco.[31]

Table 2
Effects of exposure to ETS at each stage of development

Developmental Stage	Toxic Effect
Preconception	Female infertility Altered sperm morphology and motility
Fetus	Intrauterine growth restriction Congenital malformations: neural tube defects?[a] Childhood cancers?[a] Impaired lung function lasting into childhood
Newborn and infant	Small for gestational age Reduced lung volume, impaired pulmonary function Upper and lower respiratory infections Decreased somatic growth Neurodevelopmental delays Sudden infant death syndrome Higher infant mortality
Child	Asthma Chronic cough, dyspnea, reduced pulmonary function Recurrent otitis media, effusion ADHD Cancer: lung cancer later in life Brain tumors, leukemia, and lymphoma?[a]
Adolescent	Abnormal pulmonary function Altered lipid profile Lung cancer later in life Nicotine addition

ETS consists of smoke coming from the end of a burning cigarette (sidestream smoke) and from smoker's exhalation (mainstream or secondhand smoke). ETS contains more than 250 harmful chemicals, many of which are carcinogens. There is no safe level of exposure.
[a] Evidence indicates association but further research is needed.
Data from Refs.[31–33]

Ethanol

No level of alcohol exposure is safe for the fetus. However, 8% to 30% of pregnant women report alcohol consumption during pregnancy. In the United States, the incidence of fetal alcohol syndrome (FAS) is approximately 2 to 7 per 10,000 live births.[42] Consumption of alcohol in excess is the cause of approximately 88,000 deaths annually in the United States, and binge drinking accounts for more than half of these deaths. Binge drinking is common among adolescents, and is associated with impaired driving, violent behavior, risky sexual activity, and unintended pregnancy.[43]

Sources of exposure

The most common exposure to ethanol is consumption of alcohol-containing beverages. Alcohol consumption is common during pregnancy. A recent US Centers for Disease Control and Prevention (CDC) survey shows that 7.6% (1 in 13) of pregnant women report drinking alcohol during the past 30 days, and the National Institutes of Alcohol Abuse and Alcoholism (NIAAA) notes that 20% to 30% of women report drinking during pregnancy. Surveys by the CDC show that more than 50% of US adults consumed at least 1 drink in the past month. Drinking rates among underage school children are similarly high (40% of eighth grade, >66% of 10th grade, and 75% of 12th grade). Mixing alcohol with caffeine has become prevalent among adolescents and young adults (31% of adolescents 12–17 years old, 34% of adolescents 18–24 years old).[44,45] Caffeine masks the effects of alcohol but does not affect metabolism, thus contributing to binge drinking and overdose. Caffeinated alcoholic beverages (CABs) are marketed toward adolescents and young adults; in 2010 the US Food and Drug Administration (FDA) banned the manufacture of 7 CABs, because of health risks.[43] Other sources of alcohol exposure are shown in **Table 3**. Exposure to these compounds likely results in low blood alcohol levels, but measureable alcohol concentrations are reported after use of certain medications[46] and hand sanitizers.[47,48]

Toxic effects

Alcohol crosses the placenta freely, and ethanol levels in fetal blood are at least equivalent to those found in maternal blood.[44,45] Effects of alcohol on the fetus are widespread, and often permanent. Outcome is determined by the timing of exposure, blood alcohol level, genetic background, use of other drugs, and health and nutritional status. Maternal age, parity, and socioeconomic status also contribute.[49,50] The term fetal alcohol spectrum disorder covers all diagnoses caused by fetal alcohol exposure, including FAS. Prenatal exposure to alcohol is the leading known cause of intellectual delay. FAS is the most severe outcome of alcohol exposure during pregnancy.[49,51,52] Infants with FAS typically are born with craniofacial abnormalities including smooth philtrum, thin upper lip, and short palpebral fissures. During infancy and childhood, growth deficiency and central nervous system dysfunction are common.[49] Exposure to alcohol during childhood also affects the kidney, liver, lung, immune, and musculo-skeletal systems.[53–56] Another concern regarding childhood exposure is the increased risk of later abuse of alcohol. Grant and Dawson[57] in 1998 reported that the younger the exposure to alcohol, the greater the risk of developing an alcohol use disorder in later life.

Preventive strategies

Abstaining from alcoholic beverage consumption is the most obvious means of prevention. NIAAA suggests that strict implementation of public policy regarding policing of drinking behaviors is the most effective means of reducing consumption by

Table 3
Other sources of alcohol, route of exposure, and preventive measures

Source of Exposure	Pathway of Exposure	Prevention
Alcoholic beverages	Consumption	Avoid
Food (eg, vanilla extract, wine vinegar, soy sauce)	Consumption	Avoid
Medicines	Consumption	Avoid
Mouthwash, insect repellant	Transdermal	Avoid
Herbal tinctures	Consumption	Avoid
Hand sanitizer	Inhalation, transdermal	Avoid or use in well-ventilated space
Solvents	Inhalation, transdermal	Avoid
Disinfectants, cleaning solutions, wipes, polishes	Inhalation, transdermal	Avoid
Ethanol-containing fuel, biofuels	Inhalation	Avoid
Aftershave, perfume, body spray, deodorant	Transdermal	Avoid
Occupational (eg manufacturing of plastics, rubber, medicines)	Inhalation, transdermal	Personal protective equipment

underage drinkers. For prevention of exposure to alcohol via other sources, the best advice is to read labels and to use personal protective equipment.

Plasticizers

BPA and phthalates are examples of plasticizers that function as EDCs. BPA is used in polycarbonate plastics to improve rigidity, whereas phthalates provide flexibility. BPA and phthalates are extensively used in consumer and industrial plastic product production, and are ubiquitous in the environment. BPA and phthalates are found in greater than 75% of urine samples from nationally representative populations in the United States.[58–60]

Sources of exposure

BPA is used in the production of plastic bottles and as a protective coating inside metal cans.[61] BPA is also found in water supply pipes, and in medical devices such as syringes, intravenous (IV) and urinary catheters, and dental sealants.[3,61,62] The primary source of exposure is via ingestion of food and beverages. BPA has been found in breast milk.[58,61,63] Infants and children are reported to have a higher daily intake of BPA than adults.[58,61] Phthalates are used to manufacture toys, vinyl products, plastic bags, plastic food packaging products, and detergents. Phthalates are found in solvents, lubricants, and insect repellants, medical gloves, blood and IV fluid and bags, medical tubing, coating of pharmaceuticals, and cosmetics such as hair spray and nail polish. Like BPA, the primary source of exposure to phthalates is via ingestion.[64,65] Both BPA and phthalates leach from plastic containers into food and beverages, particularly after heating. Other potential routes of exposure are inhalation (air, dust) and dermal absorption. Dibutyl phthalate (DBP) is found in cosmetics and nail polish, and levels are significantly higher in women of reproductive age.[64] Plasticizers used in medical equipment can be absorbed directly from the bloodstream after exposure via IV fluid bags and tubing; both BPA and phthalate metabolites have been found in the urine of premature infants in the neonatal intensive care unit.[61,66] **Table 4** lists potential sources of phthalate exposure.

Toxic effects

BPA is an EDC with estrogenic properties. In experimental animals, low-dose exposure is correlated with accelerated puberty, altered mammary and prostate morphology known to predispose to cancer, genital malformations, and disruption of sexual differentiation in the brain.[60,63] Although human epidemiologic data are limited, it is hypothesized that the increasing incidence of obesity, precocious puberty, infertility, genital tract anomalies, and breast cancer may be secondary to BPA exposure during early development.[63] BPA exposure is associated with recurrent miscarriages and preterm delivery in women, and low sperm count, poor motility, and increased sperm DNA breakage in men. BPA has been measured in urine and blood during pregnancy, amniotic fluid, ovarian follicular fluid, placental tissue, fetal blood, and umbilical cord blood.[63] Gestational BPA exposure is associated with anxiety, hyperactivity, and impaired emotional regulation, especially among girls.[67] Like BPA, phthalates are antiandrogenic EDCs; the most sensitive target tissue is the male reproductive tract. In animals, prenatal exposure leads to congenital anomalies such as cleft palate, and skeletal malformations. Male offspring develop hypospadias and cryptorchidism, low sperm production, and testicular-Leydig adenomas as adults. Findings are similar to testicular dysgenesis syndrome found in humans.[65] Children exposed to phthalates in utero show poor executive functioning, and behavioral problems such as depression, inattention, and impaired emotional regulation.[68]

Table 4		
Sources of phthalate exposure, and toxic effects in animal models		
Phthalate	**Source**	**Fetal Effects (Animal Model)**
DEHP	Medical tubing and IV fluid bags Food packaging Plastic toys Wall coverings, floor tiles, shower curtains Rainwear, shoes Furniture and auto upholstery	Rat: skeletal malformations, cleft palate, cryptorchidism, hypospadias, low testosterone level
DBP	Nail polish, makeup, perfume, coatings on pharmaceuticals/herbal products	Rat: skeletal malformations, cleft palate, cryptorchidism, hypospadias, low testosterone level, delayed puberty
DMP	Insecticides Adhesives Hair styling products, shampoo, aftershave	Unknown
BBP	Vinyl flooring and tile, carpet, artificial leather Adhesives and sealants Food packaging Furniture upholstery	Rat: skeletal malformations, cleft palate, cryptorchidism, hypospadias, delayed puberty
DEP	Cosmetics, nail polish, deodorant, perfume, lotion Insecticide Pharmaceuticals, herbal products	Rat: skeletal anomalies, decreased testosterone

Abbreviations: BBP, butyl benzyl phthalate; DBP, dibutyl phthalate; DEHP, di(2-ethylhexyl) phthalate; DMP, dimethyl phthalate; IV, intravenous.

Adapted from American Academy of Pediatrics Council on Environmental Health, Etzel RA, editors. Pediatric environmental health. 3rd edition. Elk Grove Village (IL): American Academy of Pediatrics; 2012.

In boys, prenatal BPA and phthalate exposures are associated with shorted anogenital distance (AGD). Decreased AGD is correlated with the other male reproductive tract anomalies, such as small scrotum, hypospadias, reduced penile length, and testicular maldescent.[64,69,70]

Preventive strategies

In 2012 to 2013, the FDA prohibited use of BPA in baby bottles, sippy cups, and infant formula containers. Dietary exposure to plasticizers may be reduced by (1) avoiding heating of plastic containers or food covered with plastic wrap in microwave ovens; (2) avoiding long-term storage in plastic containers; (3) reducing use of canned foods; (4) using glass or stainless steel containers, particularly for hot foods or liquids; (5) checking recycle codes on plastic containers (codes 3 or 7 may contain BPA); and (6) using BPA-free baby bottles.[3,64,71]

Heavy Metals

Heavy metals are members of a group of metallic elements naturally found in the Earth's crust. Some heavy metals (iron, cobalt, copper, manganese, chromium, zinc, selenium) have essential physiologic roles in humans, whereas others (lead, mercury, arsenic, and cadmium) are toxic at any level. Heavy metals are potent neurotoxins.[72] Heavy metal exposure can lead to developmental delay and serious sequelae in children. The known toxicities of lead, mercury, and arsenic are discussed later.

Sources of exposure
Exposure to heavy metals occurs from inhalation, ingestion, and handling of contaminants. Common sources are food, drinking water, motor vehicle emissions, and contaminated household products.[3]

Lead It is estimated that 4 million children are exposed to high lead levels in their homes, and that approximately half a million US children aged 1 to 5 years have lead levels greater than 5 μg/dL.[73] Children are exposed to lead through ingestion of dust from paint or soil, or from the water supply.[3]

Mercury Methylmercury is the organic form that naturally bioaccumulates in aquatic systems, and biomagnifies in the food chain. Shellfish and predator fish, such as shark and tuna, may contain high concentrations. Methylmercury is lipid soluble, crosses the placenta, and is found in breast milk.[3]

Arsenic Arsenic is one of the common metals in the Earth crust. It has been used historically as a poison, and is currently used in silicon-based computer chips, as a feed additive for poultry and swine, and as a pesticide. Contaminated drinking water is the most common source. Arsenic also readily crosses the placenta and can reach the fetus.[3,74]

Toxic effects
Lead Lead is a potent neurotoxin, and exposure in fetuses, newborns, and children leads to neurodevelopmental delay, cognitive impairment, and behavioral dysfunction. There is no safe lead exposure in developing fetuses. The exact neurotoxic mechanism of action is unknown.[75,76] Lead has been shown to affect calcium modulating and signaling in neurons in very low concentrations in vitro.[77] Lead bioaccumulates in bone, and is mobilized during pregnancy from maternal skeletal stores. Thus, the developing fetus is at risk for enhanced exposure and neurotoxicity. The effect is most pronounced in the first trimester.[76] Lead exposure has subclinical effects on the central nervous system. Blood lead concentrations, even those less than 10 μg/dL, are inversely associated with intelligence quotient scores at 3 and 5 years.[78] High blood lead level causes headaches, abdominal pain agitation, stupor, and convulsions. Symptomatic lead toxicity should be treated as an emergency. Chelation therapy is recommended for levels greater than 45 μg/dL.[3]

Mercury Mercury irreversibly inhibits selenium-dependent enzymes, which are essential for normal physiologic function. Methylmercury is a known teratogen that disrupts neuronal migration; fetuses and newborns are highly susceptible.[3,79] Children evaluated at 7 to 14 years of age after documented prenatal exposure had deficits in motor, attention, and verbal test results.[80] Long-term methylmercury toxicity leads to visual and hearing loss, paresthesias progressing to ataxia and generalized weakness, tremor and muscle spasticity, followed by coma and even death. Acrodynia is the triad of neurologic symptoms, erythematous desquamating rash on the hands and feet, and hypertension.[3,74] Thimerosal is a mercury-based preservative that has been used in the United States in multidose vaccines. The association between thimerosal-containing vaccines and autism has been discredited in multiple scientific studies.[81,82] However, all vaccines licensed by the FDA for use in children less than 6 years of age have been thimerosal free since 2001.[83]

Arsenic Arsenic is a known carcinogen that has inhibitory effects on key enzymes. Arsenic exposure can adversely affect every organ system; acute toxicity is characterized by gastrointestinal symptoms, from mild to severe depending on dose. Chronic toxicity can lead to hepatic dysfunction, bone marrow suppression, arrhythmia, cardiomyopathy, peripheral neuropathy, and intellectual dysfunction. The peripheral neuropathy resembles Guillain-Barré syndrome.[3,74,84] Fetal and early childhood exposures are linked to bronchiectasis and to lung cancer in adulthood.[85] In addition, exposure is correlated with increased risk of leukemia, aplastic anemia, and liver and kidney cancer.[86]

Preventive strategies

Lead CDC recommendations (2012) state that public health actions should be initiated when any child less than 5 years old has a blood lead level greater than 5 μg/dL. The focus on prevention of lead exposure is to eliminate dangerous lead sources from children's environments. Parent and public education is vital. The CDC's Childhood Lead Poisoning Prevention Program is committed to the Healthy People 2020 goals of eliminating blood lead levels greater than or equal to 10 μg/dL.[87,88]

Mercury Consumption of contaminated fish is the most common source of mercury poisoning. The FDA recommends limiting intake of certain fish in pregnant and breast feeding women, and in young children.

Arsenic The EPA has banned use of copper arsenate and other arsenic compounds as wood preservatives since 2003. Public health policies currently are focused on the safety of drinking water.

Solvents

Solvents are a large group of chemicals used primarily to dissolve lipids and high-molecular-weight compounds in solution. Solvents are found in the outdoors (gasoline, groundwater, downwind of dry cleaners, highways, and farms), the household (dry-cleaned clothing, cigarette smoke, vinyl shower curtains, glues and paints, personal care products), and in industry (electronic assembly; rubber, paint, textile, and other chemical manufacturing plants; automobile repair shops; gas stations; nail and hair salons; laboratories; and hospitals).[89] Millions of US workers are exposed occupationally, including women of reproductive age.

Sources of exposure

Solvents are ubiquitous in the environment. Exposure occurs via transdermal absorption, ingestion, or inhalation. As organic solvents are volatile chemicals, inhalation represents the most common route. Concentrations are much greater indoors than outdoors. Solvents are lipophilic, cross the placenta readily, and can affect developing fetuses.[90,91] Solvents are known to rapidly impart a feeling of euphoria after inhalation, and are used as recreational drugs (they are inexpensive and easily attainable). Inhalational use typically begins during childhood, peaks at age 14 to 25 years, and typically declines by late adolescence.[91,92]

Toxic effects

Solvents are known teratogens. Both animal and human epidemiologic research supports a relationship between maternal occupational exposure to solvents and congenital anomalies such as neural tube defects and congenital heart disease.[93–95] Toluene embryopathy has been reported after maternal recreational inhalation of paint or glue. Features include growth restriction, congenital anomalies, neurodevelopmental delay, and facial features resembling FAS.[96] Certain solvents, such as benzene and trichloroethylene, are known carcinogens. Although evidence is limited, prenatal and postnatal exposure to solvents has been linked to the development of childhood cancer. Two childhood cancer clusters were noted in the United States (Woburn, MA; Toms River, NJ); in both settings, drinking water was contaminated with trichloroethylene.[97,98] Acute effects of solvent inhalation include euphoria, central nervous system depression, dizziness, slurred speech, blurred vision, hallucinations, headache, respiratory irritation, and emotional lability. Overdose can lead to loss of consciousness, cardiac arrhythmias, and death. Chronic solvent abusers are at risk for leukoencephalopathy, hearing loss, cognitive impairment, cerebellar atrophy, ataxia, and hepatic and renal dysfunction.[91]

Preventive strategies
Measures that may reduce childhood exposure to solvents include (1) airing out recently dry-cleaned clothes before bringing them indoors; (2) avoiding use of cleaners, glues, and paints containing solvents; (3) use of appropriate ventilation during and after use; (3) proper storage and disposal of household chemicals following manufacturer's recommendations; and (4) limiting frequent, sustained exposure to nail salons.

Persistent Organic Pollutants

Persistent organic pollutants (POPs) are lipophilic, organic compounds that resist biological and chemical degradation. These chemicals were primarily produced during the twentieth century and are found in pesticides (eg, chlordane, dichlorodiphenyltrichloroethane [DDT], aldrin) and industrial chemicals (PCBs), and are by-products of manufacturing and waste incineration (dioxins and furans). POPs persist in the environment for years to decades, and exposures are associated with serious adverse health effects. Although these chemicals are banned in most developed countries, they remain ubiquitous in the environment.[99,100]

Sources of exposure
POPs are found in air, water, and soil, and travel long distances, leading to widespread distribution. POPs tend to volatilize in warm climates, migrate within the ecosystem, and accumulate in cold regions where they condense and remain. These compounds bioaccumulate in adipose tissue of animals with extensive body fat, such as fish and marine mammals. They biomagnify as they ascend the food chain. Exposure typically occurs via ingestion of fish, meat, and dairy products, and less commonly from dermal absorption and inhalation. The term POP typically is used to refer to the 12 chemicals (the Dirty Dozen) targeted by the Stockholm Convention in 2004. **Table 5** lists these 12 chemicals, their historical uses, and current status in the United States.[99,100]

Toxic effects
Reproductive, developmental, behavioral, neurologic, endocrine, and immunologic adverse health effects have been associated with exposure to POPs. Because POPs are lipophilic, they mobilize from adipose during pregnancy, cross the placenta, and reach the fetus.[101,102] In utero exposure affects metabolic programming and adipogenesis during early fetal development.[103] Exposure increases weight gain in animals,[104] and causes rapid growth in the first year of life in humans.[105] The mechanism by which POPs act as obesogens is unknown, but may be mediated through steroid receptors.[104] POPs are known neurotoxins. Prenatal exposure is associated with impaired neurodevelopment.[99,106] Newborn exposure through consumption of breast milk has been documented; approximately 20% of the maternal body burden may reach the infant.[100,107–110] In childhood, exposure is linked to

Table 5
The 12 POPs targeted by the Stockholm Convention, their historical use, and current US status

POP	Historical Use	Overview of US Status
Aldrin and dieldrin	Insecticides used on crops such as corn and cotton; also used for termite control	Under FIFRA: no US registrations; most uses canceled in 1969; all uses 1987 No production, import, or export allowed
Chlordane	Insecticide used on crops such fruits, vegetables, grains, potatoes, nuts, and cotton; used on home, lawn, and garden pests, and extensively to control termites	Under FIFRA: no US registrations; most uses canceled in 1978; all uses by 1988 No production (stopped in 1997), import, or export. Regulated as a hazardous air pollutant (CAA)
DDT	Insecticide used on agricultural crops, primarily cotton, and insects that carry diseases such as malaria and typhus	Under FIFRA: no US registrations; most uses canceled in 1972; all by 1989 No US production, import, or export DDE (a metabolite of DDT) regulated as a hazardous air pollutant (CAA). Priority toxic pollutant (CWA)
Endrin	Insecticide used on crops such as cotton and grains; also used to control rodents	Under FIFRA, no US registrations; most uses canceled in 1979; all uses by 1984 No production, import, or export Priority toxic pollutant (CWA)
Mirex	Insecticide used for fire ants, termites, and mealybugs. Used as a fire retardant in plastics, rubber, and electrical products	Under FIFRA, no US registrations; all uses canceled in 1977. No production, import, or export
Heptachlor	Insecticide used primarily against soil insects and termites. Also used against some crop pests and to combat malaria	Under FIFRA: most uses canceled by 1978; registrant voluntarily canceled use to control fire ants in underground cable boxes in early 2000. All pesticide tolerances on food crops revoked in 1989, no production, import, or export
Hexachlorobenzene	Fungicide used for seed treatment. Industrial chemical used to make fireworks, ammunition, synthetic rubber. Unintentionally produced during combustion and manufacture of certain chemicals. An impurity in certain pesticides	Under FIFRA, no US registrations; all uses canceled by 1985. No production, import, or export as a pesticide. Manufacture and use for chemical intermediate (as allowed under the Convention). Regulated as a hazardous air pollutant (CAA). Priority toxic pollutant (CWA)
PCBs	Used in industrial processes, including electrical transformers and capacitors, heat exchange fluids, paint additives, carbonless copy paper, and in plastics. Unintentionally produced during combustion	Manufacture and new use prohibited in 1978 (TSCA). Regulated as a hazardous air pollutant (CAA). Priority toxic pollutant (CWA)

(continued on next page)

Table 5 (continued)		
POP	**Historical Use**	**Overview of US Status**
Toxaphene	Insecticide used to control pests on crops and livestock, and to kill unwanted fish	Under FIFRA: no US registrations; most uses canceled in 1982; all uses by 1990 All tolerances on food crops revoked in 1993 No production, import, or export. Regulated as a hazardous air pollutant (CAA)
Dioxins and furans	Unintentionally produced during most forms of combustion, including burning of municipal and medical wastes, backyard burning of trash, and industrial processes. Also found as trace contaminants in certain herbicides, wood preservatives, and in PCB mixtures	Regulated as hazardous air pollutants (CAA) Dioxin in the form of 2,3,7,8-TCDD is a priority toxic pollutant (CWA)

Abbreviations: 2,3,7,8-TCDD, 2,3,7,8-Tetrachlorodibenzo-p-Dioxin; CAA, Clean Air Act; CWA, Clean Water Act; DDE-1, 1-dichloro-2,2-bis(p-chlorophenyl) ethylene; FIFRA, Federal Insecticide, Fungicide, and Rodenticide Act; TSCA, Toxic Substances Control Act.

Data from Guidotti TL, Gitterman BA. Global pediatric environmental health. Pediatr Clin North Am 2007;54:335–50; and World Health Organization. Persistent organic pollutants effect/affect on child health. WHO; 2010. Available at: www.who.int/ceh/publications/persistent_organic_pollutant/en/. Accessed February 4, 2015.

neurodevelopmental and cognitive delays,[100,109,111] and learning disabilities including ADHD.[100,112] POPs are known EDCs, and may have estrogenic, antiestrogenic, anti-androgenic, or antithyroid properties.[100] Reproductive, thyroid, and pancreatic dysfunction in children have been linked to prenatal and postnatal exposure.[100,113–115] One of the greatest concerns for humans is increased cancer risk. Certain POPs, such as dioxin, are known human carcinogens.[100] The increased burden found in the Arctic has been speculated to contribute to the increasing incidence and early onset of breast cancer.[116]

Preventive strategies

Families should be encouraged to eat fruits, vegetables, fish, and meat products that are low in fat. Organic and locally grown vegetables and fruits are optimal, but costly. Because some POPs are concentrated in the outer skins of fruits and vegetables, washing is recommended. Exposure to toxins such as PCBs via fish may be limited by avoidance of fish grown primarily in farms, and by removing the skin, which is where POPs are concentrated. Exposure may be decreased through consumer education, public health programs, legislation, and environmental health infrastructure.[100]

Volatile Organic Compounds

VOCs are hydrocarbons that are emitted as gases from certain solids or liquids. VOCs are air pollutants; the higher the volatility (or lower the boiling point), the more likely the compound is to be released into ambient air.[3] VOCs are used in many household products, and concentrations are consistently higher indoors than outdoors. Because young children spend much of their time indoors, they are at risk for enhanced exposure.[117–119]

Sources of exposure

Children are exposed primarily via inhalation, and less commonly through ingestion and dermal absorption. VOCs are emitted by a wide variety of products used in the home, office, and at school, including hairspray, dry-cleaning solutions, paints and paint strippers, cleaning supplies, glues, pesticides, building materials and furnishings, and office equipment such as printers or copiers.[117–119] The EPA has identified 3000 high-production-volume HPV chemicals in widest commercial use that have greatest potential for human exposure.[120] Children and pregnant women are exposed extensively, and CDC surveys have detected quantifiable levels of nearly 200 HPV chemicals in representative samples of the US population, including pregnant women.[121]

Toxic effects

Acute symptoms include fatigue, conjunctival and respiratory tract irritation, headache, dizziness, visual impairment, dyspnea, allergic skin reactions, and memory loss.[118] Epidemiologic studies have shown that exposure during fetal and early postnatal life is associated with impaired development, decreased lung growth, increased rate of upper respiratory tract infections, childhood asthma, and behavioral and neurocognitive deficits.[122–124] In children, VOCs can disrupt the endocrine system, interrupt gene activation, and alter brain development.[125] Certain VOCs, such as trichloroethylene, formaldehyde, and benzene, are suspected or known carcinogens.[3,118]

Preventive strategies

The EPA regulates outdoor emission of VOCs, primarily to prevent the development of ozone, which is a component of photochemical smog. The EPA does not have authority to establish indoor air quality standards. Indoor air quality can be improved by (1) increasing ventilation, especially during and after use of VOCs; (2) changing heating and air conditioning filters frequently; (3) reducing humidity; (4) following manufacturers' instructions carefully; (5) purchasing small quantities of chemicals containing VOCs; (6) using chemicals containing VOCs soon after purchase; and (7) disposing of partially full containers. Instructions from local government organizations should be followed to aid in disposal of toxic wastes.[118,119] The US Occupational Safety and Health Administration (OSHA) regulates formaldehyde, a specific VOC, as a carcinogen. OSHA has adopted an action level of 0.5 ppm in industrial settings. No standards have been established for air quality in non-industrial environments.[118]

Pesticides

Pesticides are a broad group of chemicals intended to kill unwanted insects, plants, molds, and rodents. These chemicals are often used in vicinity of households and schools, and in agriculture. Approximately 450 million kilograms (1 billion pounds) are applied annually in the United States.[126] Classifications of pesticides, level of toxicity, and mechanisms of action are shown in **Table 6**.

Sources of exposure

Residential use of pesticides is common. In children, exposure occurs through dermal absorption, inhalation, and ingestion. Many pesticides are readily absorbed through skin, and inhalation occurs from lawn and agricultural sprays. The most important source for children is the food supply.[3,127] The FDA is responsible for monitoring allowable limits of pesticides in food. In 2011, 60% of domestically sampled fruits and 36% of vegetables contained legally allowable amounts of pesticide residue, and 2% had more than the FDA limits.[128]

Table 6
Classifications of pesticides, mechanisms of action, and examples of products are illustrated
(see Table 5 for further description of organochlorine pesticides)

Classification	Mechanism of Action	Toxicity	Uses and Characteristics	Products
Organochlorine	GABA antagonist	High	Banned in United States because of health risk, bioaccumulation (see text) Lipid soluble Lindane used for lice, scabies	DDT Chlordane Lindane Aldrin
Organophosphates	Acetylcholinesterase inhibitors	High	Insect control in agriculture Banned for home use	Chlorpyrifos Malathion Parathion Phosmet
Pyrethrins and pyrethroids	Sodium channel antagonist	Low to moderate	Pest control Pediculicide Insect control in home, garden, agriculture	Permethrin Deltamethrin
Carbamates	Acetylcholinesterase inhibitors	Variable	Insect control in agriculture and home	Aldicarb Carbaryl Primicarb
Neonicotinoids	Selective for insect acetylcholine receptors	Low	Flea control for domestic animals Agriculture	Imidacloprid

Abbreviation: GABA, gamma-aminobutyric acid.
Adapted from American Academy of Pediatrics Council on Environmental Health, Etzel RA, editors. Pediatric environmental health. 3rd edition. Elk Grove Village (IL): American Academy of Pediatrics; 2012.

Toxic effects

Because most pesticides are neurotoxins, exposure in fetuses, newborns, and children may have major impacts on developing brains.[3,129] Pesticides also function as EDCs, immunotoxicants, and carcinogens in animals and humans.[3,127,130] Evidence has shown that organophosphate pesticides cross the placenta.[131] Epidemiologic data suggest an association between prenatal pesticide exposure and infertility, spontaneous abortion, preterm birth, intrauterine growth restriction, congenital anomalies, and neurodevelopmental impairment.[3,127,130,132] Children are thought to be particularly sensitive to the carcinogenic effects.[133] Although evidence supports a relationship between pesticide exposure and childhood cancer, a pathophysiologic mechanism has not been identified. Factors such as genetic predisposition likely play an important role.[133,134] Future research should focus on improved exposure assessment, evaluation of risk by age at exposure, and investigation of possible genetic-environment interactions.[133]

Prevention strategies

The EPA has regulatory authority over use and distribution of pesticides. Some of these chemicals have been banned or their use has been restricted. **Fig. 2** shows important preventive strategies that may limit exposure. As introductions of new pesticides into the environment occur, their health effects need to be observed.

Preventive Strategies: Pesticide Exposure

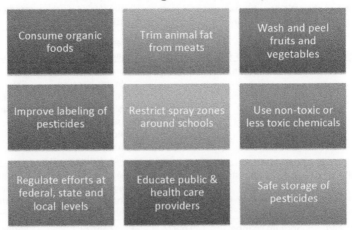

Fig. 2. Important preventive strategies that may limit exposure to pesticides. As introduction of new pesticides are introduced into the environment, their health effects need to be observed.

REFERENCES

1. Bearer CF. How are children different from adults? Environ Health Perspect 1995;103(Suppl 6):7–12.
2. Faustman EM, Sibernagel SM, Fenske RA, et al. Mechanisms underlying children's susceptibility to environmental toxicants. Environ Health Perspect 2000;108(Suppl 1):13–21.
3. American Academy of Pediatrics Council on Environmental Health, Etzel RA, editors. Pediatric environmental health. 3rd edition. Elk Grove Village (IL): American Academy of Pediatrics; 2012.
4. Perera F, Herbstman J. Prenatal environmental exposures, epigenetics, and disease. Reprod Toxicol 2011;31:363–73.
5. Dolinoy DC, Weidman JR, Jirtle RJ. Epigenetic gene regulation: linking early developmental environment to adult disease. Reprod Toxicol 2007;23(3): 297–307.
6. Bruin JE, Gerstein HC, Holloway A. Long-term consequences of fetal and neonatal nicotine exposure: a critical review. Toxicol Sci 2010;116(2):364–74.
7. Zama AM, Uzumcu M. Epigenetic effects of endocrine-disrupting chemicals on female reproduction: an ovarian perspective. Front Neuroendocrinol 2010;31: 420–39.
8. Kalfa N, Paris F, Soyer-Gobillard O, et al. Prevalence of hypospadias in grandsons of women exposed to diethylstilbestrol during pregnancy: a multigenerational national cohort study. Fertil Steril 2011;95(8):2574–7.
9. Selevan SG, Kimmel CA, Mendola P. Identifying critical windows of exposure for children's health. Environ Health Perspect 2000;108(3):451–5.
10. Blot WJ. Growth and development following prenatal and childhood exposure to atomic radiation. J Radiat Res (Tokyo) 1975;16(Suppl):82.
11. Moya J, Bearer CF, Etzel R. Children's behavior and physiology and how it affects exposure to environmental contaminants. Pediatrics 2004;113(4): 996–1006.

12. Landrigan PJ, Sonawane B, Mattison D, et al. Chemical contaminants in breast milk and their impacts on children's health: an overview. Environ Health Perspect 2002;110(6):A313–5.
13. US Environmental Protection Agency TEACH chemical summary: nitrates and nitrites. 2007. Available at: www.epa.gov/teach/chem_summ/Nitrates_summary.pdf. Accessed January 20, 2015.
14. Styles J, Jernigan TL. The basics of brain development. Neuropsychol Rev 2010;20:327–48.
15. Hawkes CP, Hourihane JO, Kenny LC, et al. Gender and gestational age-specific body fat percentage at birth. Pediatrics 2011;128(3):e645–51.
16. Wade KC. Pharmacokinetics in neonatal medicine. In: Martin RJ, Fanaroff AA, Walsh MC, editors. Fanaroff and Martin's neonatal-perinatal medicine. 10th edition. Philadelphia: Elsevier Saunders; 2015. p. 667–8.
17. Bruckner JV, Weil WB. Biological factors which may influence and older child's or adolescent's response to toxic chemicals. Regul Toxicol Pharmacol 1999;29:158–64.
18. Omiecinski CJ, Vanden Heuvel JP, Perdew GH, et al. Xenobiotic metabolism, disposition, and regulation by receptors. Toxicol Sci 2011;120(S1):49–75.
19. Knobel RB, Smith JM. Laboratory blood tests useful in monitoring renal function in neonates. Neonatal Netw 2014;33(1):35–40.
20. US Environmental Protection Agency. Implementation of requirements under the Food Quality Protection Act. 2014. Available at: www.epa.gov/pesticides/regulating/laws/fqpa/fqpa_implementation.htm. Accessed May 2, 2015.
21. Lewis RG, Fortmann RC, Camann DE. Evaluation and methods for monitoring the potential exposure of small children to pesticides in the residential environment. Arch Environ Contam Toxicol 1994;26:37–46.
22. US Environmental Protection Agency TEACH chemical summary: formaldehyde. 2007. Available at: www.epa.gov/teach/chem_summ/Formaldehyde_summary.pdf. Accessed January 21, 2015.
23. US Environmental Protection Agency: volatile organic compounds (VOCs). 2012. Available at: www.epa.gov/iaq/voc.html#Sources. Accessed January 21, 2015.
24. Hoh E, Hunt RN, Quintana PJ, et al. Environmental tobacco smoke as a source of polycyclic aromatic hydrocarbons in settled household dust. Environ Sci Technol 2012;46:4174–83.
25. Environmental Working Group executive summary. 2014. Available at: www.ewg.org/foodnews/summary.php. Accessed February 9, 2015.
26. Agocs MM, Etzel RA, Parrish RG, et al. Mercury exposure from interior latex paint. N Engl J Med 1990;323(160):1096–101.
27. Chen J. Canadian lung cancer relative risk from radon exposure for short periods in childhood compared to a lifetime. Int J Environ Res Public Health 2013;10:1916–26.
28. US Environmental Protection Agency radon fact sheet. Available at: www.epa.gov/oncampus/pdf/radonfactsheet.pdf. Accessed January 21, 2015.
29. Golub MS. Adolescent health and the environment. Environ Health Perspect 2000;108(4):355–62.
30. Waldron HA. A brief history of scrotal cancer. Br J Ind Med 1983;40(4):390–401.
31. World Health Organization report on the global tobacco epidemic 2009: implementing smoke-free environments. Available at: www.who.int/tobacco/mpower/2009/en/. Accessed January 22, 2015.
32. DiFranza JR, Aligne CA, Weitzman M. Prenatal and postnatal environmental tobacco smoke exposure and children's health. Pediatrics 2004;113(4):1007–15.

33. Office on Smoking and Health (US). The health consequences of involuntary exposure to tobacco smoke: a report of the surgeon general. Atlanta (GA): Centers for Disease Control and Prevention (US); 2006. Available at: www.ncbi.nlm. nih.gov/books/NBK44324/. Accessed April 18, 2013.

34. Dechanet C, Anahory T, Mathieu D, et al. Effects of cigarette smoking on reproduction. Hum Reprod Update 2011;17(1):76–95.

35. National Cancer Institute: secondhand smoke and cancer. 2011. Available at: www.cancer.gov/cancertopics/factsheet/tobacco/ets. Accessed January 25, 2015.

36. Leonardi-Bee J, Smyth A, Britton J, et al. Environmental tobacco smoke and fetal health: systematic review and meta-analysis. Arch Dis Child Fetal Neonatal Ed 2008;93:F351–61.

37. Feleszko W, Ruszczynski M, Jaworska J, et al. Environmental tobacco smoke exposure and risk of allergic sensitization in children: a systematic review and meta-analysis. Arch Dis Child 2014;99:985–92.

38. Braun JM, Kahn RS, Froehlich T, et al. Exposure to environmental toxicants and attention deficit hyperactivity disorder in U.S. children. Environ Health Perspect 2006;114(12):1904–9.

39. Joffer J, Burell G, Bergstrom E, et al. Predictors of smoking among Swedish adolescents. BMC Public Health 2014;14:1296.

40. World Health Organization Tobacco Free Initiative. Health effects of smoking among young people. WHO; 2015. Available at: www.who.int/tobacco/ research/youth/health_effects/en/. Accessed January 25, 2015.

41. Mays D, Gilman SE, Rende R, et al. Parental smoking exposure and adolescent trajectories. Pediatrics 2014;133(6):983–91.

42. May PA, Gossage JP, Kalberg WO, et al. Prevalence and epidemiologic characteristics of FASD from various research methods with an emphasis on recent in-school studies. Dev Disabil Res Rev 2009;15:176–92.

43. CDC fact sheet: caffeine and alcohol. 2014. Available at: www.cdc.gov/alcohol/ fact-sheets/caffeine-and-alcohol.htm. Accessed January 30, 2015.

44. Idänpään-Heikkilä J, Jouppila P, Akerblom HK, et al. Elimination and metabolic effects of ethanol in mother, fetus, and newborn infant. Am J Obstet Gynecol 1972;112(3):387–93.

45. Heller M, Burd L. Review of ethanol dispersion, distribution, and elimination from the fetal compartment. Birth Defects Res A Clin Mol Teratol 2014; 100(4):277–83.

46. Cordell RL, Pandya H, Hubbard M, et al. GC-MS analysis of ethanol and other volatile compounds in micro-volume blood samples–quantifying neonatal exposure. Anal Bioanal Chem 2013;405(12):4139–47.

47. Ali SS, Wilson MP, Castillo EM, et al. Common hand sanitizer may distort readings of breathalyzer tests in the absence of acute intoxication. Acad Emerg Med 2013;20(2):212–5.

48. Kapoor SS, Hsieh S, Wood R, et al. Alcohol exposure from hand hygiene products in preterm infants in neonatal giraffe isolette. Pediatric Academic Societies; 2013 [abstract: #2922.325].

49. Jones KL. The effects of alcohol on fetal development. Birth Defects Res C Embryo Today 2011;93(1):3–11.

50. May PA, Gossage JP. Maternal risk factors for fetal alcohol spectrum disorders: not as simple as it might seem. Alcohol Res Health 2011;34:15–26.

51. Jones KL, Smith DW. Recognition of the fetal alcohol syndrome in early infancy. Lancet 1973;2:999–1001.

52. Narr KL, Kan E, Abaryan Z, et al. A longitudinal study of the long-term consequences of drinking during pregnancy: heavy in utero alcohol exposure disrupts the normal processes of brain development. J Neurosci 2012; 32(44):15243–51.
53. Giliberti D, Mohan SS, Brown LA, et al. Perinatal exposure to alcohol: implications for lung development and disease. Paediatr Respir Rev 2013;14(1):17–21.
54. Habbick BF, Zaleski WA, Casey R, et al. Liver abnormalities in three patients with fetal alcohol syndrome. Lancet 1979;1(8116):580–1.
55. Habbick BF, Blakley PM, Houston CS, et al. Bone age and growth in fetal alcohol syndrome. Alcohol Clin Exp Res 1998;22(6):1312–6.
56. Hofer R, Burd L. Review of published studies of kidney, liver, and gastrointestinal birth defects in fetal alcohol spectrum disorders. Birth Defects Res A Clin Mol Teratol 2009;85(3):179–83.
57. Grant BF, Dawson DA. Age of onset of drug use and its association with DSM-IV drug abuse and dependence: results from the National Longitudinal Alcohol Epidemiologic Survey. J Subst Abuse 1998;10(2):163–73.
58. Mendonca K, Hauser R, Calafat AM, et al. Bisphenol A concentrations in maternal breast milk and infant urine. Int Arch Occup Environ Health 2014;87:13–20.
59. Silva MJ, Barr DB, Reidy JA, et al. Urinary levels of seven phthalate metabolites in the US population from the National Health and Nutrition Examination Survey (NHANES) 1999–2000. Environ Health Perspect 2004;112(3):331.
60. Calafat AM, Ye X, Wong L, et al. Exposure of the U.S. population to bisphenol A and 4-tertiary-octylphenol. Environ Health Perspect 2008;116(1):39–44.
61. Duty SM, Mendonca K, Hauser R, et al. Potential sources of bisphenol A in the neonatal intensive care unit. Pediatrics 2013;131(3):483–9.
62. Rubin B. Bisphenol A: an endocrine disruptor with widespread exposure and multiple effects. J Steroid Biochem Mol Biol 2011;127:27–34.
63. Vanderberg LN, Hauser R, Marcus M, et al. Human exposure to bisphenol A (BPA). Reprod Toxicol 2007;24:139–77.
64. Crinnon WJ. Toxic effects of the easily avoidable phthalates and parabens. Altern Med Rev 2010;15(3):190–6.
65. United States Environmental Protection Agency, toxicity and exposure assessment for children's health: phthalates, TEACH chemical summary. 2007. Available at: www.epa.gov/teach/chem_summ/phthalates_summary.pdf. Accessed February 9, 2015.
66. Calafat AM, Weuve J, Ye X, et al. Exposure to Bisphenol A and other phenols in the neonatal intensive care unit. Environ Health Perspect 2009;117(4):639–44.
67. Braun JM, Kalkbrenner AE, Calafat AM, et al. Impact of early-life bisphenol A exposure on behavior and executive function in children. Pediatrics 2011; 128(5):873–82.
68. Engel SM, Miodovnik A, Canfield RL, et al. Prenatal phthalate exposure is associated with childhood behavior and executive functioning. Environ Health Perspect 2010;118(4):565–71.
69. Miao M, Yuan W, He Y, et al. In utero exposure to bisphenol-A and anogenital distance of male offspring. Birth Defects Res A Clin Mol Teratol 2011;91:867–72.
70. Swan SH, Main KM, Liu F, et al, Study for Families Research Team. Decrease in anogenital distance among male infants with prenatal phthalate exposure. Environ Health Perspect 2005;113(8):1056–61.
71. US Food and Drug Administration: update on bisphenol A use in food contact applications. 2015. Available at: www.fda.gov/NewsEvents/PublicHealthFocus/ucm064437.htm. Accessed February 5, 2015.

72. Tchounwou PB, Yedjou CG, Patlolla AK, et al. Heavy metal toxicity and the environment. In: Luch A, editor. Molecular, clinical and environmental toxicology. Berlin: Springer; 2009. p. 133–64.
73. The Centers for Disease Control: Lead. 2015. Available at: www.cdc.gov/nceh/lead/. Accessed February 10, 2015.
74. Yazdani S. Mercury, arsenic, and cadmium toxicity in children. In: Roberts JR, Trousdale K, editors. Putting it into practice: pediatric environmental health training resource. Children's Environmental Health Network; 2014.
75. Gomaa A, Hu H, Bellinger D, et al. Maternal bone lead as an independent risk factor for fetal neurotoxicity: a prospective study. Pediatrics 2002;110(1):110–8.
76. Hu H, Téllez-Rojo MM, Bellinger D, et al. Fetal lead exposure at each stage of pregnancy as a predictor of infant mental development. Environ Health Perspect 2006;114(11):1730–5.
77. Markovac J, Goldstein GW. Picomolar concentrations of lead stimulate brain protein kinase C. Nature 1988;334(6177):71–3.
78. Canfield RL, Henderson CR Jr, Cory-Slechta DA, et al. Intellectual impairment in children with blood lead concentrations below 10 μg per deciliter. N Engl J Med 2003;348(16):1517–26.
79. Raymond LJ, Ralston NV. Mercury: selenium interactions and health implications. Seychelles Medical and Dental Journal 2004;7(1):72–7.
80. Debes F, Budtz-Jørgensen E, Weihe P, et al. Impact of prenatal methylmercury exposure on neurobehavioral function at age 14 years. Neurotoxicol Teratol 2006;28(3):363–75.
81. Madsen KM, Lauritsen MB, Pedersen CB, et al. Thimerosal and the occurrence of autism: negative ecological evidence from Danish population-based data. Pediatrics 2003;112(3 Pt 1):604–6.
82. Price CS, Thompson WW, Goodson B, et al. Prenatal and infant exposure to thimerosal from vaccines and immunoglobulins and risk of autism. Pediatrics 2010;126(4):656–64.
83. The Centers for Disease Control and Prevention: thimerosal and 2014–2015 seasonal flu vaccines. 2014. Available at: www.cdc.gov/flu/protect/vaccine/thimerosal.htm. Accessed February 5, 2015.
84. von Ehrenstein OS, Poddar S, Yuan Y, et al. Children's intellectual function in relation to arsenic exposure. Epidemiology 2007;18(1):44–51.
85. Smith AH, Marshall G, Yuan Y, et al. Increased mortality from lung cancer and bronchiectasis in young adults after exposure to arsenic in utero and in early childhood. Environ Health Perspect 2006;114:1293–6.
86. Khan M, Sakauchi F, Sonoda T, et al. Magnitude of arsenic toxicity in tube-well drinking water in Bangladesh and its adverse effects on human health including cancer: evidence from a review of the literature. Asian Pac J Cancer Prev 2003;4(1):7–14.
87. The CDC's Childhood Lead Poisoning Prevention Program: what do parents need to know to protect their children? 2014. Available at: www.cdc.gov/nceh/lead/acclpp/blood_lead_levels.htm. Accessed February 5, 2015.
88. The US Food and Drug Administration. Fish: what pregnant women and parents should know. 2014. Available at: www.fda.gov/Food/FoodborneIllness Contaminants/Metals/ucm393070.htm. Accessed February 5, 2015.
89. Agency for Toxic Substances & Disease Registry: Toxic Substances Portal-Toluene, Toxicological Profile for Toluene. Available at: www.atsdr.cdc.gov/toxprofiles/tp.asp?id=161&tid=29. Accessed February 5, 2015.

90. White K. Children and solvents . In: Roberts JR, Trousdale K, editors. Putting it into practice: pediatric environmental health training resource. Children's Environmental Health Network; 2014. Available at: www.cehn.org/resources/HealthCareProfessionals/PediatricTrainingResource.
91. Cruz SL, Rivera-García MT, Woodward JJ. Review of toluene action: clinical evidence, animal studies and molecular targets. J Drug Alcohol Res 2014; 3:1–8.
92. Williams JF, Storck M. Clinical report: inhalant abuse. Pediatrics 2007;119(5): 1009–17.
93. Boyer AS, Finch WT, Runyan RB. Trichloroethylene inhibits development of embryonic heart valve precursors in vitro. Toxicol Sci 2000;53(1):109–17.
94. Johnson PD, Goldberg SJ, Mays MZ, et al. Threshold of trichloroethylene contamination in maternal drinking waters affecting fetal heart development in the rat. Environ Health Perspect 2003;111(3):289–92.
95. Khattak S, K-Moghtader G, McMartin K, et al. Pregnancy outcome following gestational exposure to organic solvents. JAMA 1999;281(12):1106–9.
96. Arnold GL, Kirby RS, Langendoerfer S, et al. Toluene embryopathy: clinical delineation and developmental follow-up. Pediatrics 1994;93(2):216–20.
97. Costas K, Knorr RS, Condon SK. A case-control study of childhood leukemia in Woburn, Massachusetts: the relationship between leukemia incidence and exposure to public drinking water. Sci Total Environ 2002;300(1–3):23–35.
98. The Agency for Toxic Substances and Disease Registry. Public health assessment: Reich farm. Dover Township (PA); Ocean County (NJ): The New Jersey Department of Health and Senior Services; 2001. Available at: www.state.nj.us/health/eoh/assess/cgc_pha_fnl.pdf. Accessed January 5, 2015.
99. Guidotti TL, Gitterman BA. Global pediatric environmental health. Pediatr Clin North Am 2007;54:335–50.
100. World Health Organization. Persistent organic pollutants impact on child health. WHO; 2010. Available at: www.who.int/ceh/publications/persistent_organic_pollutant/en/. Accessed February 4, 2015.
101. Leino O, Kiviranta H, Karjalainen A, et al. Pollutant concentrations in placenta. Food Chem Toxicol 2013;54:59–69.
102. Ren A, Qiu X, Jin L, et al. Association of selected persistent organic pollutants in the placenta with the risk of neural tube defects. Proc Natl Acad Sci U S A 2011; 108:12770–5.
103. Grün F, Blumberg B. Endocrine disrupters as obesogens. Mol Cell Endocrinol 2009;304:19–29.
104. Ibrahim MM, Fjære E, Lock E, et al. Chronic consumption of farmed salmon containing persistent organic pollutants causes insulin resistance and obesity in mice. PLoS One 2011;6:e25170.
105. Valvi D, Mendez MA, Garcia-Esteban R, et al. Prenatal exposure to persistent organic pollutants and rapid weight gain and overweight in infancy. Obesity 2014;22:488–96.
106. Jacobson JL, Jacobson SW. Intellectual impairment in children exposed to polychlorinated biphenyls in 8,utero. N Engl J Med 1996;335:783–9.
107. Laug EP, Kunze FM, Prickett CS. Occurrence of DDT in human fat and milk. AMA Arch Ind Hyg Occup Med 1951;3:245–6.
108. Patandin S, Dagnelie PC, Mulder PG, et al. Dietary exposure to polychlorinated biphenyls and dioxins from infancy until adulthood: a comparison between breast-feeding, toddler, and long-term exposure. Environ Health Perspect 1999;107:45–51.

109. Hooper K, McDonald TA. The PBDEs: an emerging environmental challenge and another reason for breast-milk monitoring programs. Environ Health Perspect 2000;108:387–92.

110. Thundiyil JG, Solomon GM, Miller MD. Transgenerational exposures: persistent chemical pollutants in the environment and breast milk. Pediatr Clin North Am 2007;54:81–101.

111. Herbstman JB, Sjodin A, Kurzon M, et al. Prenatal exposure to PBDEs and neurodevelopment. Environ Health Perspect 2010;118:712–9.

112. Lee DH, Jacobs DR, Porta M. Association of serum concentrations of persistent organic pollutants with the prevalence of learning disability and attention deficit disorder. J Epidemiol Community Health 2007;61:591–6.

113. Mazhitova Z, Jensen S, Ritzen M, et al. Chlorinated contaminants, growth and thyroid function in schoolchildren from the Aral Sea region in Kazakhstan. Acta Paediatr 1998;87:991–5.

114. Longnecker MP, Gladen BC, Patterson DG Jr, et al. Polychlorinated biphenyl (PCB) exposure in relation to thyroid hormone levels in neonates. Epidemiology 2000;11:249–54.

115. Rogan WJ, Ragan NB. Evidence of effects of environmental chemicals on the endocrine system in children. Pediatrics 2003;112:247–52.

116. Fredslund SO, Bonefeld-Jorgensen EC. Breast cancer in the Arctic–changes over the past decades. Int J Circumpolar Health 2012;71:19155.

117. UL Environment: indoor air quality. Available at: greenguard.org/en/indoorAirQuality/iaq_chemicals.aspx. Accessed February 10, 2015.

118. The US EPA: an introduction to indoor air quality, volatile organic compounds. Available at: www.epa.gov/iaq/voc.html. Accessed February 4, 2015.

119. Children's Environmental Health Network: air quality. 2012. Available at: www.cehn.org/education/airquality. Accessed February 10, 2015.

120. Goldman LR. Chemicals and children's environment: what we don't know about risks. Environ Health Perspect 1998;106(Suppl 3):875–80.

121. Woodruff TJ, Zota AR, Schwartz JM. Environmental chemicals in pregnant women in the United States: NHANES 2003–2004. Environ Health Perspect 2011;119:878–85.

122. Wang S, Ang H, Tade MO. Volatile organic compounds in indoor environment and photocatalytic oxidation: state of the art. Environ Int 2007;33:694–705.

123. Weisel CP. Assessing exposure to air toxics relative to asthma. Environ Health Perspect 2002;110(Suppl 4):527–37.

124. Sherriff A, Farrow A, Golding J, et al. Frequent use of chemical household products is associated with persistent wheezing in pre-school age children. Thorax 2005;60:45–9.

125. Landrigan PJ, Lambertini L, Birnbaum LS. A research strategy to discover the environmental causes of autism and neurodevelopmental disabilities. Environ Health Perspect 2012;120:a258–60.

126. Bradman A, Barr DB, Claus Henn BG, et al. Measurement of pesticides and other toxicants in amniotic fluid as a potential biomarker of prenatal exposure: a validation study. Environ Health Perspect 2003;111(14):1779.

127. Roberts JR, Karr CJ, Council On Environmental Health. Pesticide exposure in children. Pediatrics 2012;130(6):e1765–88.

128. US Food and Drug Administration Pesticide Monitoring Program: 2011 pesticide report. Available at: www.fda.gov/downloads/Food/FoodborneIllness Contaminants/Pesticides/UCM382443.pdf. Accessed February 5, 2015.

129. Bouchard MF, Chevrier J, Harley KG, et al. Prenatal exposure to organophosphate pesticides and IQ in 7 year-old children. Environ Health Perspect 2011; 119(8):1189–95.
130. Weselak M, Arbuckle TE, Foster W. Pesticide exposures and developmental outcomes: the epidemiologic evidence. J Toxicol Environ Health B 2007;10:41–80.
131. Whyatt RM, Rauh V, Barr DB, et al. Prenatal insecticide exposures and birth weight and length among an urban minority cohort. Environ Health Perspect 2004;112(10):1125–32.
132. Rauh VA, Garfinkel R, Perera FP, et al. Impact of prenatal chlorpyrifos exposure on neurodevelopment in the first 3 years of life among inner-city children. Pediatrics 2006;118(6):e1845–59.
133. Zahm SH, Ward MH. Pesticides and childhood cancer. Environ Health Perspect 1998;106(Suppl 3):893–908.
134. Infante-Rivard C, Weichenthal S. Pesticides and childhood cancer: an update of Zahm and Ward's 1998 review. J Toxicol Environ Health B Crit Rev 2007;10(1–2): 81–99.

Childhood Asthma Management and Environmental Triggers

Jessica P. Hollenbach, PhD[a], Michelle M. Cloutier, MD[b],*

KEYWORDS

- Childhood asthma • Asthma exacerbations • Prevention • Management
- Environmental triggers • Trigger remediation

KEY POINTS

- The causes of asthma development are not known and thus asthma cannot be prevented based on the current level of understanding.
- Home environmental intervention strategies can reduce asthma morbidity in sensitized children but are probably not effective in children not sensitized to the specific allergen.
- Interventions tailored to the allergen sensitization of the child coupled with education and appropriate severity-specific asthma medication may be the most effective strategy to reduce asthma morbidity.
- Efforts to prevent environmental tobacco smoke exposure are important for everyone in the household.

INTRODUCTION

Asthma is the most common chronic disease of children, affecting more than 6.8 million children in the United States (9.3% of all children).[1] Asthma cannot be cured. Asthma cannot be prevented. However, asthma can be controlled. This article first reviews asthma epidemiology and the current understanding of the genetics of asthma. It then discusses the various proposed hypotheses for the continuing increase in asthma prevalence and risk factors for asthma. In addition, it discusses emerging work on asthma prevention and strategies to prevent asthma exacerbations.

Disclosure: The authors have nothing to disclose.
[a] Department of Pediatrics, Asthma Center, The Children's Center for Community Research, CT Children's Medical Center, University of Connecticut School of Medicine, 282 Washington Street, Hartford, CT 06106, USA; [b] Department of Pediatrics, Asthma Center, The Children's Center for Community Research, Connecticut Children's Medical Center, University of Connecticut Health Center, 282 Washington Street, Hartford, CT 06106, USA
* Corresponding author.
E-mail address: mclouti@connecticutchildrens.org

Pediatr Clin N Am 62 (2015) 1199–1214
http://dx.doi.org/10.1016/j.pcl.2015.05.011
0031-3955/15/$ – see front matter © 2015 Elsevier Inc. All rights reserved.

pediatric.theclinics.com

EPIDEMIOLOGY

In industrialized countries with Western lifestyles, lifetime asthma prevalence is high and has increased approximately 2.7 percentage points per year since 1997.[2] In the United States, the lifetime reported asthma prevalence in individuals of all ages is 13.0% (2012). Lifetime prevalence is higher in children (14%) than in adults and increases from early childhood (7.0% at 0–4 years of age) to adolescence (18.4% at 15–19 years of age), with current asthma prevalence showing a similar trend.[1] Asthma is a major public health problem costing the health care system nearly $56 billion annually, with direct health care costs estimated at $50.1 billion and indirect costs (lost productivity) contributing an additional $5.9 billion.[2]

Asthma in childhood disproportionately affects more boys than girls and underrepresented minority populations with African Americans and (some) Hispanic people having higher rates than other racial and ethnic groups. Children of Puerto Rican origin have the highest asthma prevalence of all ethnic and racial groups, whereas Mexican children have one of the lowest reported rates, making it difficult to examine prevalence when all individuals of Hispanic origin are grouped together.[2–4]

Asthma morbidity is high but hospitalization rates for asthma decreased 24% between 2003 and 2010 (National Health Interview Survey, 2001–2011).[2] Compared with adults, children are disproportionately hospitalized for asthma. Approximately 29% of the asthma hospital discharges in 2010 occurred in children less than 15 years of age even though only 21% of the US population is less than 15 years of age.[2] In 2010, asthma was responsible for 2.1 million emergency room visits, 10.6 million physician office visits, and 1.2 million hospital visits.[2]

Asthma deaths are rare in children but increase with age. In 2009, 157 children less than 15 years of age (0.2 per 100,000) died of asthma compared with 617 adults older than 85 years.[2] Black adult women have the highest mortality from asthma (2.5 per 100,000), with an age-adjusted death rate in black people that is 3.1 times higher than the rate in the white population.[2]

Genetics of Asthma

Asthma is a complex and chronic disease that depends on the interplay of genetic and environmental triggers. More than 100 candidate genetic loci have been identified using epidemiologic linkage studies.[5] This finding suggests that individuals with asthma may have many susceptibility loci, each of small effect. Multiple genome-wide association studies using population cohorts have identified several regions associated with asthma, including the 17q21 locus (ORMDL3/GSDML), IL33 on chromosome 9p24, HLA-DR/DQ on 6p21, IL1RL1/IL18R1 on 2q12, WDR36/TSLP on 5q22, and IL13 on 5q31.[5] Many of the associations have not been replicated in other populations, suggesting a role of population-specific variants in the causation of asthma and showing an important role for regulatory genes. Genomic studies using human fetal tissue suggest a complex interaction between environmental factors such as in utero smoke exposure, maternal diet, folate and vitamin D, lung structural genes, and lung function growth trajectory.[6]

African ancestry has been found to affect lung function and asthma severity. Using ancestry informative markers, lung function is inversely correlated with the percentage of African ancestry in 3 independent African American populations.[7] Genetic variation leading to an increased risk for exacerbations is also more common in African individuals.[8] Results from the GALA (Genetics of Asthma in Latino Americans) study show that individuals who are Puerto Rican have a higher degree of African and European ancestry than Mexican American individuals. It has been suggested that this difference may contribute to the high morbidity and mortality experienced by Puerto Rican compared with Mexican American individuals.[9]

Variable responses to specific therapeutic asthma medications have been reported in different ethnic groups and this variable response may also relate to the extent of African ancestry.[10] African ancestry might introduce genetic variation associated with a greater likelihood for alteration in the therapeutic response to inhaled short-acting and long-acting beta agonists (LABAs). In the SMART (Salmeterol Multicenter Asthma Research Trial) study, African American participants treated with salmeterol experienced an increase in asthma life-threatening exacerbations and death but they were also less likely to have been treated with an inhaled corticosteroid (ICS) and more likely to have been hospitalized than the other study participants.[11] Additional studies and a large meta-analysis have consistently shown that the combination of a LABA and an ICS is safe and efficacious, but the SMART study resulted in the boxed warning for all LABA-containing inhalers.[12,13]

Other studies have shown that African American individuals respond differently to combination therapies. In the BADGER (Best Add-on Therapy Giving Effective Response) trial from the Childhood Asthma Research and Education Network, African American children did not show a preferential response to a step-up from low-dose ICS to LABA and ICS combination therapy and thus the addition of a LABA to ICS therapy was no more efficacious than increasing the ICS dose.[14] In contrast, Hispanic and non-Hispanic white children responded to the addition of a LABA to their ICS therapy. In addition, Puerto Rican participants in the GALA study were less bronchodilator responsive after administration of a short-acting bronchodilator.[15]

Hypotheses on the Origins of Asthma

Epidemiologists have long sought to determine the underlying causes of childhood asthma. Since the early 1990s, asthma rates have increased worldwide and observational studies have tried to explain this increase in prevalence.[16] Proposed reasons for this increase in prevalence have included increasing pollution levels,[17] obesity, dietary changes, the hygiene effect,[18] low vitamin D levels,[19] and early exposure to acetaminophen (APAP).[20] Three of the currently most popular hypotheses are discussed here.

The hygiene hypothesis

The largest increase in asthma prevalence over the past 30 years has been observed in the Western world.[21] Given the short time frame, genetic changes are unlikely to explain this observation but improvements in public health measures, treatment of diseases, vaccination programs, and hygiene strongly associate with the increase in asthma. These improvements in public health have occurred with a corresponding decrease in exposure to noninfectious microorganisms. In 1989 Strachan[22] hypothesized that the increase in asthma and allergic disorders in industrialized nations was caused by the absence of early life exposure to viral and bacterial organisms and their products (eg, endotoxins). This theory is referred to as the hygiene hypothesis. Early life exposure to viruses and bacteria primes and trains the immune system. Elimination of this training results in a shift toward a more inflammatory immune response that has been associated with asthma and allergic disease. Studies have found that farm exposures and larger family size are associated with these early life exposures and are also associated with lower rates of asthma and atopy. In addition, the increased asthma prevalence parallels the increase in autoimmune diseases and corresponds with decreases in rates of infectious diseases. These data suggest that, in the absence of exposure to foreign microbes, the immune system sustains a hypervigilant state that results in a mismatch between the host and innocuous environmental challenges.

Because of this mismatch, the immune system turns on itself, resulting in increases in autoimmune diseases and asthma.

Although microbial exposure (such as bacterial endotoxin) is associated with protection against asthma, the hygiene hypothesis does not reconcile the observed higher asthma prevalence in inner-city, urban environments, where endotoxin exposure has been shown to be a risk factor for asthma.[23] Inner-city housing conditions have unlikely become more hygienic in the United States but asthma prevalence has increased significantly among racial and ethnic minorities living in poverty. To explain these observations, the narrow version of the hygiene hypothesis has evolved, which focuses on early life microbial exposure protecting against allergic asthma by suppressing TH_2 immune responses. It is now suggested that it is the diversity of microbial exposure that is particularly protective against asthma[24] and that this diversity, rather than endotoxin per se, may explain the protective effect of farm living.

The vitamin D hypothesis

Hypovitaminosis D is prevalent worldwide and increasing. Multiple studies have shown an increase in asthma prevalence and severity in children with asthma in association with low levels of vitamin D.[25–27] However, a recent systematic review of childhood cohort studies concluded that there was only a potential association between low vitamin D levels and asthma.[19] Vitamin D is both a hormone and a nutrient; levels of vitamin D are determined primarily by environmental mechanisms such as exposure to the sun, latitude, and skin color. Vitamin D has both in utero and postnatal effects on lung and immune system development and function, and vitamin D is thought to have an immunomodulatory role in both the innate and adaptive immune response. Several genome-wide association studies have uncovered genetic variants that associate with serum vitamin D levels in children with asthma.[28,29] Overall, studies examining the relationship between vitamin D and asthma have problems with selection bias, inadequate measuring of outcomes, and confounding.[19]

The acetaminophen hypothesis

APAP is a widely used antipyretic and analgesic that has recently been identified as a possible cause for the current increase in asthma prevalence.[30] APAP replaced aspirin in the 1990s as the antipyretic of choice when aspirin was thought to be associated with Reye syndrome. Since then, several longitudinal studies have reported an association between increased APAP use and the increased prevalence of childhood asthma.[20] Induction of asthma by APAP is biologically plausible, because APAP decreases airway antioxidant defenses through depletion of glutathione.[31] However, an alternative explanation for the APAP/asthma association may be confounding by indication. APAP is commonly used to treat fever and pain caused by respiratory tract infections, which are a known risk factor for childhood asthma. Children with asthma may have a longer duration of fever in association with respiratory tract infections, and this may have resulted in greater APAP exposure.[32,33] According to a recent systematic review and meta-analysis, there currently is insufficient evidence to support an association between APAP use in childhood and incidence of asthma.[20]

ASTHMA PATHOPHYSIOLOGY

Asthma is a chronic inflammatory disease of the airways that results from the combination of environmental exposures and genetic/biological susceptibility. Asthma has 3 major characteristics: (1) chronic airway inflammation; (2) airway obstruction that, for the most part, is reversible; and (3) airway hyperresponsiveness to a variety of stimuli. Although airway eosinophil inflammation is typical, many patients, especially those with mild asthma, have noneosinophilic disease.[34] Airflow obstruction is usually reversible but some patients develop irreversible airflow obstruction, which has been attributed to remodeling of the airway wall.

Symptoms of asthma include recurrent wheezing, cough, and shortness of breath. A diagnosis of asthma is based on the presence of these symptoms and objective confirmation of (at least partially) reversible airflow obstruction. However, some children and adults with asthma only cough and never wheeze, whereas others experience shortness of breath and never wheeze.[35] Diagnosing asthma in these individuals can be difficult unless the clinician has a high index of suspicion. Triggers for cough-variant asthma and asthma-related dyspnea are the same as for individuals with wheezing, and are discussed later.

Asthma diagnosis and approach to treatment are discussed in a 2013 article in the *Pediatric Clinics of North America*.[36]

Risk Factors and Natural History

Brief periods of a loss of asthma control, manifested by cough, wheezing, and/or shortness breath, are the result of exposure to nonspecific triggers such as strong smells or exercise, whereas moderate or severe exacerbations are usually caused by exposure to allergens or viruses, with human rhinovirus being the most important. More than 80% of children who are diagnosed with asthma at 6 years of age have a history of wheezing in the first 3 years of life.[37] The opposite is not true; half of all children who wheeze in the first year of life are wheeze free and do not go on to have recurring episodes.[38] In general, children who have mild asthma rarely progress to severe disease, but severe and frequent wheezing is a well-established risk factor for persistence and disease severity in adulthood. Boys with wheezing illnesses in early childhood are more likely to outgrow their asthma, probably because of a smaller airway structure that predisposes boys to wheezing illnesses in early life.[39]

PREVENTION STRATEGIES
Asthma Prevention

There are no effective strategies to prevent the development of asthma in children. In order for an agent/exposure to be determined to have a causal relationship, there must be evidence of a strong and consistent association, a biological gradient, biological plausibility and coherence, and a temporally correct association. At present, no agent or exposure reaches this level of evidence. The last systematic summary of the evidence supporting a causal relationship for the development of asthma was published in 2000 (Committee on the Assessment of Asthma and Indoor Air of the Institute of Medicine [IOM]).[40] House dust mite and environmental tobacco smoke (ETS) had the strongest association with asthma development but neither reached the level of causation.

Dust mite exposure and asthma development

Exposure to dust mite is associated with dust mite sensitization and dust mite sensitization is a risk factor for the development of asthma.[41] Three large studies have implemented house dust mite avoidance measures during pregnancy, at birth, and later in childhood and assessed asthma development in childhood.[42-44] Strategies to reduce house dust mite exposure, such as impermeable mite mattress covers, anti–dust mite spray, and carpet removal reduced dust mite levels and dust mite sensitization in children but effects on wheezing outcomes were short-term with no long-term benefit on the development of asthma.[45-48] Some investigators have suggested that these same strategies might also have reduced endotoxin exposure, which has been found to be protective against asthma in several studies.[49]

Respiratory tract infections and asthma development
The role of viral infections in the development of asthma has long been debated. Viral infections, particularly respiratory syncytial virus (RSV) and rhinovirus, are associated with wheezing episodes in children and children with asthma are at greater risk for more severe infection and thus greater morbidity with these infections.[50] Emerging evidence suggests that prevention of RSV infection might be protective against asthma. In a randomized controlled trial, use of a highly specific monoclonal immunoglobulin G antibody directed against the RSV fusion protein (palivizumab) glycoprotein reduced recurrent wheezing in healthy preterm infants by 50% in the first year of life.[51] Similar reductions in recurrent wheezing and the diagnosis of asthma have been observed in infants receiving ribavirin antiviral therapy and in premature infants treated with palivizumab.[52–54] These data suggest that preventing RSV lower respiratory tract infections in the first year of life may prevent asthma or wheezing.

Environmental tobacco smoke and asthma development
Multiple studies have linked ETS and asthma, and several systematic reviews of the literature have concluded that ETS exposure is a risk factor for the development of asthma in children.[55] The Surgeon General's 2006 report concluded that there was a causal relationship between parental smoking and ever having asthma in school-aged children and between parental smoking and wheezing illness in early childhood.[56] However, the evidence was only sufficient to show an association between parental ETS exposure and the onset of childhood asthma. In a survey of more than 11,000 children 4 to 6 years of age in the United Kingdom, the odds ratio for childhood wheezing in the previous 12 months increased with each additional smoker in the home. Lewis and colleagues[57] suggested that 8% of asthma in children 4 to 6 years of age could be attributable to ETS exposure at home. Quitting smoking before pregnancy reduced the risk of asthma to that of the nonsmoking population, and this is the only known effective prevention strategy.

Multiple other intervention strategies to reduce asthma development have not been successful. These strategies include breastfeeding during the first 4 to 6 months of life, maternal avoidance of allergenic foods during pregnancy, antioxidant supplementation (vitamins A and C) during pregnancy, and delayed introduction of solids.[41]

Asthma Exacerbation Prevention

In 2000 the Committee on the Assessment of Asthma and Indoor Air of the IOM reviewed and summarized the scientific evidence for the relationship between indoor air exposures and asthma exacerbations.[40] This report was updated in October 2014[58] and the results are summarized in **Box 1**. Several important new findings related to exposures that cause asthma exacerbations are highlighted here.

Dust mite and asthma exacerbations
In children sensitized to dust mite (Der p1 and Der f1 are the 2 common dust mite allergens), a dose-related association between dust mite antigen and wheeze has been found.[59] Both intervention studies[60] and prospective studies[61–63] have reported associations between dust mite exposure and asthma exacerbations. In children of unknown dust mite sensitization, most studies have found associations with exacerbations,[64,65] but not all.[66] Dust mite exposure has also been associated with fraction of exhaled nitric oxide (FeNO) measurements, suggesting a direct role in airway inflammation.

> **Box 1**
> **Summary of 2014 scientific evidence for exposures and asthma exacerbations**
>
> *Exposures with sufficient evidence to show causation of asthma exacerbations*
>
> House dust mite allergens in sensitized individuals
>
> Cat allergen in sensitized individuals
>
> Cockroach allergen in sensitized individuals (especially adults)
>
> Outdoor culturable fungal exposure in sensitized individuals
>
> Dampness or dampness-related agents in children
>
> *Exposures associated with asthma exacerbations but with insufficient evidence to show causation*
>
> Chronic ETS exposure in preschool-aged children
>
> Dog allergen in sensitized individuals
>
> Brief high-level exposures to NO_2 in conjunction with a nonspecific chemical irritant or inhaled allergen
>
> Indoor endotoxin exposure
>
> *Exposures with limited or suggestive evidence of an association with asthma exacerbations*
>
> Chronic ETS exposure in older children and adults
>
> Indoor culturable *Penicillium* in individuals with any fungal sensitization
>
> Formaldehyde
>
> Fragrance exposure
>
> Rodent and mice exposure in the home in rodent-sensitized children
>
> Synthetic bedding
>
> *Exposures with inadequate or insufficient evidence of an association with asthma exacerbations*
>
> Pesticides
>
> Houseplants
>
> Plasticizers
>
> Residential volatile organic compounds
>
> Indoor pollen exposures
>
> Low building ventilation rates

Cat allergen exposure and asthma exacerbations

Cat allergen exposure in children with asthma sensitized to cat is associated with increased asthma severity, greater rescue medication use, increased asthma symptom frequency, and/or increased FeNO.[59,61,67] This association has not been reported in cross-sectional studies[65,66] but it has been suggested that the findings were biased by cat-allergic subjects not owning cats. Other studies have found no association between cat exposure and asthma exacerbations in individuals who were atopic but not sensitized to cat.[68]

Cockroach exposure and asthma exacerbations

There is strong evidence of a causal relationship between exposure to cockroach antigen and asthma exacerbations in cockroach-sensitized adults[69,70] but the evidence in children for this association is less consistent. Bedroom cockroach exposure in sensitized children is consistently associated with asthma exacerbations in prospective studies,[71,72] whereas results from cross-sectional studies have been mixed for bedroom exposure[59,66] but positive for kitchen exposure.[64] Cockroach allergen can induce allergic sensitization and inflammation,[73] and expression of inflammatory cytokines,[74,75] suggesting a potential mechanism for asthma morbidity in sensitized and nonsensitized individuals.

Fungi and asthma exacerbations

Outdoor fungal exposures cause exacerbations of asthma in sensitized individuals, including children.[76,77] Outdoor fungal concentrations are associated with admissions to emergency rooms even after adjustment for pollen and air pollutants.[76] Two studies have reported an association between culturable airborne indoor *Penicillium* exposure and severe asthma exacerbations and asthma severity even after adjustment for outdoor fungal levels.[61,77] Indoor *Penicillium* levels have been associated with increased asthma symptoms in several other studies[78,79] but the sampling strategy was suspect because of high temporal variability so the IOM was unable to conclude that there was an association between indoor cultural *Penicillium* exposure and asthma exacerbations in children.

Dampness and asthma exacerbations

Multiple studies published in the past 15 years have shown a positive association between evident or measured dampness or mold and asthma severity or exacerbations,[80–83] and remediation of dampness sources and visible mold has been shown to reduce severe asthma exacerbations.[80,84] The specific causal agents for asthma exacerbations associated with dampness have not been identified but are thought to include fungal agents and/or other biological exposures, such as bacteria or dust mites, that thrive in dampness.

Environmental tobacco smoke exposure and asthma exacerbations

One of the major changes in the recently released update to the IOM report was the downgrading of the evidence in support of a causal relationship between ETS exposure and asthma exacerbations.[58] Citing 19 recent studies on ETS exposure and asthma exacerbations, the update concluded that the "weight of evidence no longer supports a causal relationship."[58] In preschool children for whom the evidence is the strongest and formed the basis for the 2000 IOM conclusion, more recent studies have found that high ETS exposure is not related to increased wheezing episodes or unscheduled medical visits.[85,86] Other investigators have reported an inverse relationship between current ETS and FeNO, with ETS exposure at age 4 years associated with lower forced expiratory volume in 1 second at age 7 years but not concurrent exposure at age 7 years. Other studies have also found no association between FeNO and ETS.[65,87–90] In contrast, multiple other studies in children have continued to show an association between ETS exposure and reduced lung function, increased wheezing, nocturnal symptoms, and emergency department visits.[91–96]

Asthma Exacerbation Prevention Strategies

There is significant evidence that 3 groups of intervention strategies are effective in reducing asthma symptoms and possibly asthma exacerbations. These groups are (1) a tailored in-home education and remediation of asthma triggers in sensitized individuals; (2) integrated pest management in sensitized individuals; and (3) combined elimination of moisture intrusion and leaks, and removal of mold items.[97]

Asthma Trigger Remediation

Dust mite
Multiple studies have shown the effectiveness of a comprehensive dust mite mitigation strategy on dust mite exposure in homes. The most effective strategies have included dust-impermeable pillow, mattress, and box spring covers; use of a high-efficiency particulate air (HEPA) vacuum cleaner; and removal of the carpets.[98] Sophisticated (and high-cost) interventions have included installation of central heating and use of a whole-home mechanical ventilation system with heat recovery unit, which significantly reduced humidity levels and resulted in a significant reduction in house dust mite counts. Bedroom and living room air cleaners have been shown to reduce cat and dog allergens but do not reduce dust mite levels in homes.[99] Reductions in dust mite exposure using either multiple bedroom strategies and/or sophisticated interventions have been associated with decreases in asthma symptoms. In contrast, isolated interventions, such as dust-impermeable pillow and mattress and box spring covers, have not been effective.[46,48]

Environmental tobacco smoke
Although comprehensive smoke-free laws prohibiting smoking in public places correlated with declines in smoking rates among adults, ETS exposure has declined more slowly among children.[100] In a cross-sectional study, using National Health and Nutrition Examination Survey 2003 to 2010 data, 53.3% of nonsmoking children 6 to 19 years of age with asthma were exposed to ETS.[101] Several interventions have targeted tobacco smoke cessation and reduction of secondhand smoke exposure in the home. However, most interventions designed to reduce children's ETS exposure have been ineffective.[102] The most effective strategy among children, who have minimal control over ETS exposure, was reported by Lanphear and colleagues,[103] in which HEPA filters reduced the number of unscheduled asthma visits. However, there was no difference in serum or hair cotinine between the intervention and control groups. Children are more vulnerable than adults to the effects of third-hand smoke, which can persist for weeks to months on surfaces and in settled dust. Studies of smoking outside the home have shown small decreases in urine cotinine among infants living in homes of smokers who smoked outside.[104] This finding suggests that even smoking outside the home is not an effective strategy for remediating ETS exposure.

Integrated pest management
Integrated pest management (IPM) is a prevention-based approach to pest control that reduces the need for pesticides. It is a safer, and often more effective, long-term means of reducing the presence of pest allergens in homes compared with traditional pest control methods. IPM focuses on eliminating the root causes of pests (**Table 1**) and includes (1) using small, sticky traps or glue boards in areas of the house that are more susceptible to pests, such as the kitchen, basement, or bathroom; (2) preventing pest access by caulking cracks and crevices that pests use to move or hide; (3) reducing clutter to remove pest hiding places; (4) preventing food sources by using plastic or glass containers with tight-fitting lids, washing and drying dirty dishes, storing pet foods in pest-proof containers, and using a trash can with a tight-fitting lid; and (5) removing water sources by fixing any water leaks, wiping up spills, and removing pets' water dishes at night. In New York City, IPM involves a 3-hour intervention including a home inspection, vacuuming, steam cleaning, pest exclusion activities (sealing holes), low-toxicity pesticide application, and tenant education, and costs from $400 to $500 per unit.[105]

Table 1	
Supplies needed to implement asthma exacerbation prevention strategies	
Dust mites	Dust-impermeable pillow, mattress, and box spring covers
	HEPA vacuum cleaner
	Carpet removal
IPM	Cockroach glue traps
	Mouse glue traps
	Door sweeps
	Caulk for cracks
	Plastic containers with tight lids
	Trash can with tight lid
	Roller mop
	Copper mesh to fill holes

Adapted from Asthma Regional Council of New England. The role of pest control in effective asthma management: a business case. 2009. Available at: http://asthmaregionalcouncil.org. Accessed January 26, 2015.

Moisture and mold interventions

In children with sensitization to mold, a comprehensive asthma program consisting of evaluation by an asthma specialist with development of a written asthma treatment plan, asthma education, and skill building in individualized problem solving was coupled with household interventions designed to reduce dampness and mold.[84] Specific interventions were directed at reducing water infiltration, removing water-damaged building materials, alterations to the heating/ventilation/air conditioning, lead hazard control, and environmental cleaning. Mold was cleaned from hard surfaces, mold exposure pathways were moved, rainwater intrusion was stopped, water vapor was exhausted from kitchens and bathroom, and plumbing leaks were repaired. The cost for the intervention was $3458 ± $2795 and resulted in a reduction in asthma symptoms and mold levels, and a modest reduction in health care use.

REFERENCES

1. Center for Disease Control and Prevention - National Center for Health Statistics. National Health Interview Survey Raw Data. 2009.
2. American Lung Association - Epidemiology and Statistics Unit - Research Program Services. Trends in asthma morbidity and mortality. September 2012.
3. Bloom B, Jonas LI, Freeman G. Summary health statistics for US Children. National Health Interview Survey. Vital Health Stat 10 2012;(254):1–88.
4. Centers for Disease Control and Prevention. Vital signs. 2011.
5. Lockett GA, Holloway JW. Genome-wide association studies in asthma; perhaps, the end of the beginning. Curr Opin Allergy Clin Immunol 2013;13:463–9.
6. Sharma SK, Chhabra D, Kho AT, et al. The genomic origins of asthma. Thorax 2014;69:481–7.
7. Kumar R, Seibold MA, Aldrich MC, et al. Genetic ancestry in lung function predictions. N Engl J Med 2010;363:321–30.
8. Rumpel JA, Ahmedani BK, Peterson EL, et al. Genetic ancestry and its association with asthma exacerbations among African American subjects with asthma. J Allergy Clin Immunol 2012;130:1302–6.
9. Rose D, Mannino DM, Leaderer BP. Asthma prevalence among US adults, 1998-2000: role of Puerto Rican ethnicity and behavioral and geographic factors. Am J Public Health 2006;96:880–8.

10. Ortega VE, Meyers DA. Pharmacogenetics: implications of race and ethnicity on defining genetic profiles for personalized medicine. J Allergy Clin Immunol 2014;133:16–26.
11. Nelson HS, Weiss ST, Bleecker ER, et al. The Salmeterol Multicenter Asthma Research Trial: a comparison of usual pharmacotherapy for asthma or usual pharmacotherapy plus salmeterol. Chest 2006;129:15–26.
12. Salpeter SR, Buckley MS, Ormiston TM, et al. Meta-analysis: effect of long-acting beta-agonists on severe asthma exacerbations and asthma-related deaths. Ann Intern Med 2006;144:904–12.
13. Sears MR, Ottosson A, Radner F, et al. Long-acting beta-agonists: a review of formoterol safety data from asthma clinical trials. Eur Respir J 2009;33: 21–32.
14. Lemanske RF, Mauger DT, Sorkness CA, et al. Step-up therapy for children with uncontrolled asthma receiving inhaled corticosteroids. N Engl J Med 2010;362: 975–82.
15. Naqvi M, Thyne S, Choudhry S, et al. Ethnic-specific differences in bronchodilator responsiveness among African Americans, Puerto Ricans, and Mexicans with asthma. J Asthma 2007;44:639–48.
16. Asher MI, Montefort S, Bjorksten B, et al. Worldwide time trends in the prevalence of symptoms of asthma, allergic rhinoconjunctivitis, and eczema in childhood: ISAAC phases one and three repeat multicountry cross-sectional surveys. Lancet 2006;368(9537):733–43.
17. Brauer M, Hoek G, Van Vliet P, et al. Air pollution from traffic and the development of respiratory infections and asthmatic and allergic symptoms in children. Am J Respir Crit Care Med 2002;166(8):1092–8.
18. Brooks C, Pearce N, Douwes J. The hygiene hypothesis in allergy and asthma: an update. Curr Opin Allergy Clin Immunol 2013;13(1):70–7.
19. Rajabbik MH, Lotfi T, Alkhaled L, et al. Association between low vitamin D levels and the diagnosis of asthma in children: a systematic review of cohort studies. Allergy Asthma Clin Immunol 2014;10(1):31.
20. Cheelo M, Lodge CJ, Dharmage SC, et al. Paracetamol exposure in pregnancy and early childhood and development of childhood asthma: a systematic review and meta-analysis. Arch Dis Child 2015;100(1):81–9.
21. Pearce N, Douwes J. The global epidemiology of asthma in children. Int J Tuberc Lung Dis 2006;10(2):125–32.
22. Strachan DP. Hay fever, hygiene, and household size. BMJ 1989;299(6710): 1259–60.
23. Perzanowski MS, Miller RL, Thorne PS, et al. Endotoxin in inner-city homes: associations with wheeze and eczema in early childhood. J Allergy Clin Immunol 2006;117(5):1082–9.
24. Haahtela T, Holgate S, Pawankar R, et al. The biodiversity hypothesis and allergic disease: World Allergy Organization position statement. World Allergy Organ J 2013;6(1):3.
25. Braegger C, Campoy C, Colomb V, et al. Vitamin D in the healthy European paediatric population. J Pediatr Gastroenterol Nutr 2013;56(6):692–701.
26. van Oeffelen AA, Bekkers MB, Smit HA, et al. Serum micronutrient concentrations and childhood asthma: the PIAMA birth cohort study. Pediatr Allergy Immunol 2011;22(8):784–93.
27. Hollams EM, Hart PH, Holt BJ, et al. Vitamin D and atopy and asthma phenotypes in children: a longitudinal cohort study. Eur Respir J 2011;38(6): 1320–7.

28. Lasky-Su J, Lange N, Brehm JM, et al. Genome-wide association analysis of circulating vitamin D levels in children with asthma. Hum Genet 2012;131(9): 1495–505.

29. Litonjua AA. Vitamin D deficiency as a risk factor for childhood allergic disease and asthma. Curr Opin Allergy Clin Immunol 2012;12(2):179–85.

30. Shaheen SO. Acetaminophen and childhood asthma: pill-popping at our peril? J Allergy Clin Immunol 2015;135(2):449–50.

31. Perquin M, Oster T, Maul A, et al. The glutathione-related detoxification system is increased in human breast cancer in correlation with clinical and histopathological features. J Cancer Res Clin Oncol 2001;127(6):368–74.

32. Jackson DJ, Gangnon RE, Evans MD, et al. Wheezing rhinovirus illnesses in early life predict asthma development in high-risk children. Am J Respir Crit Care Med 2008;178(7):667–72.

33. Schnabel E, Heinrich J, LISA Study Group. Respiratory tract infections and not paracetamol medication during infancy are associated with asthma development in childhood. J Allergy Clin Immunol 2010;126(5):1071–3.

34. McGrath KW, Icitovic N, Boushey HA, et al. A large subgroup of mild-to-moderate asthma is persistently noneosinophilic. Am J Respir Crit Care Med 2012;185:612–9.

35. Niimi A, Matsumoto H, Mishima M. Eosinophilic airways disorders associated with chronic cough. Pulm Pharmacol Ther 2009;22:114–20.

36. Nelson KA, Zorc JJ. Asthma update. Pediatr Clin North Am 2013;60:1035–48.

37. Guilbert TW, Morgan WJ, Zeiger RS, et al. Long-term inhaled corticosteroids in preschool children at high risk for asthma. N Engl J Med 2006;354(19):1985–97.

38. Martinez FD, Wright AL, Taussig LM, et al. Asthma and wheezing in the first six years of life. The Group Health Medical Associates. N Engl J Med 1995;332: 133–8.

39. Boezen HM, Jansen DF, Postma DS. Sex and gender differences in lung development and their clinical significance. Clin Chest Med 2004;25:237–45.

40. Institute of Medicine. Clearing the air: asthma and indoor air exposures. Washington, DC: National Academy Press; 2000.

41. Arshad SH. Primary prevention of asthma and allergy. J Allergy Clin Immunol 2005;116:3–14.

42. Custovic A, Simpson BM, Simpson A, et al. Manchester Asthma and Allergy Study: low-allergen environment can be achieved and maintained during pregnancy and in early life. J Allergy Clin Immunol 2000;105:282–8.

43. Halmerbauer G, Gartner C, Schier M, et al. Study on the Prevention of Allergy in Children in Europe (SPACE): allergic sensitization in children at 1 year of age in a controlled trial of allergen avoidance from birth. Pediatr Allergy Immunol 2002; 13(suppl 15):47–54.

44. van Strien RT, Koopman LP, Kerkhof M, et al. Mattress encasings and mite allergen levels in the prevention and incidence of asthma and mite allergy study. Clin Exp Allergy 2003;33:490–5.

45. Brunekreef B, Smit J, de Jongste JC, et al. The prevention and incidence of asthma and mite allergy (PIAMA) birth cohort study: design and first results. Pediatr Allergy Immunol 2002;13:55–60.

46. Horak FJ, Matthews S, Ihorst G, et al. Effect of mite-impermeable mattress encasings and an educational package on the development of allergies in a multinational randomized, controlled birth-cohort study-24 months results of the Study of Prevention of Allergy in Children in Europe. Clin Exp Allergy 2004;34: 1220–5.

47. Simpson A, Simpson B, Custovic A, et al. Stringent environmental control in pregnancy and early life: the long-term effects on mite, cat and dog allergen. Clin Exp Allergy 2003;33:1183–9.
48. Gehring U, de Jongste JC, Kerkhof M, et al. The 8-year follow up of the PIAMA intervention study assessing the effect of mite-impermeable mattress covers. Allergy 2012;67:248–56.
49. Sabina I, Weber J, Zutavern A, et al. Perinatal influences on the development of asthma and atopy in childhood. Ann Allergy Asthma Immunol 2014;112: 132–9.
50. Feldman AS, He Y, Moore ML, et al. Toward primary prevention of asthma: reviewing the evidence of early-life respiratory viral infections as modifiable risk factors to prevent childhood asthma. Am J Respir Crit Care Med 2015;191: 34–44.
51. Blanken MO, Rovers MM, Molenaar JM, et al, Dutch RSV Neonatal Network. Respiratory syncytial virus and recurrent wheeze in healthy preterm infants. N Engl J Med 2013;368:1791–9.
52. Chen CH, Lin YT, Yang YH, et al. Ribavirin for respiratory syncytial virus bronchiolitis reduced the risk of asthma and allergen sensitization. Pediatr Allergy Immunol 2008;19:166–72.
53. Simoes EA, Groothuis JR, Carbonell-Estrany X, et al. Palivizumab prophylaxis, respiratory syncytial virus, and subsequent recurrent wheezing. J Pediatr 2007;151:34–42.
54. Yoshihara S, Kusuda S, Mochizuki H, et al. Effect of palivizumab prophylaxis on subsequent recurrent wheezing in preterm infants. Pediatrics 2013;132: 811–8.
55. Thomson NC. The role of environmental tobacco smoke in the origins and progression of asthma. Curr Allergy Asthma Rep 2007;7:303–9.
56. U.S. Department of Health and Human Services. The Health Consequences of Involuntary Exposure to Tobacco Smoke: A Report of the Surgeon General. Atlanta (GA): US Department of Health and Human Services; Centers for Disease Control and Prevention; Coordinating, Center for Health Promotion; National Center for Chronic Disease Prevention and Health Promotion; Office on Smoking and Health; 2006.
57. Lewis SA, Antoniak M, Venn AJ, et al. Secondhand smoke, dietary fruit intake, road traffic exposures and the prevalence of asthma: a cross-sectional study in young children. Am J Epidemiol 2005;161:406–11.
58. Kanchongkittiphonn W, Mendel MJ, Gaffin JM, et al. Indoor environmental exposures and exacerbation of asthma: an update to the 2000 review by the Institute of Medicine. Environ Health Perspect 2015;123:6–20.
59. Gent JF, Belanger K, Triche EW, et al. Association of pediatric asthma severity with exposure to common household dust allergens. Environ Res 2009;109: 968–74.
60. El-Ghitany EM, Abd El-Salam MM. Association of residential dampness and mold with respiratory tract infections and bronchitis: a meta-analysis. Environ Health Perspect 2010;9:1–11.
61. Gent JF, Kezik JM, Hill ME, et al. Household mold and dust allergens: exposure, sensitization and childhood asthma morbidity. Environ Res 2012;118: 86–93.
62. Halken S, Host A, Niklassen U, et al. Effect of mattress and pillow encasings on children with asthma and house dust mite allergy. J Allergy Clin Immunol 2003; 111:169–76.

63. Nitschke M, Pilotto LS, Attewell RG, et al. A cohort study of indoor nitrogen dioxide and house dust mite exposure in asthmatic children. Occup Environ Med 2006;48:462–9.
64. Rabito FA, Carlson J, Hold EW, et al. Cockroach exposure independent of sensitization status and association with hospitalization for asthma in inner-city children. Ann Allergy Asthma Immunol 2011;106:103–9.
65. Spanier AJ, Hornung R, Lierl M, et al. Environmental exposures and exhaled nitric oxide in children with asthma. J Pediatr 2006;149:220–6.
66. Turyk M, Curtis LH, Scheff P, et al. Environmental allergens and asthma morbidity in low-income children. J Asthma 2006;43:453–7.
67. Murray CS, Poletti G, Kebadze T, et al. Study of modifiable risk factors for asthma exacerbations: virus infection and allergen exposure increase the risk of asthma hospital admissions in children. Thorax 2006;61:376–82.
68. Langley SJ, Goldthorpe S, Craven M, et al. Relationship between exposure to domestic allergens and bronchial hyperresponsiveness in non-sensitised, atopic asthmatic subjects. Thorax 2005;60:17–21.
69. Kang BH. Study on cockroach antigen as a probable causative agent in bronchial asthma. J Allergy Clin Immunol 1976;58:357–65.
70. Bernton HS, McMahon RF, Brown H. Cockroach asthma. Br J Dis Chest 1972;66:61–6.
71. Gruchalla RS, Pongracic J, Plaut M, et al. Inner City Asthma Study: relationships among sensitivity, allergen exposure, and asthma morbidity. J Allergy Clin Immunol 2005;115:478–85.
72. Rosenstreich DL, Eggleston P, Kattan M, et al. The role of cockroach allergy and exposure to cockroach allergen in causing morbidity among inner-city children with asthma. N Engl J Med 1997;336:1356–63.
73. Jeong SK, Kim HJ, Youm JK, et al. Mite and cockroach allergens activate protease-activated receptor 2 and delay epidermal permeability barrier recovery. J Invest Dermatol 2008;128:1930–9.
74. Kauffman HF. Innate immune responses to environmental allergens. Clin Rev Allergy Immunol 2006;30:129–40.
75. Matsumura Y. Role of allergen source-derived proteases in sensitization via airway epithelial cells. J Allergy (Cairo) 2012;90:365–9.
76. Atkinson RW, Strachan DP, Anderson HR, et al. Temporal associations between daily counts of fungal spores and asthma exacerbations. Occup Environ Med 2006;63:580–90.
77. Pongracic JA, O'Connor GT, Muilenberg ML, et al. Differential effects of outdoor versus indoor fungal spores on asthma morbidity in inner-city children. J Allergy Clin Immunol 2010;125:593–9.
78. Bundy KW, Gent JF, Beckett W, et al. Household airborne *Penicillium* associated with peak expiratory flow variability in asthmatic children. Ann Allergy Asthma Immunol 2009;103:26–30.
79. Inal A, Karakoc GB, Altintas DU, et al. Effect of indoor mold concentrations on daily symptom severity of children with asthma and/or rhinitis monosensitized to molds. J Asthma 2007;44:543–6.
80. Bernstein JA, Bobbitt RC, Levin L, et al. Health effects of ultraviolet irradiation in asthmatic children's homes. J Asthma 2006;43:255–62.
81. Bonner S, Matte TD, Fagan J, et al. Self-reported moisture or mildew in the homes of Head Start children with asthma is associated with greater asthma morbidity. J Urban Health 2006;83:129–37.

82. Hagmolen of Ten Have W, van den Berg MJ, van der Palen J, et al. Residential exposure to mould and dampness is associated with adverse respiratory health. Clin Exp Allergy 2007;37:1827–32.

83. Venn AJ, Cooper M, Antoniak M, et al. Effects of volatile organic compounds, damp and other environmental exposure in the home on wheezing illness in children. Thorax 2003;58:955–60.

84. Kercsmar CM, Dearborn DG, Schluchter M, et al. Reduction in asthma morbidity in children as a result of home remediation aimed at moisture sources. Environ Health Perspect 2006;114:1574–80.

85. Kattan M, Gergen PJ, Eggleston P, et al. Health effects of indoor nitrogen dioxide and passive smoking on urban asthmatic children. J Allergy Clin Immunol 2007;120:618–24.

86. Perzanowski MS, Divjan A, Mellins RB, et al. Exhaled NO among inner-city children in New York City. J Asthma 2010;47:1015–21.

87. Dinakar C, Lapuente M, Barnes C, et al. Real-life environmental tobacco exposure does not affect exhaled nitric oxide levels in asthmatic children. J Asthma 2005;42:113–8.

88. Spanier AJ, Hornung R, Kahn RS, et al. Seasonal variation and environmental predictors of exhaled nitric oxide in children with asthma. Pediatr Pulmonol 2008;43:576–83.

89. Vargas PA, Brenner B, Clark SJ, et al. Exposure to environmental tobacco smoke among children presenting to the emergency department with acute asthma: a multicenter study. Pediatr Pulmonol 2007;42:646–55.

90. Karadag B, Karakoc F, Ceran L, et al. Does passive smoke exposure trigger acute asthma attacks in children? Allergol Immunopathol (Madr) 2003;31:318–23.

91. Chapman RS, Hadden WC, Perlin SA. Influences of asthma and household environment on lung function in children and adolescents: the third national health and nutrition examination survey. Am J Epidemiol 2003;158:175–89.

92. Lawson JA, Dosman JA, Rennie DC, et al. Relationship of endotoxin and tobacco smoke exposure to wheeze and diurnal peak expiratory flow variability in children and adolescents. Respirology 2011;16:332–9.

93. Soussan D, Liard R, Aureik M, et al. Treatment compliance, passive smoking and asthma control: a three year cohort study. Arch Dis Child 2003;88:229–33.

94. Sturm R. The effects of obesity, smoking, and drinking on medical problems and costs. Health Aff (Millwood) 2002;21(2):245–53.

95. Morkjaroenpong V, Rand CS, Butz AM, et al. Environmental tobacco smoke exposure and nocturnal symptoms among inner-city children with asthma. J Allergy Clin Immunol 2002;110:147–53.

96. Wang HC, McGeady SJ, Yousef E. Patient, home residence and neighborhood characteristics in pediatric emergency department visits for asthma. J Asthma 2007;44:95–8.

97. Krieger JW, Jacobs DE, Ashley PJ, et al. Housing interventions and control of asthma-related indoor biologic agents: a review of the evidence. J Public Health Manag Pract 2010;16:S11–20.

98. Morgan WJ, Crain EF, Gruchalla RS, et al. Results of a home-based environmental intervention among urban children with asthma. N Engl J Med 2004; 351:1068–80.

99. van der Heide S, van Aalderen WM, Kauffman HF, et al. Clinical effects of air cleaners in homes of asthmatic children sensitized to pet allergens. J Allergy Clin Immunol 1999;104:447–51.

100. Marano C, Schober SE, Brody DJ, et al. Secondhand tobacco smoke exposure among children and adolescents: United States, 2003-2006. Pediatrics 2009; 124(5):1299–305.
101. Akinbami LJ, Kit BK, Simon AE. Impact of environmental tobacco smoke on children with asthma, United States, 2003-2010. Acad Pediatr 2013;13(6):508–16.
102. Priest N, Roseby R, Waters E, et al. Family and carer smoking control programmes for reducing children's exposure to environmental tobacco smoke. Cochrane Database Syst Rev 2008;(4):CD001746.
103. Lanphear BP, Hornung RW, Khoury J, et al. Effects of HEPA air cleaners on unscheduled asthma visits and asthma symptoms for children exposed to secondhand tobacco smoke. Pediatrics 2011;127(1):93–101.
104. Matt GE, Quintana PJ, Hovell MF, et al. Households contaminated by environmental tobacco smoke: sources of infant exposures. Tob Control 2004;13(1): 29–37.
105. Asthma Regional Council of New England. The role of pest control in effective asthma management: A business case. 2009. Available at: http:// asthmaregionalcouncil.org. Accessed January 26, 2015.

Children's Oral Health Assessment, Prevention, and Treatment

Christopher Okunseri, BDS, MSc, DDPHRCSE, FFDRCSI[a],*,
Cesar Gonzalez, DDS, MS[b], Brian Hodgson, DDS[b]

KEYWORDS

- Dental caries • Risk assessment • Prevention • Treatment • Pediatricians

KEY POINTS

- Oral health is part of general health and it contributes to oral health–related quality of life in children.
- The involvement of pediatricians in advocating for dental care has facilitated the awareness and prevention of dental caries in children.
- The establishment of a dental home provides a lifetime opportunity for risk assessment, treatment, oral health promotion, and prevention of caries.

INTRODUCTION

This article provides a brief introduction to the oral health of children and the barriers to dental care as well as some discussion on prevention and treatment modalities for dental caries. Also covered is the epidemiology of dental caries, caries risk assessment, and the involvement of pediatricians in advocating for and providing preventive dental care for children. Dental caries, one of the most common dental diseases, is also referred to as tooth decay or cavities by the public.[1] Dental caries is a recognized public health concern that results from the repeated interaction of oral bacteria, primarily mutans streptococci, with fermentable sugars leading to acid production that results in microscopic dissolution of minerals in dental hard tissues and the formation of opaque white (white spot lesions) or brown spots on teeth.

Early childhood caries (ECC) is the presence of 1 or more decayed (noncavitated or cavitated lesions), missing (due to caries), or filled tooth surfaces in any primary tooth

Disclosures: None.
[a] Department of Clinical Services, School of Dentistry, Marquette University, Room 356, PO Box 1881, Milwaukee, WI 53201-1881, USA; [b] Department of Developmental Sciences, School of Dentistry, Marquette University, PO Box 1881, Milwaukee, WI 53201, USA
* Corresponding author.
E-mail address: christopher.okunseri@marquette.edu

Pediatr Clin N Am 62 (2015) 1215–1226
http://dx.doi.org/10.1016/j.pcl.2015.05.010   pediatric.theclinics.com
0031-3955/15/$ – see front matter © 2015 Elsevier Inc. All rights reserved.

in a child before the age of 6 years.[2] ECC is considered severe if the smooth surfaces of the teeth are affected in children less than 3 years old.[2] Early and preventive dental care is cost-effective in reducing dental disease burden,[3,4] as well as in establishing a dental home as a foundation on which a lifetime of preventive education and oral health care can be built.[5,6] Routine or preventive dental visits are important for early diagnosis, prevention, and treatment of dental caries and for establishing and maintaining good oral health and overall well-being[1,3,4]

BARRIERS TO CHILDREN'S ORAL HEALTH

Oral health means more than taking care of the teeth; it refers to the health of the oral cavity and its supporting structures.[1] Oral health is integral to general health and it contributes to overall health and well-being.[1] Despite documented improvement in the oral health of most Americans, access to dental care continues to be a problem in the United States. Inadequate access to dental care cuts across age, gender, and socioeconomic and geographic boundaries. Children from racial and ethnic minorities and low-income families, the uninsured, poor inner-city children, and those with special needs are disproportionately affected by dental diseases and have the most inadequate access to dental care. This problem to persists even with the many years of research into the cause and prevention of common dental diseases. Oral health care remains one of the most challenging and prevalent unmet health needs among infants, toddlers, adolescents, and young adults in the United States[1] and developing countries.

Barriers to children's oral health exist, especially for Medicaid enrollees. These barriers include workforce maldistribution and/or inadequate numbers of dentists,[7] low Medicaid reimbursement rates, and high administrative burden.[8] In addition, there is a severe shortage of minority dentists to serve the growing racial/ethnic minority Medicaid enrollees. As Okunseri and colleagues[9] have reported, minority dentists are more likely to accept new Medicaid patients. Furthermore, studies have documented that children from low-income families have lower odds of receiving comprehensive dental care and higher odds of having acute dental disease than children from middle-income and upper-income families.[10,11] To remedy these problems, professional organizations and government agencies continue to work towards expanding the workforce and developing various alternatives, such as school-based sealant and fluoride varnish application programs. These programs are usually managed by dental professionals, including dental hygienists and assistants. In addition, pediatricians and family physicians conduct oral health risk assessment and provide preventive care that includes anticipatory guidance in their offices.

EPIDEMIOLOGY OF DENTAL CARIES

Most children are susceptible to dental caries throughout their lives. However, with the knowledge of epidemiology, dental care providers and researchers have a better understanding of the distribution and determinants of dental caries in different population groups. They also have the opportunity to engage in anticipatory guidance and risk assessment, and to use different modalities of caries prevention. Although different classifications and indices of caries have been used in epidemiologic studies, the facts related to who is affected and by how much in different populations still remains easy to comprehend. Understanding dental caries epidemiology is crucial to providing appropriate clinical care and to identifying relevant public health measures to control the disease. However, because of some of the limitations associated with epidemiologic studies, clinicians are encouraged to engage in caries risk assessment.

In the last 20 years or so, epidemiologic studies have documented an overall decline in dental caries prevalence caused by population exposure to fluoride in water, tooth-pastes, mouth rinses, and in topical products applied in dental offices. In addition, improved oral hygiene, increased awareness of the relevance of dietary influence on caries, and changing patterns of refined sugar consumption have contributed to this decline.[1] Findings from epidemiologic studies continue to be used to support health care planning and resource allocation as well as in the monitoring of Healthy People 2020 objectives related to oral health.

The National Health and Nutrition Examination Survey (NHANES) 1988 to 1994 and 1999 to 2004 shows that the prevalences of untreated dental caries for children 2 to 5 years old and 6 to 11 years old were 19.1% versus 20.1% and 25.5% versus 25.0% in the primary dentition, respectively.[12] Disparities in dental caries burden per-sisted in all NHANES surveys. For example, NHANES 2009 to 2010 showed that prev-alence of untreated caries was significantly higher among non-Hispanic black children (19%), compared with non-Hispanic white children (11%) aged 3 to 5 years.[13] In terms of poverty status, children aged 3 to 5 years and 6 to 9 years living in families at or below 100% of the federal poverty level had a significantly higher number of untreated dental caries compared with those living above the poverty level.[13]

CARIES RISK ASSESSMENT

Risk refers to the probability that some unwanted event might occur. Caries risk as-sessments are as important as the specific diagnosis of the disease. The identification and mitigation of risk is the foundational component of the nonsurgical management of dental caries.[14] According to the guidelines published by the American Academy of Pediatric Dentistry (AAPD) on caries risk assessment for infants, children, and adoles-cents, risk assessment is considered a part of the standard of care for treating children.[15] Recent initiatives to include members of the medical profession in identi-fying patients at risk for dental caries have greatly assisted in the mitigation of some of the risk factors and it is hoped will lead to better outcomes for the population.[16] Educating medical colleagues in dental caries prevention, risk assessment, and referral is important to overall reduction in caries incidence and achieving excellent oral health in children.

Numerous researchers have identified caries risk factors documented by AAPD.[17–20] These risk factors include mother/caregiver with active cavities; parent/caregiver of low socioeconomic status; child with more than 3 between-meal, sugar-containing snacks or beverages per day; child put to bed with a bottle contain-ing natural or added sugar; child with special health care needs; and recent immigrant children.[15] In 1981, Berkowitz and colleagues[20] found similar oral bacteria in a mother and her child, and their research indicated that mothers with high salivary levels of *Streptococcus mutans* were 9 times more likely than mothers with low levels to trans-mit their oral bacteria to their children.[21] Kohler[21], 1988 showed that children colonized by *S mutans* at an age younger than 2 years had significantly more decayed, filled sur-faces (decayed, filled surface of 5.0 vs decayed, filled surface of 0.3) than children who were not colonized at that age.[22] Southward and colleagues[22] showed that parents with abscessed teeth were significantly more likely to have children with urgent oral care needs. Thitasomakul and colleagues[23] also showed that mothers with greater than or equal to 10 decayed teeth had children with higher incidences of cavities.

Parents/caregivers from low socioeconomic backgrounds have consistently been associated with dental caries.[23–27] Low socioeconomic status can lead to poorer food choices high in sugar content.[28,29] The classic Vipeholm caries studies[30–32] show that the frequency and not necessarily the total amount of sugar consumption is more predictive of having dental caries, thus supporting that children with greater than 3 between-meal sugar-containing snacks or beverages per day are at increased risk for dental caries. In addition, putting a child to bed with a bottle containing natural or added sugar has been documented as a risk factor for dental caries. The sugar consumed through a bottle when a child is put to bed tends to remain on the teeth for prolonged periods of time, which allows an extended period of bacterial acid generation with limited oral clearance and poor salivary buffering. The result is a greater amount of mineral dissolution from the teeth, eventually leading to cavity formation.

The AAPD's 2007 symposium on patients with special health care needs enumerates many reasons why children with special health care needs are considered to be at higher risk for dental caries.[33] These reasons include increased focus on the intensive medical attention required for their overall general health, limited oral muscle coordination and retention of foods in the oral cavity longer than healthy children, difficulty of parents/caregivers in providing adequate oral hygiene, and the requirement for special dietary formulations resulting in more frequent feedings.

PREVENTION OF DENTAL CARIES

Following caries risk assessment, the treatment of clinically evident dental caries involves both nonsurgical and surgical management. Greater emphasis is placed on nonsurgical management methods before surgical intervention when lesions are not cavitated,[34] which has great potential not only to reduce morbidities associated with the delivery of dental care (local anesthesia, removal of both diseased and sound tooth structure, possible sedation/general anesthesia) but also to reduce the risk of future disease, something that surgical restoration alone does not do.

As part of the nonsurgical approach, dentists have traditionally engaged in the distribution of written information to their patients in the form of brochures/pamphlets, or public dental advertising in magazines, radio, and even television. Some providers also show videos in their offices in an attempt to educate both parents and children. This traditional approach has the expectation of altering the behavior of both parents and children, mostly within the high-risk populations. However, this approach relies on a 1-way communication from the expert (provider) to the patient and has sometimes proved to be unsuccessful.[35–37]

A different approach has shown promising results: brief counseling. This approach involves brief motivational interviewing with follow-up by phone. This approach relies on a 2-way communication and tries to engage the parent in a healthy discussion. It has been reported that, when the counselor does most of the talking, counseling usually fails.[38] Clinical studies involving brief counseling have reported a potential benefit with the use of this technique.[39,40] Weinstein and colleagues,[41] in a 2004 study, compared traditional health education (pamphlet and video) with a brief motivational interview counseling intervention (pamphlet and video plus 1 counseling session and 6 follow-up telephone calls from a lay health counselor). Results after 1 and 2 years showed a positive impact for the brief counseling group. At 1 year, children in the counseling group had 0.71 new carious lesions compared with 1.91 in the traditional group. The data were similar for the second year.[40] Motivational interviewing is an approach that has shown promising results in the improvement of the oral health of those children at risk. In 2002, a survey of dental schools in Canada and the United States concluded that instruction in interpersonal communications skills was not adequate.[41] However, some dental schools are already teaching counseling skills similar to motivational interviewing.[41]

Other preventive approaches used both at the dental office and home include pit-and-fissure sealants, fluoride varnish, amorphous calcium phosphates, and xylitol. Sealants are a thin plastic coating placed on the chewing surfaces of posterior teeth and are considered safe, cost-effective, and easy to apply.[42–44] As long as they remain intact, they have been shown to reduce caries on these surfaces by 40% to 100%, especially in high-risk populations.[43,45–47] The American Dental Association (ADA) has published recommendations on the use of sealants as both a preventive and therapeutic service on noncavitated and inactive carious lesions.[48]

Despite strong evidence-based reports about the effectiveness of this caries preventive technique, pit-and-fissure sealants continue to be under prescribed, particularly among those at high risk for experiencing caries. That population include children from lower-income families and certain racial and ethnic groups.[49] The national oral health objectives for dental sealants, as stated in Healthy People 2010, includes increasing the proportion of children who have received dental sealants on their molar teeth to 50%.[27] However, national data collected from 1999 to 2002 indicated that sealant prevalence on permanent teeth among children aged 6 to 11 years was only 30.5%.[28]

Another nonsurgical approach is fluoride application from various sources. Once dietary issues have been adequately addressed, fluoride stabilizes the apatite mineral, has bactericidal properties,[50,51] and results in the remineralization of new tooth minerals, making it significantly more resistant to further decay. The mineral apatite is the base mineral in the structure of teeth. It can exist in multiple forms, but in the human body chiefly exists in 3 forms: carbonated apatite, hydroxyapatite, and hydroxyfluorapatite. The major apatite present in a newly erupted tooth is carbonated apatite, which has a critical pH (the pH at which the mineral is saturated with respect to the solution) of approximately 6.5. The normal pH of the saliva is close to the normal physiologic pH of the body: between 7 and 7.4. On fermentation of carbohydrates, the cavity-causing families of bacteria (mutans streptococci and lactobacilli) cause a shift in the plaque pH to less than 4.5, resulting in dissolution of the tooth mineral. Hydroxyapatite is a much more stable crystal than carbonated apatite at pHs of less than 6.5. This process results in a preferential reformation of hydroxyapatite mineral. Hydroxyapatite's critical pH is approximately 5.5. Thus, this maturation of the enamel, the replacement of carbonate ions with hydroxide ions, results in a mineral that requires 10 times as much acid to dissolve it than the original mineral.

Fluoride's ability to replace other ions in the hydroxyapatite mineral of which teeth are composed results in increased resistance to the dissolution of the teeth in the oral cavity.[50] Fluoride incorporation into the tooth structure, either pre-eruptively or post-eruptively greatly helps in reducing the risk of caries in individuals, but post-eruptive fluoride incorporation seems to provide the greatest benefit.[50] However, if the fluoride ion is present in the plaque and saliva, the substitution of hydroxide with fluoride is a significantly more stable mineral than hydroxyapatite, and hydroxyfluorapatite is preferentially reformed in the tooth. The critical pH of hydroxyfluorapatite is approximately 4.8. Therefore, with fluoride incorporation, it takes almost 100 times more acid to dissolve the hydroxyfluorapatite than the original carbonated apatite.[51] With the demineralization and remineralization process continuing throughout the day, the maintenance of low levels of fluoride in the plaque and oral fluids throughout the day has the greatest effect at reducing caries incidence. If the patient lives in a location with nonfluoridated public water supplies (either municipally provided or via a private well) the AAPD and the American Academy of Pediatrics (AAP) recommend supplementation with fluoride tablets.[52,53]

Xylitol is another product routinely prescribed in dental offices for caries prevention. Xylitol is a natural sweetener that is obtained from birch wood, corn stalks, and other sources. Multiple studies have suggested that this sugar alcohol assists in the arrestment of the caries process and can reduce the transmissibility of mutans streptococci. Difficulties in compliance with the required daily dosage (5–10 g/d in 3–5 divided doses) contribute to the lack of effectiveness with this product. In addition, concerns with osmotic diarrhea also reduce the frequency of recommendation. Dosages of up to 45 g/d for children 7 to 16 years old resulted in no significant increase in gastrointestinal disturbances compared with no xylitol consumption.[54] Compliance with the dental benefits of 5 to 10 g/d has a very low risk of gastrointestinal distress.

Amorphous calcium phosphates have been shown to both decrease demineralization and increase remineralization of early carious lesions, most likely because of the common ion effect on the equilibrium of the apatite crystal.[55] Other reports indicate that the calcium phosphopeptide–amorphous calcium phosphate (CPP-ACP) also affects the bacteria related to dental caries.[56] However, a more recent report indicates that long-term low levels of fluoride are more effective at caries prevention than CPP-ACP.[57]

TREATMENT OF DENTAL CARIES

It is sometimes challenging to prevent all carious lesion so restoring carious teeth seems to be the ideal approach to improving the oral health of children. The surgical methods for the treatment of carious lesions have changed little since the nineteenth century, with removal of carious tissues with either hand or rotary instruments followed by the placement of a filling material to restore the tooth to anatomic and morphologic shape and function. When the caries process was less clearly understood, the philosophic approach espoused by Dr G. V. Black (considered the father of restorative dentistry) was to err on the side of surgical intervention because of the high frequency of small lesions rapidly progressing to large lesions. This philosophy was dominant for the larger part of the twentieth century. With the introduction of fluoride as a preventive agent, both in municipal water supplies and in over-the-counter oral products, the rate of progression of dental diseases decreased precipitously. Despite this slowing of the disease process, the philosophic model of aggressive surgical intervention did not rapidly dissipate. However, the second half of the twentieth century saw recommendations to rethink the aggressive surgical model and promote a more conservative approach.[58]

The invasiveness of surgical treatment varies from minimally invasive (limited removal of affected tooth structure) to traditional techniques (removal of all caries-affected tissues). One of the least invasive treatments for non-cavitated carious lesion is sealant placement, but there is much hesitance on the part of dental practitioners to place a sealant over an active cavitated lesion.[57] Studies have shown that there is a significant reduction or elimination of viable bacteria in sealed, actively carious lesions.[59–61] Teeth affected by dental caries resulting in cavitated lesions have 2 layers of dentin that have been identified: a superficial, denatured, and highly bacterially contaminated layer that cannot be repaired, and a deeper affected layer that has been demineralized but not yet highly infected with bacteria.[62] This deeper affected dentin layer has been clinically shown to be remineralizable (healable) if it is effectively sealed from any further source of fermentable carbohydrate. The inner, healable layer of dentin is normally not sensitive to palpation with instruments because of the occlusion of the distal dentinal tubules that results from the advancement of the caries process.[63,64] Restorative techniques that purposefully retain this healable layer of dentin often do not require the administration of local anesthetics because of the retention of the dentinal tubule–occluded layer.[65] The purposeful retention of carious dentin underneath restorations has been recognized for several years and is referred to as an indirect pulp cap procedure. Research has shown that in teeth with a healthy pulp, indirect pulp cap–restored teeth have better long-term outcomes than teeth in which total caries removal was completed and a pulpotomy (removal of the coronal portion of the nerve only) performed.[66]

Assessment of the vitality of the pulpal (nerve) tissues inside the teeth is crucial to the treatment planning of any type of restorative procedure on a caries-affected tooth. The nerve remains vital for an extended period of time during the caries process but, as the lesion approaches the pulp, the degree of injury and inflammation in the pulpal tissue increases. Pain and sensitivity elicited by food or drink, which resolves quickly after the removal of the stimulus and that can be controlled with over-the-counter analgesics, are all subjective findings that point to the diagnosis of reversible pulpitis, an inflammatory condition of the pulp that can resolve if further caries progress is arrested. Pain that is spontaneous, prolonged, and cannot be adequately controlled with over-the-counter analgesics is an ominous sign for the long-term health of the pulp. These symptoms indicate either irreversible pulpitis (inflammation that cannot be resolved by the body) and/or necrosis of the pulpal tissues. Treatments for irreversible pulpitis/pulpal necrosis involve complete root canal therapy or extraction of the affected tooth/teeth.[66]

As the size of the caries lesion increases, the mechanical properties of the tooth and the restorative materials used to restore the tooth become less advantageous for long-term retention of the tooth. Large fillings in primary teeth often result in fracture of the remaining tooth structure, the filling, or both. Full coverage of these teeth is then recommended, most often with prefabricated stainless steel crowns. These crowns are some of the most highly successful restorations that can be placed on primary teeth and are often the best choice for restoring large cavities and/or teeth that have received direct pulpal therapy.[67] A recently introduced procedure of placing stainless steel crowns, the Hall technique, has been introduced, this combines the benefits of sealing cavities to arrest their progression with the strength and durability of the stainless steel crown.[68] These crowns are cemented without any mechanical tooth preparation and can be placed without the need for local anesthetics. Placement of these crowns depends heavily on an accurate diagnosis of the pulpal tissues, and they should not be placed when a diagnosis of irreversible pulpitis or pulpal necrosis has been made. Current research indicates that these crown procedures have similar outcomes to traditional crown placement that involves local anesthesia, mechanical removal of the decay, preparation of the tooth, and cementation of the crown.[69]

When too much tooth structure has been lost, or an abscess is present that cannot be resolved with pulpal therapy, the extraction of the tooth is the only possible remaining treatment. The loss of primary incisor teeth does not result in space loss issues, but may lead to speech delays.[70] Premature loss of posterior teeth can lead to significant spacing issues in the permanent dentition caused by mesial drifting of the unsupported posterior teeth. Placement of space-maintaining devices is recommended for the premature loss of posterior teeth.[71] Access to dental care continues to be a problem because many public health clinics are overwhelmed with children with ECC and/or dental emergencies.[72] The traditional standard of care involving restoring teeth has proved to be insufficient to stop the caries process.[73,74] Untreated tooth decay causes pain, discomfort, and suffering, and ultimately leads to problems with eating, speaking, socializing, and attending to learning.

INVOLVEMENT OF PEDIATRICIANS

Tooth decay is a chronic and infectious disease that is avoidable with early preventive measures, sustainable home care, and appropriate periodic dental visits. The AAPD emphasizes the importance of initiating professional oral health intervention in infancy and continuing through adolescence and beyond.[6] The involvement of pediatricians has facilitated the promotion and prevention of dental caries, especially for young children who otherwise would not readily go to a dental office. In addition, many states now have policies that allow pediatricians to be reimbursed for the provision of fluoride varnish treatment to children's teeth. Furthermore, *Bright Futures in Practice: Oral Health*, developed by the Maternal and Child Health Bureau and Health Resources and Services Administration, provides information regarding practice guidelines for pediatricians performing activities such as dental screening, anticipatory guidance, and referral.[75,76] Overall, advances in the understanding of the nature and clinical course of dental caries is leading to a maturation of the profession, with early detection as well as medical intervention and treatment of the lesion before surgical intervention.

REFERENCES

1. US Department of Health and Human Services. Oral health in America: a report of the Surgeon General. Rockville (MD): US Department of Health and Human Services, National Institute of Dental and Craniofacial Research, National Institutes of Health; 2000.
2. American Academy of Pediatric Dentistry. Policy on early childhood caries (ECC): classifications, consequences, and preventive strategies. Reference manual 36: 6:14/15. Available at: http://www.aapd.org/media/Policies_Guidelines/P_ECCClassifications.pdf. Accessed January10, 2015.
3. Savage MF, Lee JY, Kotch JB, et al. Early preventive dental visits: effects on subsequent utilization and costs. Pediatrics 2004;114(4):e418–23.
4. Lee JY, Bouwens TJ, Savage MF, et al. Examining the cost-effectiveness of early dental visits [review]. Pediatr Dent 2006;28(2):102–5 [discussion: 192–8].
5. American Academy of Pediatric Dentistry. Policy on the dental home. Pediatr Dent 2008;30(suppl):22–3.
6. Guideline on periodicity of examination, preventive dental services, anticipatory guidance/counseling, and oral treatment for infants, children, and adolescents. Adopted 1990, Revised 1992, 1996, 2000, 2003, 2007, 2009. Available at: http://www.aapd.org/media/Policies_Guidelines/G_Periodicity.pdf. Accessed August 20, 2009.
7. Mertz EA, Grumbal K. Identifying communities with low dentist supply in California. J Public Health Dent 2001;61:172–7.
8. United States General Accounting Office. Oral health: dental disease is a chronic problem among low-income populations. United States General Accounting Office (GAO), report to congressional requester. Washington, DC: GAO/HEHS-00–72, Washington, DC: 2000. Available at: http://www.gao.gov/new.items/he00072.pdf. Accessed February 1, 2015.
9. Okunseri C, Bajorunaite R, Abena A, et al. Racial/ethnic disparities in the acceptance of Medicaid patients in dental practices. J Public Health Dent 2008;68(3): 149–53.
10. Mouradian WE, Wehr E, Crall JJ. Disparities in children's oral health and access to dental care. JAMA 2000;284:2625–31.
11. Edelstein BL. Disparities in oral health and access to care: findings of national surveys. Ambul Pediatr 2000;1(Suppl):141–7.

12. Dye BA, Tan S, Smith V, et al. Trends in oral health status: United States, 1988-1994 and 1999-2004. Vital Health Stat 2007;11(248):1–92.

13. Dye BA, Li X, Thornton-Evans G. Oral health disparities as determined by selected Healthy People 2020 oral health objectives for the United States, 2009–2010. NCHS data brief, no 104. Hyattsville (MD): National Center for Health Statistics; 2012.

14. Berg J. Medical management of dental caries. J Calif Dent Assoc 2014;42(7): 443–7.

15. AAPD. Guideline on caries-risk assessment and management for infants, children, and adolescents. Available at: http://www.aapd.org/media/Policies_ Guidelines/G_CariesRiskAssessment.pdf. Accessed January 19, 2014.

16. Hale KJ, American Academy of Pediatrics, Section on Pediatric Dentistry. Oral health risk assessment timing and establishment of the dental home. Pediatrics 2003;111:1113–6.

17. Berkowitz RJ, Jordan H. Similarity of bacteriocins of *Streptococcus mutans* from mother and infant. Arch Oral Biol 1975;20:725–30.

18. Davey AL, Rogers AH. Multiple types of the bacterium *Streptococcus mutans* in the human mouth and their intra-family transmission. Arch Oral Biol 1984;29: 453–60.

19. Berkowitz RJ, Jones P. Mouth-to-mouth transmission of the bacterium *Streptococcus mutans* between mother and child. Arch Oral Biol 1985;30:377–9.

20. Berkowitz RJ, Turner J, Green P. Maternal salivary levels of *Streptococcus mutans* and primary oral infection in infants. Arch Oral Biol 1981;26:147–9.

21. Köhler B, Andréen I, Jonsson B. The earlier the colonization by mutans streptococci, the higher the caries prevalence at 4 years of age. Oral Microbiol Immunol 1988;3:14–7.

22. Southward LH, Robertson A, Edelstein BL, et al. Oral health of young children in Mississippi Delta child care centers: a second look at early childhood caries risk assessment. J Public Health Dent 2008;68(4):188–95.

23. Thitasomakul S, Piwat S, Thearmontree A, et al. Risks for early childhood caries analyzed by negative binomial models. J Dent Res 2009;88(2):137–41.

24. Vargas CM, Crall JJ, Schneider DA. Sociodemographic distribution of pediatric dental caries: NHANES III, 1988-1994. J Am Dent Assoc 1998;129(9):1229–38.

25. Dye BA, Arevalo O, Vargas CM. Trends in paediatric dental caries by poverty status in the United States, 1988–1994 and 1999–2004. Int J Paediatr Dent 2010; 20(2):132–43.

26. Tellez M, Sohn W, Burt BA, et al. Assessment of the relationship between neighborhood characteristics and dental caries severity among low-income African-Americans: a multilevel approach. J Public Health Dent 2006;66(1):30–6.

27. Dos Santos Junior VE, de Sousa RMB, Oliveira MC, et al. Early childhood caries and its relationship with perinatal, socioeconomic and nutritional risks: a cross-sectional study. BMC Oral Health 2014;14:47.

28. Chi DL, Masterson EE, Carle AC, et al. Socioeconomic status, food security, and dental caries in US children: mediation analysis of data from the National Health and Nutrition Examination Survey, 2007-2008. Am J Public Health 2014;104: 860–4.

29. Mello JA, Gans KM, Risica PM, et al. How is food insecurity associated with dietary behaviors? An analysis with low-income, ethnically diverse participants in a nutrition intervention study. J Am Diet Assoc 2010;110(12):1906–11.

30. Sharkey JR, Nalty C, Johnson CM, et al. Children's very low food security is associated with increased dietary intakes in energy, fat, and added sugar

among Mexican-origin children (6-11 y) in Texas border *Colonias*. BMC Pediatr 2012;12:16.
31. Gustafsson BE, Quensel CE, Swenander Lanke L, et al. The Vipeholm Dental Caries Study. The effects of different levels of carbohydrate intake in 436 individuals observed for five years. Acta Odontol Scand 1954;11:232–364.
32. Duggal MS, Toumba KJ, Amaechi BT, et al. Enamel demineralisation in situ with varying frequency of carbohydrate consumption with and without fluoride toothpaste. J Dent Res 2001;80:1721–4.
33. Arcella D, Ottolenghi L, Polomeni A, et al. The relationship between frequency of carbohydrates intake and dental caries: a cross-sectional study in Italian teenagers. Public Health Nutr 2002;5(4):553–60.
34. American Academy of Pediatric Dentistry. Symposium on lifetime oral health care for patients with special needs. Pediatr Dent 2007;29(2):92–152.
35. Tsang P, Qi F, Shi W. Medical approach to dental caries: fight the disease, not the lesion. Pediatr Dent 2006;28(2):188–91.
36. Johnsen DC. Characteristics and backgrounds of children with nursing caries. Pediatr Dent 1982;4:218–24.
37. Benitez C, O'Sullivan D, Tinanoff N. Effect of a preventive approach for the treatment of nursing bottle caries. J Dent Child 1994;61:46–9.
38. Tinanoff N, Daley NS, O'Sullivan DM, et al. Failure of intense preventive efforts to arrest early childhood and rampant caries: three case reports. Pediatr Dent 1999; 21:160–3.
39. Miller WR, Rollnick S. Motivational interviewing: preparing people for change. 2nd edition. New York: Guilford Press; 2002.
40. Harrison R, Wong T. An oral health program for an urban minority population of preschool. Community Dent Oral Epidemiol 2003;31:392–9.
41. Weinstein P, Harrison R, Benton T. Motivating parents to prevent caries in their young children. J Am Dent Assoc 2004;135:731–8.
42. Yoshida T, Milgrom P, Coldwell S. How do U.S. and Canadian dental schools teach interpersonal communication skills? J Dent Educ 2002;66(11):1281–8.
43. Simonsen RJ. Pit and fissure sealant: review of the literature. Pediatr Dent 2002; 24(5):393–414.
44. Griffin SO, Griffin PM, Gooch BF, et al. Comparing the costs of three sealant delivery strategies. J Dent Res 2002;81(9):641–5.
45. Quiñonez RB, Downs SM, Shugars D, et al. Assessing cost-effectiveness of sealant placement in children. J Public Health Dent 2005;65(2):82–9.
46. Chi DL, Van der Goes DN, Ney JP. Cost-effectiveness of pit-and-fissure sealants on primary molars in Medicaid-enrolled children. Am J Public Health 2014;104(3): 555–61.
47. Ahovuo-Saloranta A, Forss H, Walsh T, et al. Sealants for preventing dental decay in the permanent teeth. Cochrane Database Syst Rev 2013;(3):CD001830.
48. Feigal RJ, Donly KJ. The use of pit and fissure sealants. Pediatr Dent 2006;28: 143–50.
49. Beauchamp J, Caufield PW, Crall JJ, et al. Evidence-based clinical recommendations for the use of pit-and-fissure sealants. J Am Dent Assoc 2008;139(3): 257–67.
50. Centers for Disease Control and Prevention. Oral health: preventing cavities, gum disease, and tooth loss. 2007. Available at: www.cdc.gov/nccdphp/publications/ aag/oh.htm. Accessed January 8, 2008.
51. Featherstone JDB. The science and practice of caries prevention. J Am Dent Assoc 2000;131:887–99.

52. Fejerskov O, Kidd E. Dental caries. The disease and its clinical management. 2nd edition. Oxford (United Kingdom): Blackwell Munksgaard; 2008.
53. AAPD. Guideline on fluoride therapy. 2014. Available at: http://www.aapd.org/media/Policies_Guidelines/G_FluorideTherapy.pdf. Accessed January 26, 2015.
54. AAP. Oral health policies. 2015. Available at: http://www2.aap.org/oralhealth/pact/ch6_sect3b.cfm. Accessed January 26, 2015.
55. Akerblom HK, Koivukangas T, Puukka R, et al. The tolerance of increasing amounts of dietary xylitol in children. Int J Vitam Nutr Res 1982;22:53–66.
56. Shen P, Cai F, Nowicki A, et al. Remineralization of enamel subsurface lesions by sugar-free chewing gum containing casein phosphopeptide-amorphous calcium phosphate. J Dent Res 2001;80(12):2066–70.
57. Pukallus ML, Plonka KA, Holcombe TF, et al. A randomized controlled trial of a 10 percent CPP-ACP cream to reduce mutans streptococci colonization. Pediatr Dent 2013;35(7):550–5.
58. Meyer-Lueckel H, Wierichs RJ, Schellwien T, et al. Remineralizing efficacy of a CPP-ACP cream on enamel caries lesions in situ. Caries Res 2015;49:56–62.
59. Hume WR. Need for change in standards of caries diagnosis–perspective based on the structure and behavior of the caries lesion [review]. J Dent Educ 1993; 57(6):439–43.
60. Chapko MK. A study of the intentional use of pit and fissure sealants over carious lesions. J Public Health Dent 1987;47(3):139–42.
61. Besic FC. The fate of bacteria sealed in dental cavities. J Dent Res 1943;22(5): 349–54.
62. Oong EM, Griffin SO, Kohn WG, et al. The effect of dental sealants on bacteria levels in caries lesions. J Am Dent Assoc 2008;139(3):271–8.
63. Fusayama T. Two layers of carious dentin; diagnosis and treatment. Oper Dent 1979;4(2):63–70.
64. Mjor IA, editor. Reaction patterns in human teeth. Boca Raton (FL): CRS Press; 1983. p. 86–103.
65. Frencken JE. The state-of-the-art of ART restorations. Dent Update 2014;41(3): 218–20, 222–4.
66. Coll JA. Indirect pulp capping and primary teeth: is the primary tooth pulpotomy out of date? Pediatr Dent 2008;30:230–6.
67. AAPD. Guideline on management of the developing dentition and occlusion in pediatric dentistry. Available at: http://www.aapd.org/media/Policies_Guidelines/G_DevelopDentition.pdf. Accessed January 20, 2015.
68. Messer LB, Levering NJ. The durability of primary molar restorations: II. Observations and predictions of success of stainless steel crowns. Pediatr Dent 1988; 10(2):81–5.
69. Innes NP, Evans DJP, Stirrups DR. The Hall technique; a randomized controlled clinical trial of a novel method of managing carious primary molars in general dental practice: acceptability of the technique and outcomes at 23 months. BMC Oral Health 2007;7:18.
70. Ludwig KH, Fontana M, Vinson LA, et al. The success of stainless steel crowns placed with the Hall technique: a retrospective study. J Am Dent Assoc 2014; 145(12):1248–53.
71. Riekman GA, ElBadrawy HE. Effect of premature loss of primary maxillary incisors on speech. Pediatr Dent 1985;7:119–22.
72. AAPD. Pulp therapy for primary and young permanent teeth. Available at: http://www.aapd.org/media/Policies_Guidelines/G_Pulp.pdf. Accessed January 26, 2015.

73. Raadal M, Espelid I, Mejare I. The caries lesion and its management in children and adolescents. In: Koch G, Poulsen S, editors. Pediatric dentistry: a clinical approach. Copenhagen (Denmark): Munksgaard; 2001. p. 173–212.
74. Raadal M. Management of early carious lesions in primary teeth. In: Hugoson A, et al, editors. Consensus conference on caries in the primary dentition and its clinical management. Jönköping (Sweden): The Institute for Postgraduate Dental Education; 2002. p. 48–57.
75. Maternal and Child Health Bureau, Health Resources and Services Administration. Bright futures in practice: oral health 1996. Available at: http://www.brightfutures.org/oralhealth/about.html. Accessed February 1, 2015.
76. Pierce KM, Rozier RG, Vann WF Jr. Accuracy of pediatric primary care providers' screening and referral for early childhood caries. Pediatrics 2002;109:E82.

Epigenetics and Understanding the Impact of Social Determinants of Health

CrossMark

Daniel A. Notterman, MD[a],*, Colter Mitchell, PhD[b]

KEYWORDS

- Epigenetics • Methylation • Health disparity • Social disparity • Telomere • DNA

KEY POINTS

- Epigenetic factors, especially DNA methylation, and telomere length are currently being examined as biological mechanisms linking social factors and health.
- Social deprivation is associated with a wide range of epigenetic change in children and young adults.
- Epigenetic markers are associated with obesity and eating disorders, mental health, and asthma.
- Research is still too new to provide actionable evidence for a causal mechanism linking social experiences and child health through epigenetics and telomere length.
- Research exploring the overlap between social and natural environmental links to epigenetics and health is desperately needed.

SOCIAL DETERMINANTS OF CHILD HEALTH

The health consequences of material deficiency (eg, extreme malnutrition or lack of water or inadequate clothing and shelter) have been long known.[1] However, recently, a new, more broadly applicable research agenda emphasizing social factors and health has emerged.[2] The term social determinant of health often refers to any nonmedical factor directly influencing health, including values, attitudes, knowledge,

Funding for some of the research reported in this paper was provided by the Eunice Kennedy Shriver National Institute of Child Health and Human Development (R01 HD076592). In addition, this work was supported by the Eunice Kennedy Shriver National Institute of Child Health and Human Development through Grants R01HD36916, R01HD39135, and R01HD40421 and by a consortium of private foundations of the Fragile Families and Child Wellbeing Study.

[a] Lewis Thomas Laboratory, Department of Molecular Biology, Princeton University, Princeton, NJ 08544, USA; [b] Institute of Social Research, University of Michigan-Ann Arbor, 426 Thompson Street, 2264 ISR, Ann Arbor, MI 48106, USA
* Corresponding author.
E-mail address: DAN1@princeton.edu

Pediatr Clin N Am 62 (2015) 1227–1240
http://dx.doi.org/10.1016/j.pcl.2015.05.012
0031-3955/15/$ – see front matter © 2015 Elsevier Inc. All rights reserved.

and behaviors. However, it can also refer to more external sources of influence such as family, neighborhood, and social network context. A large and convincing literature over the last several decades shows that health across the life span is strongly linked to social disadvantage.[1-4]

For example, neighborhoods can influence health through their physical and geographic characteristics, such as air and water quality, lead paint exposure, proximity to both health-promoting and health-suppressing features (ie, hospitals and nutritious food stores vs toxic factories and fast food), access to green space, and so on.[2,5,6] Additionally, more social aspects of neighborhoods such as strong cohesion are associated with far better health and safety.[7,8]

Recent evidence demonstrates that the chronic stress of social disadvantage, socioeconomic inequality, and racial discrimination act through a variety of biological pathways to influence health, including neuroendocrine, developmental, immunologic, and vascular mechanisms.[2,9] In response to stressful events, cortisol, cytokines, and other intermediates are released, and if there is long-term, repetitive or chronic exposure, these substances may damage key physiologic systems.[9,10] It is thought that this mechanism of physiologic strain accelerates the onset or progression of chronic illnesses.[11]

One of the largest and most consistently replicated areas of research demonstrates the negative effects of social disadvantage in childhood on later child and adult health, socio-emotional wellbeing, and cognitive ability.[12-16] This body of work indicates that childhood social disadvantage operates through a variety of complex mechanisms to result in dramatically different developmental outcomes, which are often apparent even in childhood, but which are typically more fully manifest in adulthood. Indeed, there is evidence that early childhood disadvantage appears to leave a biological residue, which in turn has effects on development, health, and wellbeing.[16,17]

Social Determinants of Child Mental Health

There is strong evidence that the mental health of children, adolescents, and young adults is affected by social factors at personal, family, community, and national levels.[11,18] In particular, the evidence is good that paired with a safe and supportive social environment, such as family and schools, children need positive peer networks in order to have healthy mental health development. Even national-level social determinants of health such as national wealth, income inequality, and access to education were associated with a range of mental health outcomes in young people.[18]

Social Determinants of Asthma

Lung function, allergy, and asthma appear to have a strong links to early life stress and social disadvantage.[19] Due to the large health inequalities in this area, social stressors have been used extensively to explain racial disparities in childhood asthma.[20] Indeed, recent research suggests that the social context in which children are raised may be equal to the natural environmental effects in asthma disease risk.[21]

BIOLOGICAL UNDERPINNINGS OF SOCIAL DETERMINANTS

Early life experience gets under the skin in ways that affect the health, wellbeing, and child development. Although the most extensive research shows strong biological effects of physical and emotional abuse (and other similarly extreme childhood events) on health and developmental consequences, more recent research shows that less obvious but more regular adversities of early childhood also have a lasting influence on later health and development.[22,23] Recent work has begun to focus on epigenetics as a key biological mechanism linking early life experience and health.

DESCRIPTION OF EPIGENETICS

Despite having the same DNA, different cell types have distinct gene expression patterns in order to perform different functions.[24] One mechanism of this differential gene expression is through epigenetic changes, which some have argued may also explain some of the variation in behavioral phenotypes of people.[25] One key aspect of the epigenome is that, unlike the DNA sequence, it may be modified by environmental or pharmaceutical interventions. This provides the potential for reversing the effect of adverse life events on later health and wellbeing.[17] Epigenetic changes, or marks, refer to alterations in DNA or histone structure that do not affect the sequence of DNA but may affect gene expression and therefore cellular function. The effect on cellular function may be sustained, and under many circumstances, it can be transmitted to subsequent generations of cells.

Recall that DNA is organized as a linear molecule, in which the 4 nucleotides (adenine, A; thymine, T; guanine, G; cytosine, C) form the core of the DNA molecule, and sugar phosphates form the backbone of the DNA (**Fig. 1**). In people, nuclear DNA is organized into 46 chromosomes: 22 autosomes and 1 sex chromosome from each parent. The flow of information in a cell has been termed the central dogma (**Fig. 2**), in which information flows from DNA to messenger RNA (mRNA), to protein. Genes are arrayed along the chromosomes, and a gene can be viewed as consisting of the arrangement of base sequences that specifies a complementary mRNA, and, therefore, a specific protein, together with those nearby DNA sequences that determine when and to what extent the gene is transcribed into RNA.

Fig. 3 provides a schematic of a typical gene as it appears in DNA. Bases that code specific amino acids are organized in blocks termed, exons. Between the exons are the introns, which are composed of bases that do not specify specific amino acids but may contain control regions. Because of the orientation of the DNA strands, 1 side of the gene is termed the 5′ end, and the other, the 3′ end. At the 5′ end of the gene is a sequence of bases termed the promoter/enhancer, which is enriched for cytosine and guanine bases. Binding of the promotor by a series of transcription factors activates transcription, the process by which RNA polymerase syntheses a complementary strand of mRNA. Soon after the new primary RNA copy of the gene is synthesized, the introns are removed, and the exons are stitched together. After several more steps, the mRNA is used by the ribosome as a template for synthesis of a polypeptide chain, the basic structure of all proteins.

This arrangement provides for several points at which gene regulation can adjust the synthesis of proteins to meet the needs of the cell. Transcriptional control is a key form of regulation, through which the amount of mRNA synthesized from a particular gene is increased or decreased as necessary.

Upon receipt of an appropriate signal, the cell can deploy or withdraw specific transcription factors within minutes, thereby rapidly modulating the transcription of specific genes. This type of signaling response is rapid, and easily reversible. On the other hand, epigenetic changes to DNA generally take days to years to occur, and as mentioned, they tend to be stable.

DNA METHYLATION

The promotor regions of genes are enriched for sequences containing cytosine alternating with guanine (5′-CG-3′ abbreviated CpG). Areas in which the proportion of CpG

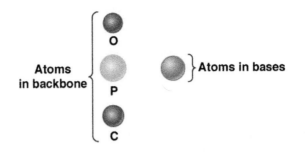

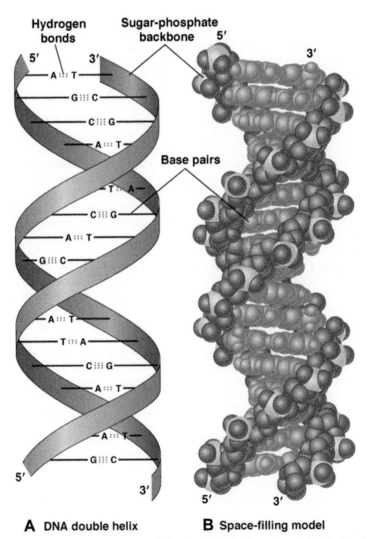

A DNA double helix **B** Space-filling model

Fig. 1. (*A*) A schematic representation of the double helical structure of DNA. A, adenosine; C, cytosine; G, guanine; T, thymidine. The strips represent the helical structure formed by the phosphodiester bonds (the double helix), and the horizontal bars represent paired bases. (*B*) A space-filling model of the DNA double helix. The color-coded atoms are shown at the top of the figure. (*From* Hardin J, Bertoni G, Kleinsmith LJ. Becker's World of the cell. 8th edition. San Francisco (CA): Benjamin Cummings; 2006. ©2012. Reprinted by permission of Pearson Education, Inc., New York, New York.)

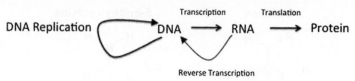

Fig. 2. The central dogma of molecular biology, modified to include reverse transcription.

is greater than statistically predicted are termed CpG islands. Wherever a CpG occurs, the C is susceptible to being modified by the enzyme DNA methyltranferase through the addition of a methyl (CH_3) group (forming 5-methylcytosine) **(Fig. 4)**. A promoter containing a group of CpG sequences that have been methylated is less able to bind relevant transcription factors, and this attenuates or halts transcription. Because the addition of a methyl group to cytosine is a covalent reaction, it may be an enduring change; furthermore, the DNA replication apparatus has mechanisms for ensuring that the corresponding CpG is methylated in newly synthesized DNA.

Clusters of CpG residues are not only found in promoters, but also interspersed within genes, and along intergenic regions. The role played in cellular physiology by methylation of these other CpG sites is the subject of considerable research, and may be more important in controlling transcription than the CpG islands.

The methylation of DNA is just 1 way in which a cell can create an epigenetic mark. DNA is tightly coiled around highly basic proteins called histones. One effect of this winding is to greatly compress the DNA, allowing it to be packaged into a cell nucleus. Fully extended, the DNA of a chromosome would extend about 75 mm, but in its coiled state, it is about 5 μm (compression of about 15,000 fold). Often, when DNA is tightly wound on a nucleosome, the DNA regulatory sites (such as the promoter) become inaccessible to transcription signals, and the affected genes become silent. Histone proteins have several sites at which they can be covalently modified, principally by methylation or acetylation. The effect of these covalent changes may be to slightly

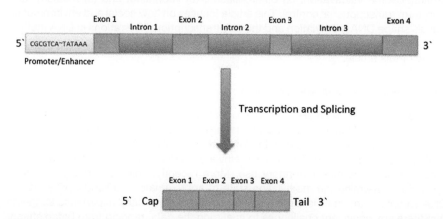

Fig. 3. Schematic of a typical human gene. The 5' end of the gene contains a promoter/ enhancer region that is enriched for CpG sequence. The promoter also contains a special sequence, TATTAAA, which is a target for the transcription factors to bind. Several other sequences may intervene between the CpG island and the TATTAAA. Introns are shown in blue, and exons in orange. During transcription and splicing, an RNA copy of the gene is made, and the introns are excised. A 5' cap and a 3' tails are added to the final mRNA copy of the gene.

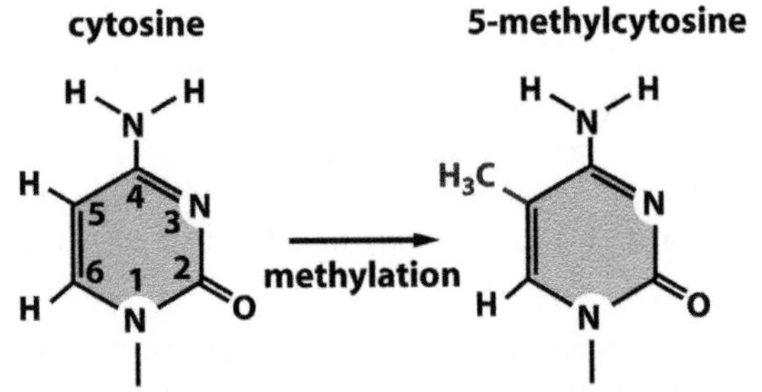

cytosine   5-methylcytosine

Fig. 4. 5-methylcytosine is formed by the addition of a methyl (–CH₃) group to cytosine. (*From* Alberts B, Johnson A, Lewis J, et al. Molecular biology of the cell. 5th edition. New York: Garland Science; 2008; with permission.)

relax the DNA, thereby freeing regulatory sites for interactions with various transcriptional activator proteins. These histone changes are also termed epigenetic marks. As is the case with DNA methylation, the cell is able to duplicate the histone marks on newly synthesized histones that are destined for daughter cells. Thus, histone-based epigenetic marks are heritable, even though they are not coded in the DNA.

It is important to note that although epigenetic marks are heritable from parent cell to daughter cell, this is often misunderstood to mean that in multicellular organisms, such as people, epigenetic marks are transferred directly from parent to child. Rather, during the process of gamete formation, most epigenetic marks are cleared, and each generation develops a new set of epigenetic marks. However, under appropriate circumstances environmental signals (including those supplied through maternal behavior) may result in patterns of epigenetic marks in the offspring that reflect those also found in the parent.

At the biochemical level, epigenetics affects transcription and ultimately the protein repertoire of a cell. The epigenetic mechanism serves 4 essential cellular roles: (1) X-chromosome inactivation, (2) differentiation, (3) imprinting, and (4) medium- and long-term transcriptional control. This article focuses on how social and environmental signals shape DNA methylation and thereby transcription. Aberrations in DNA methylation are frequently associated with cancer, but this phenomenon is not within the scope of this article.

MEASUREMENT OF DNA METHYLATION

Although it is likely that marks based in both DNA and histones are important epigenetic signals of adversity and stress, for technical reasons, most of the social science research to date has involved detecting changes only in DNA methylation. Determining whether a specific CpG site is methylated is relatively simple, and several approaches are in routine laboratory use. More recently, chip technology has been applied to determine the methylation state of approximately 500,000 CpG sites per DNA sample. Although the technology is straightforward, early experience suggests that there are significant challenges to analyzing the data, ranging from batch effects (artifacts induced by day-to-day variation in laboratory procedures) to the statistical challenges implicit in large numbers of repeated measures in a limited number of samples. Furthermore, although it is relatively straightforward to identify which CpG sites are hyper- or hypomethylated under a certain condition, it is much more difficult to associate this observation with a specific functional significance. This is because the biological effect of a change in methylation status at a particular CpG or cluster of CpGs is often unknown or unpredictable. Although work with both rodents and people has demonstrated the value of methylation changes in explaining how environmental inputs are translated to durable behavioral effects, this work has, so far, depended upon measurement of the methylation state of specific sites with known or clearly predictable functions. How methylation profiles across hundreds of thousands of sites should be correlated with underlying social inputs and health or behavior states remains an important topic for research. Furthermore, because the methylation state of differentiated tissues is highly specific, it is not clear how methylation profiles developed in circulating blood cells or saliva cells will provide information about changes in DNA from less accessible tissue such as brain, cells of the autonomic nervous system, or specific immune cells. All of these questions require extensive additional research.

DESCRIPTION OF TELOMERES

During DNA replication, the fact that DNA is replicated from the 5' to the 3' direction means that the end of 1 strand of the chromosome shortens with each cycle of chromosomal replication and cellular division. To prevent loss of genetically important information, chromosomes are capped by repetitive DNA sequences $(TTAGGG)_n$ and associated proteins, termed telomeres.[26] In addition, the presence of the telomere prevents fusion of adjoining chromosomal ends. Over time, with each cell division, the telomere ends become shorter, and so the telomere has been referred to as a mitotic clock. Associated with progressive telomere shortening, the cell activates pathways that prevent further cell division (replicative senescence). Stem cells maintain telomere length by activating an enzyme, telomerase. Telomerase consists of both a protein catalytic unit (TERT) and an RNA template unit (TERC), used to specify the sequence of the newly synthesized telomeric bases. Most specialized cells do not express, or express very low levels of telomerase, so their telomeres progressively shorten with the age of the organism (**Fig. 5**).

Mutations in telomere-associated proteins produce a number of serious hereditary diseases in humans. Dyskeratosis congenita (dystrophic nails, oral leukoplakia, and skin depigmentation) in infancy is followed by bone marrow failure, occasionally, pulmonary fibrosis, cirrhosis, and increased susceptibility for cancer. First attributed to a mutation in a gene on the X-chromosome, dyskerin (*DKC1*), several other telomere-associated mutations have subsequently been associated with the disorder and related conditions. Patients with dyskeratosis congenita have abnormally short telomeres through life.[27]

Accelerated telomere shortening is also associated with a number of acquired disease processes, including cancer associated with chronic inflammation, such as esophageal cancer with Barrett esophagitis, colon cancer with ulcerative colitis, and lung cancer. Several population-based and clinical studies have also correlated telomere length shortening with coronary artery disease. Because cancer and coronary disease are the major causes of death in older individuals, and telomere shortening is a consequence of normal aging (see **Fig. 5**), some have postulated that aging (or the diseases of aging) is related to telomere shortening. In this model, telomere shortening beyond a critical limit results in senesce of various cell populations, impeding for example, repair, and immune surveillance. Although it is clear that, on average, telomere length decreases as people age, this association does not establish a cause-and-effect relationship, and many questions regarding the role of telomere shortening on the age-associated changes in cellularity and reparative ability remain to be elucidated.

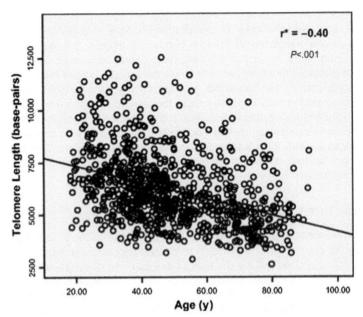

Fig. 5. Correlation between leukocyte telomere length and age. (*From* Njajou OT, Cawthon RM, Damcott CM, et al. Telomere length is paternally inherited and is associated with parental lifespan. Proc Natl Acad Sci U S A 2007;104:12136; with permission.)

As described subsequently, an emerging literature also links accelerated telomere shortening with stress, including both environmental stress such as malnutrition or violence, and social stress, such as perceived racism, depression, and absence of a father. Despite much literature that replicates this basic observation, it is not clear whether telomere attrition contributes mechanistically to the health effects associated with chronic stress, or whether it is merely a biomarker that reflects these effects.

The mechanism by which stress modulates telomere shortening is not well understood. Some research suggests that the physiologic correlates of stress (ie, activation of the hypothalamic–pituitary–adrenal [HPA] axis, inflammation) impose an increased oxidative burden on the cell, which damages the telomere, resulting in accelerated telomere attrition.[28] Other studies point to depressed telomerase function, also associated with stress, as contributing to reduced average telomere length.[29] The evidence for either mechanism is not strong. Understanding how stress affects telomere length is an urgent research priority, because without better knowledge of the biological mechanisms that link stress and other moderators of wellness and health to telomere length, it is not possible to articulate a convincing model to explain either the causes or the consequences of the observed disparities in telomere length.

MEASUREMENT OF TELOMERE LENGTH

Several approaches are used to determine the average telomere length in a sample of DNA. The classic approach is the terminal restriction fragment (TRF) length Southern blot assay. In many laboratories, a rapid quantitative real-time polymerase chain reaction(qRT-PCR) is used to compare the amount of telomere DNA (TTAGGG) in a sample with the amount of another, control gene. Often results are expressed as a ratio of telomere to control DNA (T/S ratio),[30] but more recently investigators have used internal control oligomers to report the length of the telomere in base pairs.[31] Using this method, the authors' laboratory has observed that the average telomere length in a sample of women (average age 34.2 years) is 6.12 kb, and in a sample of 2818 children (average age 9.28 years), it is 9.66 kb. Between boys and girls, the telomere length was 9.70 and 9.88 kb, respectively (P = ns) (Schneper L, personal communication, 2015). Several other approaches are occasionally employed, and all produce roughly similar results. Recent reports have used DNA derived from saliva to measurement telomere length. Although saliva telomere length is significantly longer than telomere length derived from peripheral blood mononuclear cells (the usual source) across an individual, the 2 sample types produce highly correlated measurements.[16]

SOCIAL DETERMINANTS OF EPIGENETIC MARKS

Research on epigenetic regulation of gene activity related to behavior and the influence of the social environment on epigenetic regulation began about a decade ago.[25] Despite this relative novelty, there is now evidence that life experiences (and especially early life experiences) can directly influence genetic function by altering the epigenetic patterns in specific loci on the genome.[32] It is important to note that the vast majority of work looking at environmental influences on DNA methylation or DNA methylation effects on health has been done on animals (especially mice, rats, and voles). Animals studies have shown that the strong effect of mother's nurturing on rat pups' ability to handle stress and form attachments is associated in part with increases in CpG methylation of the promoters regions of the glucocorticoid and estrogen receptor genes and the BDNF gene.[33] Another line of research shows that animals that have been stressed either through social isolation, nutritional deprivation, or contextual uncertainty also exhibit changes in methylation, typically decreasing methylation at the promoter regions of central nervous system (CNS) genes.[34]

In addition to parenting quality, other environmental or life experiences are related to methylation. For example, using buccal cells, a study recently found that adversity (such as physical abuse) in infancy and preschool was related to methylation pattern differences in adolescents.[22] Adverse early life experiences have also been tied to differences in epigenetic patterns for genes related to mental health,[35] drug addiction,[36] and obesity.[37]

SOCIAL DETERMINANTS OF TELOMERE LENGTH

Telomere length appears to be a biomarker of social stress. Telomere shortening has been associated with depression, harsh parenting, paternal absence, and perceived racism. Stress-related telomere shortening could evoke physiologic weathering in a way similar to aging.[38] Research suggests several possible behavioral mediators of the negative association between stress and telomere length, including smoking, mental illness (particularly depression), caregiver stress, and obesity.[39] Considering the strong association between social deprivation and these mediators, it is not surprising that some measures of social standing and social deprivation have also been found to be associated with telomere length.[16,40]

The telomere length literature has focused almost exclusively on adults, although several studies have used retrospective reports to measure childhood conditions, and 1 prospective study has examined the association between childhood conditions between ages 5 and 10 and telomere length, and a second study determined that the duration of exposure to institutional care between 22 and 54 months was negatively associated with telomere length.[26,39] Recently, the authors reported that the association between children's social environment and telomere length is moderated by specific variants or alleles in dopaminergic and serotonergic pathways. Involved genes associated with serotonergic transmission are HTT and TPH2 and with dopaminergic transmission are COMT, DAT, DRD2, and DRD4 (**Fig. 6**).[16]

EPIGENETIC ASSOCIATION WITH CHILD MENTAL HEALTH

A growing body of evidence suggests that DNA methylation plays an important role in mental health disorders also.[41] For example, exposure to third trimester depressed maternal mood is associated with methylation status of a CpG-island of *NR3C1* in newborns and altered HPA stress reactivity at age 3 months.[42] The association is indicative of a potential epigenetic mechanism linking maternal depression and newborn physiology. A second example suggests that depression is associated with higher methylation levels in the 5-hydroxytryptamine transporter (5-HTT, or SLC6A4) gene.[43] This work also ties back into the larger work on 5-HTTLPR and

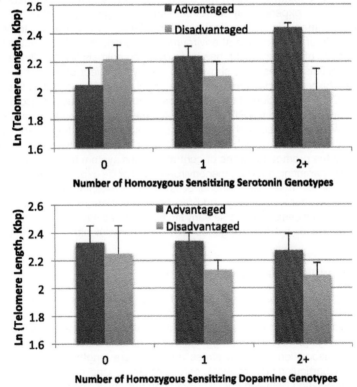

Fig. 6. ln(telomere length) by environment type (advantaged vs disadvantaged) and serotonin pathway (upper) and dopamine pathway (lower) homozygous genotype counts. For the serotonin pathway genotypes, the environment effect is borderline for 0 genotypes ($P = .09$), not significant for 1 genotype ($P = .32$), and significant for 2 + genotypes ($P = .02$). For the dopamine pathway genotypes, the environment difference is not significant for 0 genotypes ($P = .63$), significant for 1 genotype ($P = .05$), and borderline for 2 + genotypes ($P = .08$). This indicates that specific alleles in neurotransmitter pathways moderate the effect of social stress on telomere length. (*From* Mitchell C, Hobcraft J, McLanahan SS, et al. Social disadvantage, genetic sensitivity, and children's telomere length. Proc Natl Acad Sci U S A 2014;16:5947; with permission.)

depression[44] by showing that both genetic (the S allele of 5-HTTLPR) and epigenetic factors (methylation of the 5-HTTLPR promoter) may interact with environmental states to moderate risk of depression. However, this research area is nascent, and therefore the mechanisms that lead to changes in methylation or how that methylation modifies biology to influence mental health are still unknown.

EPIGENETIC ASSOCIATION WITH ASTHMA

Like the rest of the epigenetic literature, the work on asthma and allergy exploits both candidate gene and genome-wide approaches.[45] The candidate gene approach was the first method and still most common, but epigenome-wide data are becoming more available. For example, the 17q12 to 21 locus is one of the most widely replicated genetic loci for asthma. Interestingly, the effect of polymorphisms at this locus seems to be suppressed in females by higher levels of methylation of this locus,[46] which would tend to reduce expression of the risk allele. Another interaction between a genetic variant, this time in Il-4R, and the extent of methylation of a related CpG site has recently been described. The Il-4R gene variant (rs rs3024685) is not independently associated with risk of asthma, but the combination of this variant with a high level of methylation increased asthma risk by approximately 47-fold.[47] The biochemical mechanism underlying this effect remains to be better defined, but interactions between genetic variants (the genome) and the extent of methylation (the epigenome) may underlie many examples in which conventional rules of genetics fail to account for observed phenotypes. These studies show how polymorphisms and epigenetic regulation are interrelated and how future studies should be structured to examine these interactions. Not surprisingly most of the environmental exposures in this literature implicate the natural environment rather than the social environment.[45] However, in many cases, the social and natural environments are highly correlated; thus more research is needed to evaluate possible indirect and potentially spurious associations.

CURRENT RECOMMENDATIONS

Substantial evidence indicates that pathways initiated by childhood social adversity can be interrupted. Studies show that high-quality early development interventions, including center-based programs to nurture and stimulate children and to support and educate parents, greatly ameliorate the effects of social disadvantage on children's cognitive, emotional/behavioral, and physical development; the first 5 years of life appear to be most crucial, although opportunities for intervention continue throughout childhood and adolescence.[48-50] However, the extent to which these improvements are based on or related to epigenetic changes has not yet been evaluated, although there is great interest in pursuing these mechanisms. Therefore, although the early epigenetic literature cannot support specific recommendations, the authors expect that in the next few years the mechanistic link between early social adversity, early childhood development, and interventions to enhance development will begin to come into focus. Ideally, this research will be longitudinal, collaborative, and may involve very large data sets and new statistical methods based on bioinformatics.

Finally, although not explored in this article, a major limitation of this area is the lack of integrated research in social and natural environmental effects on epigenetics. Social and natural environment are highly correlated and yet are rarely discussed together. To what extent one might explain the effects of the other environment type on methylation patterns has not fully been explored. This might be a particularly useful way to expand available data and research.

REFERENCES

1. Rosen G. The history of public health. Baltimore, MD: Johns Hopkins University Press; 1993.
2. Braveman P, Egerter S, Williams DR. The social determinants of health: coming of age. Annu Rev Public Health 2011;32:381–98.
3. Adler NE, Ostrove JM. Socioeconomic status and health: what we know and what we don't. Ann N Y Acad Sci 1999;896(1):3–15.
4. Williams DR, Mohammed SA, Leavell J, et al. Race, socioeconomic status, and health: complexities, ongoing challenges, and research opportunities. Ann N Y Acad Sci 2010;1186(1):69–101.
5. Williams DR, Collins C. Racial residential segregation: a fundamental cause of racial disparities in health. Public Health Rep 2001;116(5):404.
6. Sallis JF, Glanz K. The role of built environments in physical activity, eating, and obesity in childhood. Future Child 2006;16(1):89–108.
7. Morenoff JD, Sampson RJ, Raudenbush SW. Neighborhood inequality, collective efficacy, and the spatial dynamics of urban violence. Criminology 2001;39(3):517–58.
8. Ross CE. Neighborhood disadvantage and adult depression. J Health Soc Behav 2000;41(2):177–87.
9. Wolfe B, Evans W, Seeman TE, editors. The biological consequences of socioeconomic inequalities. New York: Russell Sage Foundation; 2012.
10. Seeman T, Epel E, Gruenewald T, et al. Socio-economic differentials in peripheral biology: cumulative allostatic load. Ann N Y Acad Sci 2010;1186(1):223–39.
11. Shonkoff JP, Garner AS. The lifelong effects of early childhood adversity and toxic stress. Pediatrics 2012;129(1):e232–46.
12. Bradley RH, Corwyn RF. Socioeconomic status and child development. Annu Rev Psychol 2002;53:371–99.
13. Cohen S, Janicki-Deverts D, Chen E, et al. Childhood socioeconomic status and adult health. Ann N Y Acad Sci 2010;1186:37–55.
14. Guo G, Harris KM. The mechanisms mediating the effects of poverty on children's intellectual development. Demography 2000;37(4):431–47.
15. Jack PS, Deborah AP, editors. From neurons to neighborhoods: the science of early childhood development. Washington, DC: National Acadamies Press; 2000.
16. Mitchell C, Hobcraft J, McLanahan SS, et al. Social disadvantage, genetic sensitivity, and children's telomere length. Proc Natl Acad Sci U S A 2014;111(16):5944–9.
17. Miller GE, Chen E, Fok AK, et al. Low early-life social class leaves a biological residue manifested by decreased glucocorticoid and increased proinflammatory signaling. Proc Natl Acad Sci U S A 2009;106(34):14716–21.
18. Viner RM, Ozer EM, Denny S, et al. Adolescence and the social determinants of health. Lancet 2012;379(9826):1641–52.
19. Wright RJ. Epidemiology of stress and asthma: from constricting communities and fragile families to epigenetics. Immunol Allergy Clin N Am 2011;31(1):19–39.
20. Gee GC, Payne-Sturges DC. Environmental health disparities: a framework integrating psychosocial and environmental concepts. Environ Health Perspect 2004;112(17):1645–53.
21. Wright RJ. Moving towards making social toxins mainstream in children's environmental health. Curr Opin Pediatr 2009;21(2):222–9.
22. Essex MJ, Boyce WT, Hertzman C, et al. Epigenetic vestiges of early developmental adversity: childhood stress exposure and DNA methylation in adolescence. Child Development 2013;84(1):58–75.

23. Kishiyama MM, Boyce WT, Jimenez AM, et al. Socioeconomic disparities affect prefrontal function in children. J Cogn Neurosci 2009;21(6):1106–15.

24. Razin A. CpG methylation, chromatin structure and gene silencing-a three-way connection. EMBO J 1998;17(17):4905–8.

25. Szyf M. Early life, the epigenome and human health. Acta Paediatr 2009;98(7): 1082–4.

26. Shalev I, Entringer S, Wadhwa PD, et al. Stress and telomere biology: a lifespan perspective. Psychoneuroendocrinology 2013;38(9):1835–42.

27. Vulliamy T, Marrone A, Goldman F, et al. The RNA component of telomerase is mutated in autosomal dominant dyskeratosis congenita. Nature 2001; 413(6854):432–5.

28. von Zglinicki T. Oxidative stress shortens telomeres. Trends Biochem Sci 2002; 27(7):339–44.

29. Epel ES, Blackburn EH, Lin J, et al. Accelerated telomere shortening in response to life stress. Proc Natl Acad Sci U S A 2004;101(49):17312–5.

30. Cawthon RM. Telomere measurement by quantitative PCR. Nucleic Acids Res 2002;30(10):e47.

31. O'Callaghan NJ, Fenech M. A quantitative PCR method for measuring absolute telomere length. Biol Proced Online 2011;13:3.

32. Champagne FA. Epigenetic influence of social experiences across the lifespan. Dev Psychobiol 2010;52(4):299–311.

33. Champagne FA, Weaver IC, Diorio J, et al. Maternal care associated with methylation of the estrogen receptor-alpha1b promoter and estrogen receptor-alpha expression in the medial preoptic area of female offspring. Endocrinology 2006;147(6):2909–15.

34. Meaney MJ. Epigenetics and the biological definition of gene x environment interactions. Child Development 2010;81(1):41–79.

35. Galea S, Uddin M, Koenen K. The urban environment and mental disorders: epigenetic links. Epigenetics 2011;6(4):400–4.

36. Renthal W, Nestler EJ. Epigenetic mechanisms in drug addiction. Trends Mol Med 2008;14(8):341–50.

37. Campion J, Milagro F, Martinez JA. Epigenetics and obesity. Prog Mol Biol Transl Sci 2010;94:291–347.

38. Geronimus AT. The weathering hypothesis and the health of African-American women and infants: evidence and speculations. Ethn Dis 1992;2(3):207–21.

39. Shalev I, Moffitt TE, Sugden K, et al. Exposure to violence during childhood is associated with telomere erosion from 5 to 10 years of age: a longitudinal study. Mol Psychiatry 2013;18(5):576–81.

40. Carroll JE, Diez-Roux AV, Adler NE, et al. Socioeconomic factors and leukocyte telomere length in a multi-ethnic sample: findings from the multi-ethnic study of atherosclerosis (MESA). Brain Behav Immun 2013;28:108–14.

41. Toyokawa S, Uddin M, Koenen KC, et al. How does the social environment 'get into the mind'? Epigenetics at the intersection of social and psychiatric epidemiology. Soc Sci Med 2012;74(1):67–74.

42. Oberlander TF, Weinberg J, Papsdorf M, et al. Prenatal exposure to maternal depression, neonatal methylation of human glucocorticoid receptor gene (NR3C1) and infant cortisol stress responses. Epigenetics 2008;3(2):97–106.

43. Olsson CA, Foley DL, Parkinson-Bates M, et al. Prospects for epigenetic research within cohort studies of psychological disorder: a pilot investigation of a peripheral cell marker of epigenetic risk for depression. Biol Psychol 2010;83(2):159–65.

44. Mitchell C, Notterman D, Brooks-Gunn J, et al. Role of mother's genes and environment in postpartum depression. Proc Natl Acad Sci U S A 2011;108(20): 8189–93.
45. Durham AL, Adcock IM. Epigenetic regulation of asthma and allergic diseases. Epigenetic aspects of chronic diseases. London: Springer; 2011. p. 147–61.
46. Naumova AK, Al Tuwaijri A, Morin A, et al. Sex- and age-dependent DNA methylation at the 17q12-q21 locus associated with childhood asthma. Hum Genet 2013;132(7):811–22.
47. Soto-Ramirez N, Arshad SH, Holloway JW, et al. The interaction of genetic variants and DNA methylation of the interleukin-4 receptor gene increase the risk of asthma at age 18 years. Clin Epigenetics 2013;5(1):1.
48. Campbell F, Conti G, Heckman JJ, et al. Early childhood investments substantially boost adult health. Science 2014;343(6178):1478–85.
49. Hoagwood K, Burns BJ, Kiser L, et al. Evidence-based practice in child and adolescent mental health services. Psychiatr Serv 2001;52(9):1179–89.
50. Morrison J, Pikhart H, Ruiz M, et al. Systematic review of early childhood interventions in European countries (1990-2013) that aimed to address health and development. Eur J Public Health 2014;24(suppl 2).

Addressing Childhood Obesity

Opportunities for Prevention

Callie L. Brown, MD[a], Elizabeth E. Halvorson, MD[b],
Gail M. Cohen, MD, MS[b,c], Suzanne Lazorick, MD, MPH[d,e],
Joseph A. Skelton, MD, MS[b,c,f],*

KEYWORDS

- Etiology • Prevention • Obesity • Risk factors • Pediatric • Genetics • Overweight

KEY POINTS

- Childhood obesity is a complex medical issue, representing the interplay of physical and environmental factors.
- The neuroendocrine control of weight includes multiple situations where genetic variation can influence a person's weight status.
- The unhealthy evolution of food and activity environments has placed children at a higher risk for obesity and associated weight problems than they have ever been.

INTRODUCTION

The prevalence of obesity in the United States remains dangerously high, at nearly 10% among infants and toddlers, 17% of children and teens, and more than 30% of adults.[1] Although the prevalence has stabilized somewhat over the past few years,[1]

The authors have no other financial disclosures to make.
Support: Supported in part by a grant from NICHD/NIH Mentored Patient-Oriented Research Career Development Award K23 HD061597 (J.A. Skelton) and from the Health Recourses and Service Administration National Research Service Award (NRSA) grant T32 HP14001 (C.L. Brown).
[a] Department of Pediatrics, University of North Carolina at Chapel Hill, 301B, S. Columbia Street, Chapel Hill, NC 27599, USA; [b] Department of Pediatrics, Wake Forest School of Medicine, Medical Center Boulevard, Winston-Salem, NC 27157, USA; [c] Brenner FIT (Families in Training) Program, Brenner Children's Hospital, Medical Center Boulevard, Winston-Salem, NC 27157, USA; [d] Department of Pediatrics, Brody School of Medicine, East Carolina University, Greenville, NC 27834, USA; [e] Department of Public Health, East Carolina University, Greenville, NC 27834, USA; [f] Division of Public Health Sciences, Department of Epidemiology and Prevention, Wake Forest School of Medicine, Winston-Salem, NC, USA
* Corresponding author. Department of Pediatrics, Wake Forest School of Medicine, Medical Center Boulevard, Winston-Salem, NC 27157.
E-mail address: jskelton@wakehealth.edu

Pediatr Clin N Am 62 (2015) 1241–1261
http://dx.doi.org/10.1016/j.pcl.2015.05.013
pediatric.theclinics.com

rates of severe obesity have continued to climb, particularly in high-risk populations.[2] Intervening during childhood is important due to the persistence of obesity into adulthood with associated increased morbidity and mortality.[3-6] Comorbidities often affect children before they reach adulthood, requiring increased diligence in evaluating and treating these conditions[7-9] and leading to increased health care expenditures.[10,11] The personal and emotional face of childhood obesity is also serious: daily quality of life can be significantly worsened by obesity.[12] The psychosocial complications of obesity include depression, body dissatisfaction, unhealthy weight control behaviors, stigmatization, and poor self-esteem.[12]

Groups have advocated for the prevention of obesity for some time, yet efforts to advance preventative interventions may have been limited by the difficulties and expense of long-term studies of a complex problem and increasing focus on treatments. Despite the progress over the past 20 years, there is not a clear solution or one-size-fits-all approach. The body of literature on proved prevention interventions is not robust, although cross-sectional and associational studies have identified risk factors to address, and practical experience has provided a foundation on which to work with children and families. Childhood obesity is incredibly complex and reflects numerous systems that have an impact on a child's health. Repetition of concepts can aid in approaching an issue as complex as childhood obesity; the ecological model of childhood obesity (**Fig. 1**) provides a broad framework for understanding the mediators and moderators of childhood obesity. This overview highlights evidence-based factors on which clinicians can focus efforts to effectively prevent the development of childhood obesity. This article reviews both general and age-specific risk factors for pediatric obesity and discusses specific strategies for intervention at the level of the pediatrician, school, government, and family.

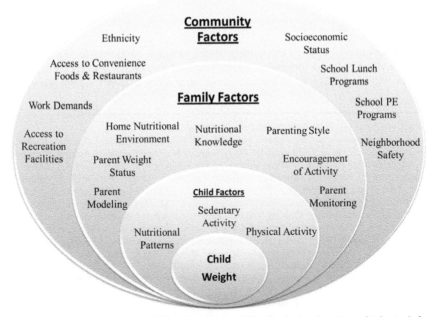

Fig. 1. Ecological model of childhood obesity. PE, physical education. (*Adapted from* Davison KK, Birch LL. Childhood overweight: a contextual model and recommendations for future research. Obes Rev 2001;2(3):161; with permission.)

RISK FACTORS
Genetic Risk Factors

Obesity is commonly known to run in families. The genetic contribution to this obser-vation is difficult to discern, however, because families usually share not only genetic material but also environments and habits. Obesity in children correlates with obesity in their parents, and the level of obesity in children increases when both parents are obese as well as with increasing levels of obesity in the parents.[13] It has been shown that parental overweight is the most significant risk factor for childhood overweight.[14] Children's food choices and eating behaviors are learned from parents at very young ages and influence eating behaviors as children get older.[15,16]

Although a vast majority of cases of childhood obesity are exogenous, a small proportion may have endogenous causes. The following genetic disorders, both syndromic as well as monogenic in origin, predispose children to obesity:

- Syndromes: trisomy 21 syndrome; Prader-Willi syndrome; Albright hereditary os-teodystrophy; Cohen syndrome; Bardet-Biedl syndrome; Alström syndrome; and Wilms tumor, aniridia, genitourinary anomalies, and mental retardation (WAGR).[17,18]
- Monogenic disorders: leptin deficiency, leptin receptor mutations, proopiomela-nocortin deficiency, preproconvertase deficiency, and melanocortin 4 receptor mutations.[17]
- Hormonal disorders: hypothyroidism, growth hormone deficiency, Cushing syndrome, hypothalamic obesity, polycystic ovary syndrome, and hyperprolactinemia.[17]

Environmental/Societal Risk Factors

A child's living environment, both in the home as well as in the community, can contribute to a higher risk of development of obesity:

- Living in lower-income, predominantly white, or non–mixed-race neighborhoods.[19]
- Parents' perceptions of the food and physical activity environments in their neighborhoods
- Difficulty getting to a main food store or difficulty purchasing fruits and vegeta-bles there (food desert)
- Increased distance from parks
- Perceived danger of their neighborhood[19]
- Food insecurity, although the evidence is mixed[19,20]

Behavioral Risk Factors

Nutrition and diet
Although it might seem logical that increased total energy intake should be associated with a higher risk of childhood obesity, the evidence does not support this relation-ship.[14,21] Similarly, the relationship between dietary fat intake and childhood obesity is not clearly established.[21] A lower intake of dairy products or calcium is associated with childhood obesity, but the data regarding intake of fruits and vegetables are mixed and do not indicate a strong association with childhood weight status.[21,22] Beverage choice may increase risk for childhood obesity: fruit juice, especially in large quantities[21]; SSBs[21,23]; and sodas[21,24,25] are all positively associated with childhood obesity.

Some specific eating behaviors have been associated with childhood obesity. Skip-ping breakfast[21,26,27]; eating meals away from home, especially fast food[21]; quicker eating pace[28]; larger portion sizes[21]; and eating in the absence of hunger[28] are all positively associated with childhood obesity. No consistent association has been identified with frequent snacking,[21,29] whereas eating meals as a family is inversely associated with childhood obesity.[20,21]

Although there can be conflicting evidence, or less-than-clear associations, clinicians can be confident in addressing intake of unhealthy foods, such as fast food, SSBs, high-fat proteins, and processed snacks, and encourage intake of healthy items, in particular fruits, vegetables, lean meats, and sugar-free beverages. Underneath the intake of these foods are the habits behind them, which clinicians should be cognizant of during an interaction: foods eaten away from home, eating in the absence of hunger, snacking, and family meals. Awareness of these issues can assist clinicians in working with families to prevent the development of unhealthy habits and build healthy ones to prevent excessive weight gain.

Physical activity

Overall, decreased physical activity among children is associated with obesity.[14,21,30,31] Prospective studies objectively measuring physical activity have yielded inconsistent results; however, studies of either self-reported or parent-reported physical activity have demonstrated an inverse relationship between physical activity and both childhood and future adult obesity.[30] An inverse relationship exists between some specific activity-related behaviors and childhood obesity, including sports team participation and active commuting to school.[32]

Physical inactivity and sedentary behaviors are likely associated with childhood obesity,[21,25,30] although the effect size may be small.[14] Some prospective studies have found that more hours engaged in sedentary behavior, specifically watching TV or playing video games, was associated with an increased risk of becoming obese in the future[21,30]; however, other studies found no association between sedentary behavior and childhood obesity.[33] Increased screen time, including television[33] and electronic devices,[34] is also associated with childhood obesity. Although increased sedentary time and decreased physical activity are both associated with childhood obesity, they may not be inversely proportional. Regardless, efforts to lower the former and increase the latter are key to preventing obesity development.

Sleep

Although there is less evidence regarding sleep, it seems that shorter sleep duration is associated with childhood obesity.[20,35] Some prospective studies have borne out this association, both in the short term in young children[36] and in the long term, persisting into adulthood.[37] In combination with other positive household routines (eating as a family and limiting screen time), obtaining adequate sleep has a strong inverse relationship with obesity among preschool-aged children.[38]

Stress

The short- and long-term effects of stress on the development of obesity are an emerging area for research. There are several types of stress that can affect a child: personal, parental, and family. Each of these can increase a child's risk for obesity independently or in concert. Although the data are somewhat mixed, it is likely that there is a positive association between chronic stress and the risk of childhood obesity.[39] This can manifest during childhood[40] and may persist into adulthood.[41] In many studies, parental stress is associated with obesity in children; this relationship is strengthened when a parent experiences stress from more than 1 source.[39] Similarly, stress within the family is also associated with childhood obesity (**Box 1**).[39]

Box 1
Review of risk factors for pediatric obesity

- Genetic syndromes, monogenic disorders, or hormonal disorders
- Living in neighborhoods that are lower income, predominantly non–mixed race, perceived as dangerous, or at an increased distance from parks and foods stores
- Increased intake of SSBs, fast food, and processed snacks
- Decreased physical activity
- Shorter sleep duration
- Increased personal, prenatal, or family stress

DEVELOPMENTAL APPROACH TO OBESITY PREVENTION

Many of the risk factors discussed previously, related to diet, physical and sedentary activity, and sleep, apply to children of many different ages. Other risk factors for pediatric obesity may apply at distinct development stages, offering specific opportunities for intervention by a primary care provider. These stage-specific risk factors have been identified as early as the prenatal period. Although obesity in either parent may increase a child's risk, as discussed previously, a mother's prepregnancy body mass index (BMI) and gestational weight gain have been directly associated with obesity in infancy and early childhood.[42–45] Maintaining gestational weight gain within the Institute of Medicine (IOM) guidelines[46] (**Table 1**) is especially important for women who are overweight or obese at the time of conception and should be an important component of prenatal counseling. Both over- and undernutrition at this stage are thought to affect fetal programming and predispose to future obesity and metabolic disorders.[17,47] One recent meta-analysis identified a moderate association between delivery via cesarean section and offspring obesity, with persistence of the association into adulthood.[48] In addition, maternal exposure to tobacco[43,49,50] and caffeine[51] have both been associated with obesity at various points during gestation and throughout a child's life.

Additional risk factors become evident in infancy. High birth weight and rapid infant weight gain correlate with future childhood obesity,[43] although they may be difficult to address specifically as modifiable risk factors. Many studies have attempted to determine optimal dietary intake during infancy, but the results are conflicting. Although many studies suggest that breastfeeding is protective against the development of obesity,[43,52,53] others show no relationship.[54,55] These differing results may be due to confounders present in the study; for example, it has been shown that lower protein content in infant formula is protective against obesity at 6 years, so studies on breastfeeding may differ based on the types of formula used by control infants. Results have also been mixed when assessing the effects of duration of breastfeeding.[43] It has been suggested that it is an infant's degree of self-regulation while breastfeeding rather than the composition of breast milk that may be protective, so that bottle-feeding either formula or pumped breast milk may be associated with increased risk.[56]

Complementary foods represent another important dietary change during infancy, and both the timing of introduction and food selection may have an impact on future risk of obesity. Early introduction of solids (defined as ages <3–5 months depending on the study) may be associated with increased childhood overweight.[57] Similarly, 1 systematic review concludes that higher intake of protein and energy during infancy can be associated with increased BMI,[58] although other studies conclude that no

Table 1
Anticipatory guidance and specific interventions by age and developmental stage

	Nutrition	Physical Activity/ Other	Specific Interventions

Prenatal period	• Avoid over- and undernutrition during pregnancy
	• Avoid caffeine
		• Avoid tobacco	• Weight gain per IOM guidelines:
			   Underweight: 28–40 lb
			   Normal weight: 25–35 lb
			   Overweight: 15–25 lb
			   Obese: 11–20 lb

Newborn– 6 mo	• Exclusive breastfeeding until 6 mo • Only breast milk or formula, no SSBs • Be mindful of child's feeding cues • Allow child to feed at own pace • Stop feeding when child is done • Do not put to sleep while feeding • No television, especially while feeding	• Tummy time • No screen time or television	• Avoid broad-spectrum antibiotics if possible
6–12 mo	• Continued breastfeeding until 12 mo and beyond • Introduce solids when developmentally ready (sit, open mouth on cue, close mouth around spoon) • Encourage fruits and vegetables • Finger foods with soft table foods • Wide variety of textures and flavors • Continue to offer foods that a child has previously not liked • Structured meal and snack times	• No screen time or television	• Avoid broad-spectrum antibiotics if possible
12–24 mo	• Limited SSBs • Eat together as a family at structured meal and snack times • Sit at table for all snacks, drinks, and meals • Prepare foods in a variety of ways • Limit eating at restaurants, especially fast food • Let child choose how much of offered food to eat • Encourage positive parent modeling • Provide perspective on portion size	• <1 h of Screen time per day	• Consider early bottle weaning • Avoid broad-spectrum antibiotics if possible • Avoid restrictive or emotional feeding habits

(continued on next page)

Table 1
(*continued*)

	Nutrition	Physical Activity/ Other	Specific Interventions
24–48 mo	• Realistic expectations for table manners • 3 Meals a day at set times • No grazing between meals except for scheduled snacks	• <2 h of Screen time per day	• Avoid restrictive or emotional feeding habits
4–12 y	• Set some basic rules, then allow child to choose after-school snack	• At least 60 min of moderate to vigorous physical activity daily	• Consider technological interventions
13–18 y	• Allow child to take re-sponsibility for choosing and eating meals away from home • Expect child to be hungry at dinner • Teach how to plan and prepare meals and snacks	• 60 min Physical activity daily	• Consider technological interventions • Involve peer groups in interventions

specific complementary foods are associated with increased risk.[59] Overall, the available evidence makes it difficult to establish firm guidelines for infants' dietary intake.

Other exposures in infancy have also been investigated. Use of broad-spectrum antibiotics, especially with repeated exposures prior to 23 months of age, has a small but significant association with obesity in early childhood.[60] Studies have yielded mixed results for family socioeconomic status, maternal parity, and maternal marital status.[43] Finally, temperament traits identified as early as infancy, especially early negativity and lack of self-regulation, may predispose to later obesity.[61,62]

Child temperament and parental feeding practices remain important predictors of obesity for toddlers and preschool-aged children. The concerning character traits are thought to be similar to those seen in infancy, in particular poor self-regulation and distress to limitations.[62] Part of the mechanism of this association may reflect parental response to the child's temperament, especially if parents initiate restrictive feeding practices given concerns over self-regulation or use emotional feeding habits, such as providing obesogenic foods to soothe a negative child.[59,62] Children are typically weaned from the bottle as toddlers; the timing of this transition may affect obesity risk. At earlier ages (between 12 and 36 months), there is an association between current bottle use and obesity, but this was not seen at later ages (37–60 months).[63] Furthermore, an intervention centered on bottle-weaning effectively reduced total caloric intake in children but did not change overweight status,[64] so the degree to which prolonged bottle use contributes to obesity risk is unclear.

Although sedentary behavior and screen time are concerns for children of all ages, 1 systematic review suggests that preschool children are most amenable to interventions addressing this risk factor.[65] Weight gain in this age group is known to be highly predictive of later obesity, with an earlier adiposity rebound (at <5 years old) associated with both BMI and adiposity at age 15 years.[66] Therefore, this is an important age group to target as effective interventions are identified.

Most studies of obesity in school-aged children focus on interventions delivered within the school system (discussed later). Some research has shown, however, that children with overweight and obesity actually gain more weight during the summer months than during the school year,[67,68] suggesting that interventions outside of school should also be investigated. The primary difference noted between the school year and summertime is in the level of physical activity.[68] One intervention that has shown success in increasing physical activity in this age group, as well as adolescents, is exergaming, or use of electronic games designed to promote physical exercise.[69] Although the video game experience makes activity more entertaining for children, use of exergames in several studies was found to increase energy expenditure and time spent on physical activity and to reduce waist circumference.[69] These findings suggest that targeting known risk factors during the summer months may be especially important for obesity prevention at this age.

Use of technology for obesity prevention continues to be important in the adolescent age group. Technology-based interventions targeting both diet and exercise have been shown effective in this population, although there is wide variation among studies.[70] Peer groups also take on increased importance during adolescence, and research has attempted to determine how this influences the risk of obesity. Peers are able to influence diet and activity levels in both positive and negative ways,[71,72] so the inclusion of the peer group in interventions targeting adolescents is important.[72]

Adolescence is a time of significant biological changes, notably puberty. Although there is a clear association between early puberty and obesity, it is difficult to determine cause and effect because prepubertal BMI influences the timing of puberty.[47] Some studies have demonstrated an effect of early puberty on subsequent adiposity and fat distribution, but results have been mixed.[47] Severe obesity in adolescence has been directly associated with poor health outcomes in adulthood,[5] which makes prevention in this age group especially important. In addition, because they represent the next generation of parents, establishment of healthy lifestyle habits in the adolescent population has the potential to decrease the obesity risk of subsequent generations (**Box 2**).

ROLE OF THE PRIMARY CARE PROVIDER

Primary care providers play a unique role in the prevention of obesity because they see the same patients and families, often from birth, on a regular basis (**Box 3**). This gives them the opportunity to provide anticipatory guidance and counseling that can influence families' nutrition and physical activity habits. As discussed previously, it is well established that there are strong familial links to obesity, both genetic[13,14] and

---

Box 2
Review of developmental approach to obesity prevention

- Prenatal: appropriate gestational weight gain, no tobacco exposure
- Infancy: minimizing rapid weight gain, later introduction of solid foods, avoiding broad-spectrum antibiotics as possible
- Toddlers: encouraging self-regulation of feeding and lots of physical activity
- School-aged children: exergaming, use of technology-based interventions to improve nutrition and physical activity
- Adolescents: including peer groups in interventions

> **Box 3**
> **Review of the primary care provider's role in preventing obesity**
>
> - Measure height and weight and calculate BMI at least annually, observe for trends such as a rapid increase in BMI
> - Offer anticipatory guidance about nutrition and physical activity at every well child check
> - Use motivational interviewing to help families to make healthier choices
> - Advocate for children on a local and national level

environmental.[16] These influences do not dictate fate, however. By recognizing risk factors early in a child's life, primary care providers can help families make positive changes that improve a child's weight trajectory.[73]

Pediatricians should screen for obesity by measuring height and weight and calculating BMI at least annually.[74–76] By following children closely over time, physicians are in a position to detect weight problems by observing trends, such as a rapidly increasing BMI, even before a child becomes overweight. When a child is discovered to be overweight or at risk for becoming overweight, physicians should provide brief counseling and suggest weight control interventions.[74,76] The authors recommend that clinicians use motivational interviewing techniques **(Fig. 2)**[74,77–80] when counseling patients and their families about making life changes.

Primary care providers offer anticipatory guidance about nutrition and physical activity at each well child check. This anticipatory guidance should be age appropriate and can significantly shape how and what parents feed their children. All children, even those of a healthy weight, benefit from counseling about general health and wellness, and this does not need to be framed around weight. Recommended anticipatory guidance for each age range is outlined in **Table 1**.[21,30,74,81–92]

Primary care providers should advocate for their patients and families; to build community-wide efforts to prevent obesity, clinicians can look to successful models in other areas to support their efforts. The chronic care model[93] provides a useful framework for pediatricians to provide care to children who are overweight or obese. The chronic care model recognizes that families' self-management is dependent on support both from the medical system and their surrounding environment, such as school, work, and the community. Ideally, primary care physicians should be connected with numerous community resources, such as nutrition and exercise programs.[74,93] The chronic care model has been successfully implemented by health-related organizations, such as Kaiser Permanente, that provided education for providers in motivational interviewing, and WellPoint, that distributed parental toolkits to families in clinic.[74]

Advocating for children's health and health care is an important role for pediatricians to embrace on both local and national levels; examples of areas for advocacy include

- Third-party reimbursement to ensure that children continue to have access to services necessary for obesity prevention and treatment, such as yearly BMI screening and well visits with their primary care provider
- Funding for research to prevent childhood obesity
- Promotion of healthy foods and beverages and physical activities in schools and day cares
- Maintenance of safe neighborhoods that encourage physical activity
- Availability of healthy food[24]

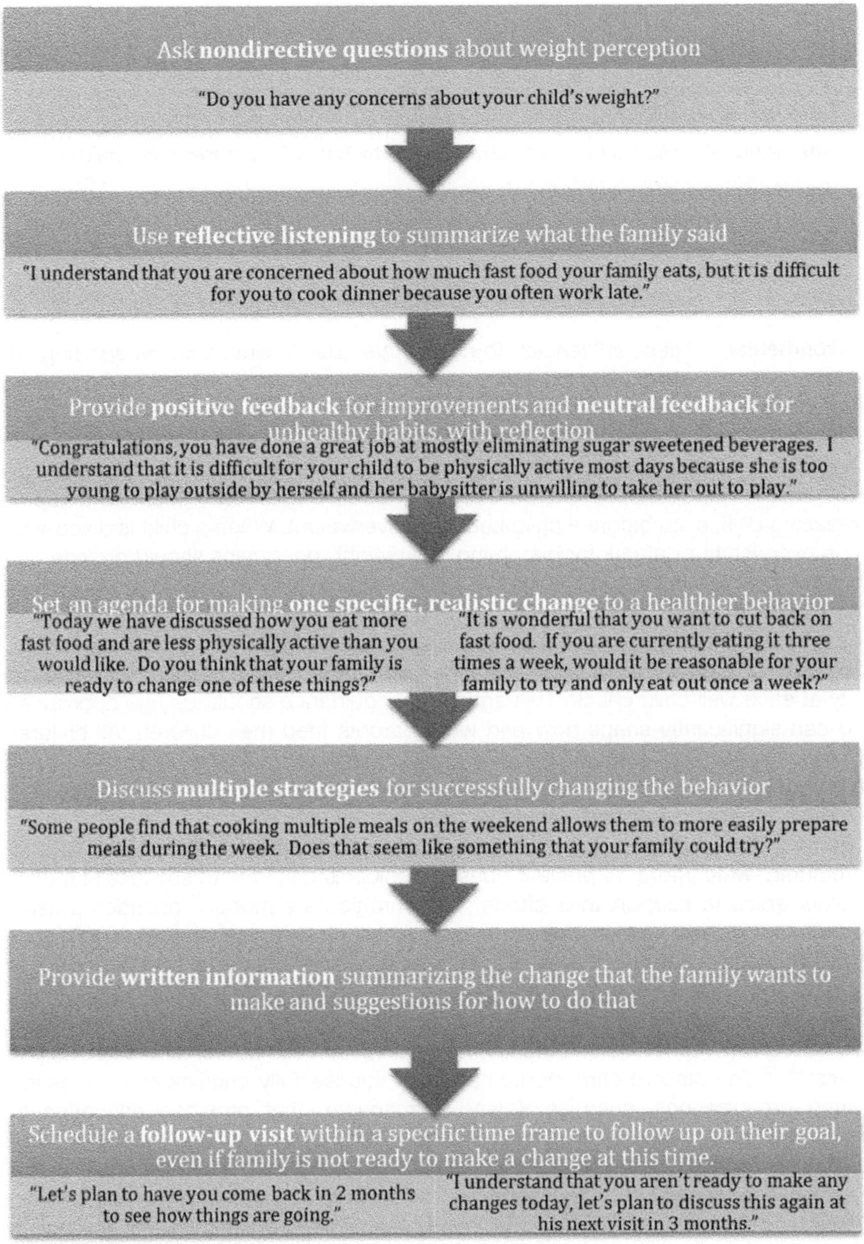

Ask **nondirective questions** about weight perception

"Do you have any concerns about your child's weight?"

Use **reflective listening** to summarize what the family said

"I understand that you are concerned about how much fast food your family eats, but it is difficult for you to cook dinner because you often work late."

Provide **positive feedback** for improvements and **neutral feedback** for unhealthy habits, with reflection

"Congratulations, you have done a great job at mostly eliminating sugar sweetened beverages. I understand that it is difficult for your child to be physically active most days because she is too young to play outside by herself and her babysitter is unwilling to take her out to play."

Set an agenda for making **one specific, realistic change** to a healthier behavior

"Today we have discussed how you eat more fast food and are less physically active than you would like. Do you think that your family is ready to change one of these things?"

"It is wonderful that you want to cut back on fast food. If you are currently eating it three times a week, would it be reasonable for your family to try and only eat out once a week?"

Discuss **multiple strategies** for successfully changing the behavior

"Some people find that cooking multiple meals on the weekend allows them to more easily prepare meals during the week. Does that seem like something that your family could try?"

Provide **written information** summarizing the change that the family wants to make and suggestions for how to do that

Schedule a **follow-up visit** within a specific time frame to follow up on their goal, even if family is not ready to make a change at this time.

"Let's plan to have you come back in 2 months to see how things are going."

"I understand that you aren't ready to make any changes today, let's plan to discuss this again at his next visit in 3 months."

Fig. 2. Motivational interviewing to help families make positive changes to prevent obesity. (*Data from* Barlow SE; Expert Committee. Expert committee recommendations regarding the prevention, assessment, and treatment of child and adolescent overweight and obesity: summary report. Pediatrics 2007;120 Suppl 4:S164–92.)

POLICY AND ENVIRONMENTAL INTERVENTIONS

Using the socioecologic model as a guide[94] on a societal level, policy and environmental interventions have the potential to exert the farthest-reaching influence in thwarting obesity.[95] Policy changes can address physical, economic, social, or communication factors and may range in scope of efforts that target:

- A whole population: national or state legislation; industry-wide improvements; social marketing), or
- Population subsets or large groups: state or regional ordinances, or
- Local or smaller groups: single organization or community[96]

Policies can be formal documented standards or laws or informal practices (eg, a medical office giving patients stickers vs candy). The overarching goals are for policies to prevent obesity by (1) increasing awareness of and actions to change attitudes and norms to support healthy energy balance; (2) making healthy options for physical activity and nutrition readily available and, where possible, the default choices; and (3) reducing barriers to making healthy choices.

For maximal impact, policy changes should be informed by the existing science of obesity prevention and established theories of behavior change, such as social cognitive theory,[97] self-determination theory,[98] and/or the transtheoretical model of behavior change,[99] and subsequently evaluated by rigorous studies demonstrating both feasibility and effectiveness. Optimally, studies of policy are thoroughly evaluated with application of appropriate methods such as the Reach, Effectiveness, Adoption, Implementation, and Maintenance framework.[100] Where large studies have not been completed, efforts should be evidence informed and practice tested.[101] Once enacted, there should be ongoing monitoring of fidelity and accountability of policies for effectiveness and use of resources, with attention to social factors that contribute to inequality in access to healthy choices. Although the body of literature assessing polices for obesity prevention is growing, there are still many areas actively under study or for which evidence is inadequate for a definitive recommendation for wide-scale adoption.[96,102]

Select examples illustrative of policies with growing support and/or evidence and ranging in scope are shown in **Table 2** and for specific settings in which children spend substantial time are shown in **Table 3**.

Notable recent progress in the policy arena has occurred in standards for food programs affecting children, including application of the 2010 United States Department of Agriculture (USDA) Dietary Guidelines for Americans to schools[107] and science-based nutrition standards for meals offered in day care and after-school programs through the pending Child and Adult Care Food Program. These changes are largely a result of passage of the Healthy, Hunger-free Kids Act of 2010 that was motivated in large part to curb the obesity epidemic.[108] The Act included several components to ensure meals served to children include more fruits and vegetables, whole grains, and less sugar and fat while also promoting breastfeeding and increasing access to healthy beverages (water or low-fat or fat-free milk). Related changes are evident in the revised food package offered to participant in the Women, Infants, and Children (WIC) program since 2007 and broadening of educational messages and materials supported by the Supplemental Nutrition Assistance Program Education (SNAP-Ed) programs to include emphasis on energy balance and obesity prevention.

Despite progress in recent decades, there remain many areas for which evidence is insufficient or policies are lacking, emerging, or facing challenges.[95] Although there are signs of growing partnership, remaining barriers include involvement of the food

Table 2 Policy examples: ranging in scope	
Scope	**Examples of Policies or Environmental Strategies**
Site specific	• Banks, stores, professionals give incentives for children that do not contribute to unhealthful habits or energy imbalance (examples: stickers instead of candy; balloons instead of cookies)[c] • Corner stores and quick marts offer low fat/sugar snacks, fruits, and vegetables[b] • Entertainment venues offer healthful options, water; allow outside (home-packed) foods[c] • Point of decision prompts (elevator vs stairs initiatives; menu, cafeteria, or buffet signage and prompts)[a]
Local	• Establish shared-use agreements for physical activity space and equipment[b] • Promote ways to allow active transport to and from school (bike lanes and racks, crossing guards, group walks to school)[b] • Emphasize maintaining or re-establishing time for recess, physical activity, physical education[b] • Support school and community gardens, partnerships with local farmers[c] • Access to safe, free drinking water in recreation environments[b]
State	• Subsidies for schools/childcare sites for provision of healthy foods[a] • Incentives for grocers in rural or urban areas[c] • Mechanism for small vendors (farmers markets) to take Supplemental Nutrition Assistance Program (SNAP) (food stamps) cards[c] • Medicaid coverage for dietician services and preventive counseling[c] • Support for increasing sites and access for recreation[a]
National	• Healthy and Hunger Free Kids Act, including standards for meals in school (eg, the National School Lunch Program)[a] • Changes to WIC food package and SNAP policies[a] • Changes to SNAP-Ed guidance for educational programs[a] • Menu labeling for restaurants[b] • Laws addressing advertising to children[c] • Food and beverage industry incentives[c]
International	• Published guidelines for member states for population-level strategies for obesity prevention across settings[103]

[a] Evidence or existing systematic review to support.
[b] Emerging strategy but more data needed.[96]
[c] Sample policy change needing pilot data and further study.[96]

industry, marketing, and entertainment venues along with pervasive social and cultural attitudes and influences. Resistance may exist due to factors, such as economic pressures or underlying fundamental political or philosophic tension between government versus individual/parent rights and freedom of choice. Some barriers may be reduced as more evidence demonstrates links between academic performance and health/obesity status or health behaviors (to support policy changes in the school setting) or the economic benefits of a healthier population/workforce to factors, such as defense preparedness and economic measures (to support changes in business and industry).

Pediatricians, primary care providers, and any professional or individual with an interest in obesity prevention for children can actively support efforts in policy or environmental changes through lending expertise, providing advocacy or local support, or by leading and role modeling in the work setting and community (**Box 4**).

THE FAMILY

Although environmental pressures at the national and community level contribute greatly to a child's risk of obesity, according to Schor, "families are the most central

Table 3
Examples of policies and programs in settings where children spend substantial time

General efforts may target	• Education about energy balance and negative health effects of obesity • Promotion of more opportunities for and enjoyment of physical activity (PA) • Offering age-appropriate portion sizes following USDA guidelines • Assuring program staff are knowledgeable and appropriately trained • Establishing and implementing local wellness polices • Improving quality and time in physical education (PE); working to designate PE as a core subject	
Setting	**Example Program**	**Description**
Childcare	• Nutrition and Physical Activity Self-Assessment for Child Care (NAP SACC; www.goNAPSACC.org)[a]	• Self-assessment, action planning, and educational tools to help early care and education programs set goals and make improvements to their nutrition and PA practices.
Elementary school	• Coordinated Approach to Child Health (CATCH, www.CATCHinfo.org), based on evidence from the Child and Adolescent Trial for Cardiovascular Health[a] • SPARK program to improve PE (www.SPARKPE.org)[a]	• Multifaceted intervention in elementary schools grades K–5: implemented in the classroom, cafeteria, PE, and families to foster healthy behaviors in diet and PA[104] • Toolkit and training for schools to improve and increase PA time in PE
Middle school	• Motivating Adolescents with Technology to Choose Health (MATCH; www.MATCHwellness.org)[b]	• Combined multidisciplinary educational-behavioral wellness intervention embedded in curriculum in 7th graders taught by classroom teachers over 4–5 mo to build skills in healthy choices[105]
After school	• SPARK after school[b] (www.SPARKPE.org) • Move More North Carolina: Recommended Standards for After-School Physical Activity[b]	• As for SPARK, targeting after-school settings • Recommended standards for after-school programs to increase and enhance quality of PA time[106]

[a] Evidence or existing systematic review to support the strategies included in this program.
[b] Addresses components with supporting evidence but further studies needed.

and enduring influence in children's lives… The health and well-being of children are inextricably linked to their parents' physical, emotional and social health, social circumstances, and child-rearing practices."[109] Inclusion of the family is established as the gold standard of treatment.[74] The same can and should be said for the

Box 4
Review of policy and environmental interventions to prevent obesity

• Improve attitudes and norms to support healthy energy balance
• Make healthy options for physical activity and nutrition easy and the default choices
• Reduce barriers to making healthy nutrition and physical activity choices
• Substantial progress has been made—policy changes are underway and are being evaluated

prevention of obesity. As discussed previously, a child's risk of obesity is greatly influenced by parental weight status. Although the genetic contribution to a child's weight is great, the environmental influence is likely greater: parental obesity can predict genetic susceptibility, but a child's environment can determine the expression and severity of that risk.[110] Despite any genetic predisposition to obesity, the environment is likely the greatest potentially modifiable determinant of obesity, with the family being the most proximate of that environment. Determining exact familial components contributing to a child's weight is difficult, however, given the changing nature of families over the past few decades and the complexity of studying and conceptualizing families.[111] As currently understood, family-related risk factors for childhood obesity include[112]

- Minority ethnic and cultural background
- Single-parent household
- Lower maternal education
- Parent obesity status and family history of obesity
- Poverty: receipt of supplemental food assistance
- Higher levels of television viewing of family, particularly during meals, and amounts and locations (bedrooms) of television viewing
- Restrictive parental feeding practices

Of these risk factors (of a total of 22 studied), parental feeding practices and parent BMI were most associated with child weight status (child sleep duration was also determined significantly associated).[112] These findings are preliminary, because the extensive, long-term studies necessary to link risk with later obesity development have not yet been performed. Clinicians should customize risk assessments to each family, knowing that sound anticipatory guidance can be safely provided to all families regardless of weight status and risk for later obesity.

Parenting styles and the risk of childhood obesity have been investigated extensively, although there are many areas still in need of study. As with many aspects of complex problems, such as childhood obesity, long-term definitive studies are lacking. Research over the past decade, however, has provided useful information about this interaction.[113–117] Parenting styles are based on 2 dimensions of parenting: (1) demandingness, or demand for child self-control, and (2) responsiveness, or sensitivity and emotional involvement. With a 2 × 2 table, this gives 4 distinct parenting styles: authoritative, authoritarian, permissive, and neglectful (**Table 4**). Authoritative parents had children with the lowest prevalence of obesity in Rhee's study of 1st graders, whereas authoritarian, or strict disciplinarian, parents had children with the highest prevalence of obesity, more than even permissive or neglectful parents.[117] These findings are important, because parents of children with obesity could be

Table 4
Parenting styles

	High Expectations for Self-Control	Low Expectations for Self-Control
High Sensitivity	Authoritative: respects child's opinions but with clear boundaries	Permissive: minimal discipline, indulgent of child
Low Sensitivity	Authoritarian: strict, significant discipline	Neglectful: no boundaries or discipline, minimally involved with child

Data from Refs.[115–117]

Box 5
Review of the family's role in preventing pediatric obesity

- Include the entire family in obesity prevention and treatment
- Act as positive role models to children regarding healthy nutrition, physical activity, and emotional and social health
- Practice authoritative, not authoritarian, parenting styles
- Have a nonrestrictive approach to early childhood feeding
- Provide structure
- Have regular family meals

---

more likely to institute dieting or restrictive behaviors to help their children lose weight. Although this has not been proved or extensively studied, it provides guidance to clinicians and parents encouraging an authoritative approach to parenting, specifically feeding, their children. A nonrestrictive approach to early childhood feeding, while providing structure and healthy meals, is important for parents of young children to ensure healthy eating habits.

The bulk of parenting research and prevention of childhood obesity relates to early childhood feeding, although many principles can likely be extended to older age groups. Analysis of an older study identified the importance of healthy parenting skills, even if the focus is not obesity or weight-related behaviors.[73] Brotman and colleagues[73] reviewed outcomes of children at high risk for behavioral problems and high risk for obesity. These children and their parents were part of an intervention aimed to improve parenting skills at age 4, then followed for 3 to 5 years. The intervention group had significantly lower prevalence of obesity as well as healthier nutrition and activity habits than control groups, despite the intervention not having a focus on nutrition, activity, or weight. Another representation of the importance of family is the influence of regular family meals, which seem to improve the nutritional status and weight of children[118] and bleeds over to improve family relationships and decrease risky behaviors.[119] Positive interaction between members during family meals may contribute just as much to these positive outcomes as changes in nutritional intake.[118]

Despite this promising research, there are no clear answers on how to become an obesity-resistant family. Future research must account for the complexity of families and may use established approaches, such as family systems theory, which views the family as more than the sum of its parts and respects its complex dynamics and function.[111] Increasing focus on family dynamics and communication will be key to successfully preventing childhood obesity within the context of the family (**Box 5**).

SUMMARY

Childhood obesity is a complex medical issue, representing the interplay of physical and environmental factors. The neuroendocrine control of weight includes multiple situations where genetic variation can influence a person's weight status. Unfortunately, the unhealthy evolution of food and activity environments has placed children at a higher risk for obesity and associated weight problems than they have ever been. Although significantly more research is needed to optimize these strategies, interventions at the level of the pediatrician, school, government, and family have shown success in the prevention of childhood obesity.

REFERENCES

1. Ogden CL, Carroll MD, Kit BK, et al. Prevalence of childhood and adult obesity in the United States, 2011–2012. JAMA 2014;311(8):806–14.
2. Skinner AC, Skelton JA. Prevalence and trends in obesity and severe obesity among children in the United States, 1999–2012. JAMA Pediatr 2014;168(6): 561–6.
3. Field AE, Cook NR, Gillman MW. Weight status in childhood as a predictor of becoming overweight or hypertensive in early adulthood. Obes Res 2005; 13(1):163–9.
4. Guo SS, Wu W, Chumlea WC, et al. Predicting overweight and obesity in adulthood from body mass index values in childhood and adolescence. Am J Clin Nutr 2002;76(3):653–8.
5. Inge TH, King WC, Jenkins TM, et al. The effect of obesity in adolescence on adult health status. Pediatrics 2013;132(6):1098–104.
6. Whitaker RC, Wright JA, Pepe MS, et al. Predicting obesity in young adulthood from childhood and parental obesity. N Engl J Med 1997;337(13):869–73.
7. Kim G, Caprio S. Diabetes and insulin resistance in pediatric obesity. Pediatr Clin North Am 2011;58(6):1355–61, ix.
8. Cook S, Kavey RE. Dyslipidemia and pediatric obesity. Pediatr Clin North Am 2011;58(6):1363–73, ix.
9. Mencin AA, Lavine JE. Advances in pediatric nonalcoholic fatty liver disease. Pediatr Clin North Am 2011;58(6):1375–92, x.
10. Wang YC, McPherson K, Marsh T, et al. Health and economic burden of the projected obesity trends in the USA and the UK. Lancet 2011;378(9793): 815–25.
11. Cawley J. The economics of childhood obesity. Health Aff 2010;29(3):364–71.
12. Vander Wal JS, Mitchell ER. Psychological complications of pediatric obesity. Pediatr Clin North Am 2011;58(6):1393–401, x.
13. Garn SM, Clark DC, Lowe CU, et al. Trends in fatness and the origins of obesity. Pediatrics 1976;57(4):443–56.
14. Agras WS, Mascola AJ. Risk factors for childhood overweight. Curr Opin Pediatr 2005;17(5):648–52.
15. Birch LL, Fisher JO. Development of eating behaviors among children and adolescents. Pediatrics 1998;101(3 Pt 2):539–49.
16. Birch LL, Davison KK. Family environmental factors influencing the developing behavioral controls of food intake and childhood overweight. Pediatr Clin North Am 2001;48(4):893–907.
17. Savona-Ventura C, Savona-Ventura S. The inheritance of obesity. Best Pract Res Clin Obstet Gynaecol 2014;29(3):300–8.
18. Mason K, Page L, Balikcioglu PG. Screening for hormonal, monogenic, and syndromic disorders in obese infants and children. Pediatr Ann 2014;43(9): e218–24.
19. Ohri-Vachaspati P, DeLia D, DeWeese RS, et al. The relative contribution of layers of the Social Ecological Model to childhood obesity. Public Health Nutr 2014;1–12 [Epub ahead of print].
20. Ogata BN, Hayes D. Position of the academy of nutrition and dietetics: nutrition guidance for healthy children ages 2 to 11 years. J Acad Nutr Diet 2014;114(8): 1257–76.
21. Davis MM, Gance-Cleveland B, Hassink S, et al. Recommendations for prevention of childhood obesity. Pediatrics 2007;120(Suppl 4):S229–53.

22. Field AE, Gillman MW, Rosner B, et al. Association between fruit and vegetable intake and change in body mass index among a large sample of children and adolescents in the United States. Int J Obes Relat Metab Disord 2003;27(7): 821–6.
23. Pan L, Li R, Park S, et al. A longitudinal analysis of sugar-sweetened beverage intake in infancy and obesity at 6 years. Pediatrics 2014;134(Suppl 1):S29–35.
24. Lee V. Promising strategies for creating healthy eating and active living environments. Convergence Partnership; 2011.
25. Seo DC, King MH, Kim N, et al. Predictors for persistent overweight, deteriorated weight status, and improved weight status during 18 months in a school-based longitudinal cohort. Am J Health Promot 2014. [Epub ahead of print].
26. Gleason PM, Dodd AH. School breakfast program but not school lunch program participation is associated with lower body mass index. J Am Diet Assoc 2009; 109(2):S118–28.
27. Timlin MT, Pereira MA, Story M, et al. Breakfast eating and weight change in a 5-year prospective analysis of adolescents: project EAT (Eating Among Teens). Pediatrics 2008;121(3):e638–45.
28. Obregón AM, Pettinelli PP, Santos JL. Childhood obesity and eating behaviour. J Pediatr Endocrinol Metab 2015;28(5–6):497–502.
29. Larson N, Story M. A review of snacking patterns among children and adolescents: what are the implications of snacking for weight status? Child Obes 2013;9(2):104–15.
30. Must A, Tybor D. Physical activity and sedentary behavior: a review of longitudinal studies of weight and adiposity in youth. Int J Obes (Lond) 2005;29: S84–96.
31. Chaput JP, Lambert M, Mathieu ME, et al. Physical activity vs sedentary time: independent associations with adiposity in children. Pediatr Obes 2012;7(3): 251–8.
32. Drake KM, Beach ML, Longacre MR, et al. Influence of sports, physical education, and active commuting to school on adolescent weight status. Pediatrics 2012;130(2):e296–304.
33. Tremblay MS, LeBlanc AG, Kho ME, et al. Systematic review of sedentary behaviour and health indicators in school-aged children and youth. Int J Behav Nutr Phys Act 2011;8(1):98.
34. Chahal H, Fung C, Kuhle S, et al. Availability and night-time use of electronic entertainment and communication devices are associated with short sleep duration and obesity among Canadian children. Pediatr Obes 2013;8(1):42–51.
35. Appelhans BM, Fitzpatrick SL, Li H, et al. The home environment and childhood obesity in low-income households: indirect effects via sleep duration and screen time. BMC Public Health 2014;14(1):1160.
36. Bell JF, Zimmerman FJ. Shortened nighttime sleep duration in early life and subsequent childhood obesity. Arch Pediatr Adolesc Med 2010;164(9):840–5.
37. Al Mamun A, Lawlor DA, Cramb S, et al. Do childhood sleeping problems predict obesity in young adulthood? Evidence from a prospective birth cohort study. Am J Epidemiol 2007;166(12):1368–73.
38. Anderson SE, Whitaker RC. Household routines and obesity in US preschool-aged children. Pediatrics 2010;125(3):420–8.
39. Wilson SM, Sato AF. Stress and paediatric obesity: what we know and where to go. Stress Health 2014;30(2):91–102.
40. Evans GW, Fuller-Rowell TE, Doan SN. Childhood cumulative risk and obesity: the mediating role of self-regulatory ability. Pediatrics 2012;129(1):e68–73.

41. Fuemmeler BF, Dedert E, McClernon FJ, et al. Adverse childhood events are associated with obesity and disordered eating: results from a US population-based survey of young adults. J Trauma Stress 2009;22(4):329–33.

42. Heerman WJ, Bian A, Shintani A, et al. Interaction between maternal prepregnancy body mass index and gestational weight gain shapes infant growth. Acad Pediatr 2014;14(5):463–70.

43. Weng SF, Redsell SA, Swift JA, et al. Systematic review and meta-analyses of risk factors for childhood overweight identifiable during infancy. Arch Dis Child 2012;97(12):1019–26.

44. Yu Z, Han S, Zhu J, et al. Pre-pregnancy body mass index in relation to infant birth weight and offspring overweight/obesity: a systematic review and meta-analysis. PLoS One 2013;8(4):e61627.

45. Lau EY, Liu J, Archer E, et al. Maternal weight gain in pregnancy and risk of obesity among offspring: a systematic review. J Obes 2014;2014:524939.

46. Institute of Medicine. Weight gain during pregnancy: reexamining the guidelines. Washington, DC: The National Academies Press; 2009.

47. Adair LS. Child and adolescent obesity: epidemiology and developmental perspectives. Physiol Behav 2008;94(1):8–16.

48. Li H, Zhou Y, Liu J. The impact of cesarean section on offspring overweight and obesity: a systematic review and meta-analysis. Int J Obes (Lond) 2012;37(7):893–9.

49. Møller SE, Ajslev TA, Andersen CS, et al. Risk of childhood overweight after exposure to tobacco smoking in prenatal and early postnatal life. PLoS One 2014;9(10):e109184.

50. Oken E, Levitan E, Gillman M. Maternal smoking during pregnancy and child overweight: systematic review and meta-analysis. Int J Obes (Lond) 2007;32(2):201–10.

51. Li D, Ferber J, Odouli R. Maternal caffeine intake during pregnancy and risk of obesity in offspring: a prospective cohort study. Int J Obes (Lond) 2015;39(4):658–64.

52. Imai CM, Gunnarsdottir I, Thorisdottir B, et al. Associations between infant feeding practice prior to six months and body mass index at six years of age. Nutrients 2014;6(4):1608–17.

53. Oddy WH, Mori TA, Huang R-C, et al. Early infant feeding and adiposity risk: from infancy to adulthood. Ann Nutr Metab 2014;64(3–4):262–70.

54. Vehapoglu A, Demir AD, Turkmen S, et al. Early infant feeding practice and childhood obesity: the relation of breast-feeding and timing of solid food introduction with childhood obesity. J Pediatr Endocrinol Metab 2014;27(11–12):1181–7.

55. Jing H, Xu H, Wan J, et al. Effect of breastfeeding on childhood BMI and obesity: the China family panel studies. Medicine 2014;93(10):e55.

56. Li R, Fein SB, Grummer-Strawn LM. Do infants fed from bottles lack self-regulation of milk intake compared with directly breastfed infants? Pediatrics 2010;125(6):e1386–93.

57. Pearce J, Langley-Evans S. The types of food introduced during complementary feeding and risk of childhood obesity: a systematic review. Int J Obes (Lond) 2013;37(4):477–85.

58. Pearce J, Taylor M, Langley-Evans S. Timing of the introduction of complementary feeding and risk of childhood obesity: a systematic review. Int J Obes (Lond) 2013;37(10):1295–306.

59. Grote V, Theurich M. Complementary feeding and obesity risk. Curr Opin Clin Nutr Metab Care 2014;17(3):273–7.

60. Bailey LC, Forrest CB, Zhang P, et al. Association of antibiotics in infancy with early childhood obesity. JAMA Pediatr 2014;168(11):1063–9.
61. Anzman-Frasca S, Stifter CA, Birch LL. Temperament and childhood obesity risk: a review of the literature. J Dev Behav Pediatr 2012;33(9):732–45.
62. Bergmeier H, Skouteris H, Horwood S, et al. Associations between child temperament, maternal feeding practices and child body mass index during the preschool years: a systematic review of the literature. Obes Rev 2014;15(1):9–18.
63. Bonuck KA, Huang V, Fletcher J. Inappropriate bottle use: an early risk for overweight? Literature review and pilot data for a bottle-weaning trial. Matern Child Nutr 2010;6(1):38–52.
64. Bonuck K, Avraham SB, Lo Y, et al. Bottle-weaning intervention and toddler overweight. J Pediatr 2014;164(2):306–12.e1–2.
65. Wahi G, Parkin PC, Beyene J, et al. Effectiveness of interventions aimed at reducing screen time in children: a systematic review and meta-analysis of randomized controlled trials. Arch Pediatr Adolesc Med 2011;165(11):979–86.
66. Hughes AR, Sherriff A, Ness AR, et al. Timing of adiposity rebound and adiposity in adolescence. Pediatrics 2014;134(5):e1354–61.
67. Moreno JP, Johnston CA, Chen TA, et al. Seasonal variability in weight change during elementary school. Obesity (Silver Spring) 2015;23(2):422–8.
68. Baranowski T, O'Connor T, Johnston C, et al. School year versus summer differences in child weight gain: a narrative review. Child Obes 2014;10(1):18–24.
69. Lamboglia CM, da Silva VT, de Vasconcelos Filho JE, et al. Exergaming as a strategic tool in the fight against childhood obesity: a systematic review. J Obes 2013;2013:438364.
70. Chen JL, Wilkosz ME. Efficacy of technology-based interventions for obesity prevention in adolescents: a systematic review. Adolesc Health Med Ther 2014;5:159.
71. Badaly D. Peer similarity and influence for weight-related outcomes in adolescence: a meta-analytic review. Clin Psychol Rev 2013;33(8):1218–36.
72. Salvy SJ, De La Haye K, Bowker JC, et al. Influence of peers and friends on children's and adolescents' eating and activity behaviors. Physiol Behav 2012; 106(3):369–78.
73. Brotman LM, Dawson-McClure S, Huang KY, et al. Early childhood family intervention and long-term obesity prevention among high-risk minority youth. Pediatrics 2012;129(3):e621–8.
74. Barlow SE, Expert C. Expert committee recommendations regarding the prevention, assessment, and treatment of child and adolescent overweight and obesity: summary report. Pediatrics 2007;120(Suppl 4):S164–92.
75. Whitlock EP, Williams SB, Gold R, et al. Screening and interventions for childhood overweight: a summary of evidence for the US Preventive Services Task Force. Pediatrics 2005;116(1):e125–44.
76. Whitlock EP, O'Connor EA, Williams SB, et al. Effectiveness of weight management interventions in children: a targeted systematic review for the USPSTF. Pediatrics 2010;125(2):e396–418.
77. Resnicow K, Davis R, Rollnick S. Motivational interviewing for pediatric obesity: conceptual issues and evidence review. J Am Diet Assoc 2006;106(12): 2024–33.
78. Schwartz RP, Hamre R, Dietz WH, et al. Office-based motivational interviewing to prevent childhood obesity: a feasibility study. Arch Pediatr Adolesc Med 2007;161(5):495–501.
79. Schwartz RP. Motivational interviewing (patient-centered counseling) to address childhood obesity. Pediatr Ann 2010;39(3):154–8.

80. Whitlock EP, O'Conner EA, Williams SB, et al. Effectiveness of primary care interventions for weight management in children and adolescents: An Updated, Targeted Systematic Review for the USPSTF [Internet]. Rockville (MD): Agency for Healthcare Research and Quality (US); 2010.

81. Birch LL, Fisher JO, Davison KK. Learning to overeat: maternal use of restrictive feeding practices promotes girls' eating in the absence of hunger. Am J Clin Nutr 2003;78(2):215–20.

82. Krebs NF, Jacobson MS. Prevention of pediatric overweight and obesity. Pediatrics 2003;112(2):424–30.

83. Owen CG, Martin RM, Whincup PH, et al. Effect of infant feeding on the risk of obesity across the life course: a quantitative review of published evidence. Pediatrics 2005;115(5):1367–77.

84. Robinson TN, Kiernan M, Matheson DM, et al. Is parental control over children's eating associated with childhood obesity? results from a population-based sample of third graders. Obes Res 2001;9(5):306–12.

85. Satter E. The feeding relationship: problems and interventions. J Pediatr 1990; 117(2):S181–9.

86. Strong WB, Malina RM, Blimkie CJ, et al. Evidence based physical activity for school-age youth. J Pediatr 2005;146(6):732–7.

87. Tan CC, Holub SC. Maternal feeding practices associated with food neophobia. Appetite 2012;59(2):483–7.

88. Ekstein S, Laniado D, Glick B. Does picky eating affect weight-for-length measurements in young children? Clin Pediatr 2010;49(3):217–20.

89. Hagan JF, Shaw JS, Duncan PM. Bright futures: guidelines for health supervision of infants, children, and adolescents. Elk Grove Village (IL): American Academy of Pediatrics; 2008.

90. Eneli IU, Crum PA, Tylka TL. The trust model: a different feeding paradigm for managing childhood obesity. Obesity (Silver Spring) 2008;16(10):2197–204.

91. Krebs NF, Himes JH, Jacobson D, et al. Assessment of child and adolescent overweight and obesity. Pediatrics 2007;120(Suppl 4):S193–228.

92. Agras WS, Hammer LD, McNicholas F, et al. Risk factors for childhood overweight: a prospective study from birth to 9.5 years. J Pediatr 2004;145(1):20–5.

93. Bodenheimer T, Wagner EH, Grumbach K. Improving primary care for patients with chronic illness: the chronic care model, Part 2. JAMA 2002;288(15):1909–14.

94. Davison KK, Birch LL. Childhood overweight: a contextual model and recommendations for future research. Obes Rev 2001;2(3):159–71.

95. Institute of Medicine, Committee of Accelerating Progress in Obesity Prevention, Glickman D. Accelerating progress in obesity prevention: solving the weight of the nation. Washington, DC: National Academies Press; 2012.

96. Brennan LK, Brownson RC, Orleans CT. Childhood obesity policy research and practice: evidence for policy and environmental strategies. Am J Prev Med 2014;46(1):e1–16.

97. Bandura A. Social foundations of thought and action. Englewood Cliffs (NJ): Prentice-Hall, Inc; 1986.

98. Deci EL, Ryan RM. Self-determination theory: a macrotheory of human motivation, development, and health. Can Psychol 2008;49(3):182.

99. Prochaska JO, Velicer WF. The transtheoretical model of health behavior change. Am J Health Promot 1997;12(1):38–48.

100. Glasgow RE, Vogt TM, Boles SM. Evaluating the public health impact of health promotion interventions: the RE-AIM framework. Am J Public Health 1999;89(9): 1322–7.

101. Leeman J, Sommers J, Leung MM, et al. Disseminating evidence from research and practice: a model for selecting evidence to guide obesity prevention. J Public Health Manag Pract 2011;17(2):133–40.
102. Katz DL, O'Connell M, Yeh MC, et al. Public health strategies for preventing and controlling overweight and obesity in school and worksite settings. MMWR Recomm Rep 2005;54(RR-10):1–12.
103. World Health Organization. Population-based approaches to childhood obesity prevention. Geneva: WHO; 2012.
104. Luepker RV, Perry CL, McKinlay SM, et al. Outcomes of a field trial to improve children's dietary patterns and physical activity: the Child and Adolescent Trial for Cardiovascular Health (CATCH). JAMA 1996;275(10):768–76.
105. Lazorick S, Crawford Y, Gilbird A, et al. Long-term obesity prevention and the Motivating Adolescents with Technology to CHOOSE Health™ program. Child Obes 2014;10(1):25–33.
106. Moore JB, Schneider L, Lazorick S, et al. Rationale and development of the move more north carolina: recommended standards for after-school physical activity. J Public Health Manag Pract 2010;16(4):359–66.
107. McGuire S. US Department of Agriculture and US Department of Health and Human Services, Dietary Guidelines for Americans, 2010. Washington, DC: US Government Printing Office, January 2011. Adv Nutr 2011;2(3):293–4.
108. S.3307, 111th Congress of the United States (2009–10). Healthy, Hunger-Free Kids Act of 2010.
109. Schor EL, American Academy of Pediatrics Task Force on the Family. Family pediatrics: report of the task force on the family. Pediatrics 2003;111(6 Pt 2): 1541–71.
110. Barsh GS, Farooqi IS, O'Rahilly S. Genetics of body-weight regulation. Nature 2000;404(6778):644–51.
111. Skelton JA, Buehler C, Irby MB, et al. Where are family theories in family-based obesity treatment?: conceptualizing the study of families in pediatric weight management. Int J Obes (Lond) 2012;36(7):891–900.
112. Dev DA, McBride BA, Fiese BH, et al. Behalf Of The Strong Kids Research T. Risk factors for overweight/obesity in preschool children: an ecological approach. Child Obes 2013;9(5):399–408.
113. Baumrind D. Current patterns of parental authority. Developmental Psychology Monographs 1971;4:101–3.
114. Baumrind D. Rearing competent children. In: Damon W, editor. Child development today and tomorrow. San Francisco (CA): Jossey-Bass; 1989. p. 349–78.
115. Maccoby E, Martin J. Socialization in the context of the family: parent-child interaction. In: Hetherington E, editor. Handbook of child psychology: socialization, personality and social development. New York: Wiley; 1983. p. 1–101.
116. Rhee K. Childhood overweight and the relationship between parent behaviors, parenting style, and family functioning. Ann Am Acad Pol Soc Sci 2008;615: 11–37.
117. Rhee KE, Lumeng JC, Appugliese DP, et al. Parenting styles and overweight status in first grade. Pediatrics 2006;117(6):2047–54.
118. Hammons AJ, Fiese BH. Is frequency of shared family meals related to the nutritional health of children and adolescents? Pediatrics 2011;127(6):e1565–74.
119. Skeer MR, Ballard EL. Are family meals as good for youth as we think they are? A review of the literature on family meals as they pertain to adolescent risk prevention. J Youth Adolesc 2013;42(7):943–63.

Legal Care as Part of Health Care

The Benefits of Medical-Legal Partnership

Johnna S. Murphy, MPH[a],*, Ellen M. Lawton, JD[b],
Megan Sandel, MD, MPH[c]

KEYWORDS

- Medical-legal partnership • Social determinants • Health • Legal needs • Clinics

KEY POINTS

- Despite legal needs being so common in low-income families and having such a strong impact on health and well-being, information about legal needs and hardships is not considered in most health care practices; access to legal expertise and interventions is not often integrated into practice.
- Emerging practices highlight the proposition that aligning legal and health care through medical-legal partnership can help communities/health care institutions lower barriers to basic needs to improve access to care.
- The medical-legal partnership approach in the clinic setting combines the knowledge, training, and resources of health care, public health, and legal professionals and staff to address and prevent the social determinants of health caused by legal needs.

MANY SOCIAL DETERMINANTS ARE LEGAL NEEDS WITH LEGAL REMEDIES

Many of the social determinants of health can be traced back to laws that are unfairly applied or underenforced. Lack of access to public services and benefits constitute legal problems that affect individual and population health. The impact of the denial of benefits and unfair application of the law is especially common in vulnerable populations, including low-income families. For example, pest infestation, which is linked to asthma rates in rental housing, violates local and state sanitary codes. If the sanitary

The article is an original work, has not been previously published, and is not under consideration for publication elsewhere. The authors have read and approved the article for journal submission.
[a] Division of General Pediatrics, Boston Medical Center, 88 East Newton Street, Vose Hall 3, Boston, MA 02118, USA; [b] National Center for Medical-Legal Partnership, Department of Health Policy and Management, Milken Institute School of Public Health, The George Washington University, 2175 K Street, NW, 513A, Washington, DC 20037, USA; [c] Pediatrics, Boston University School of Medicine, Boston Medical Center, 88 East Newton Street, Vose Hall 3, Boston, MA 02118, USA
* Corresponding author.
E-mail address: johnna.murphy@bmc.org

code is not enforced, then asthma rates can worsen. When families are wrongfully denied nutritional benefits like the Supplemental Nutrition Assistance Program (SNAP), they are at risk for malnutrition and other poor health outcomes.[1] Therefore, when these laws are not properly enforced, families risk health consequences.

Studies have shown a significant correlation between legal needs and health. Indeed, the overlap between rates of legal needs for low-income populations and poor health outcomes for low-income populations reinforces the axis between legal needs and poor health. Hardships associated with poverty (including hunger,[2] safety,[3] and substandard housing[4]) directly influence health.[5] These social determinants of health require some level of legal care/intervention to prevent poor health outcomes. The civil legal problems of low-income families, such as protection from abusive relationships, safe and healthy housing, access to necessary health care benefits and services, and family law issues, such as child support and custody, constitute basic human needs. Emerging practices highlight the proposition that aligning legal and health care through medical-legal partnership (MLP) can help communities/health care institutions lower barriers to basic needs improve access to care.[6]

PREVALENCE OF LEGAL NEEDS IN LOW-INCOME POPULATIONS

With 1 in 6 people living in poverty, the need for more/new impactful/powerful strategies to address the links between poverty and health is overwhelming.[7] Studies show that most vulnerable individuals have at least one civil legal problem that negatively affects their health; national[8] and state[9] data suggest that most low-income people experience at least 2 legal needs, and most of these needs are not addressed. This translates to more than 50 million Americans who have some sort of legal need, usually derived from the most basic human needs as detailed earlier.

Small-scale/preliminary/pilot studies indicate that legal needs are widely distributed, of long duration, and detrimental to patient health. For example, at a clinic in Tucson, Arizona, providers screened and referred 104 low-income patients for a single legal matter; at the subsequent legal intake, 170 discrete legal matters were identified, ranging from housing concerns to health insurance coverage to finances. Pediatric providers at a Baltimore hospital found similar results when surveying parents about legal concerns, with employment and education being the most prevalent. Like health needs, legal needs occur along a continuum; some problems can be successfully resolved with social resources and referrals that are guided by trained legal experts; but other legal needs can escalate to legal crises if not addressed early by legal experts. For example, families at risk of eviction for nonpayment of rent, perhaps because of job loss, may be able to rely temporarily on community safety-net resources for rental payments. But a family who has longer-term income struggles may require a lawyer to negotiate a payment plan with their landlord or secure other resources or benefits.

BRIDGING THE DIVIDE: THE LEGAL AND HEALTH CARE SYSTEMS/COMMUNITIES

Legal needs that address social determinants of health have traditionally been addressed by the legal community, with minimal input or feedback from the health care community beyond the provision of basic evidence for people with disabilities seeking public benefits. In 2012, 8100 publicly funded civil legal aid attorneys and paralegals handled legal problems for more than 800,000 low-income and vulnerable people; a significant number of those problems were legal issues linked to health most frequently related to safety and domestic violence; safe housing, including unlawful evictions and landlord-tenant issues; and income maintenance concerns, including obtaining and maintain disability benefits.[10] Despite those linkages between health and legal needs, the impact of legal interventions on individual and family health is not tracked.[11]

Despite legal needs being so common in low-income families and having such a strong impact on health and well-being, information about legal needs and hardships is not considered in most health care practices; access to legal expertise and interventions is not often integrated into practice. This circumstance might be because health care staff do not consider these concerns to be related to health; but given the emerging understanding of social determinants of health, it is more likely that physicians and other clinical staff do not have the time, staff expertise or capacity, or resources needed to respond to legal concerns. Some clinics have staff, whether clinical, paraprofessional, or volunteer, who might try to navigate the legal issues faced by their vulnerable families; but they are not trained to address the underlying legal problems or they risk exacerbating the legal problem. Amid this constellation of emerging awareness of legal needs, alongside confronting the dramatic lack of community legal resources to support vulnerable families, the MLP approach has flourished as a strategy to build capacity inside the 4 walls of the health care clinic while bridging with a community partner who holds singular expertise to address, and eliminate, the social determinants of health.

ACCESSING LEGAL SUPPORT

National studies continually document both the inability of low-income people to ascertain when they have a legal need that requires a legal expert as well as the utter lack of sufficient resources for people with legal needs.

Barriers to civil legal aid access include patients not thinking their concerns were a legal issue, being unaware of how to access legal resources, and perceiving legal assistance will not be helpful. With the exception of one family, most of the families who did access legal support found it ineffective.[12]

THE MEDICAL-LEGAL PARTNERSHIP RESPONSE

The MLP approach in the clinical settings combines the knowledge, training, and resources of health care, public health, and legal professionals and staff to address and prevent the social determinants of health caused by legal needs.

The partnership between clinical and legal staff established through MLP facilitates the identification and correction of potential legal barriers to individual and family health. Attorneys and paralegals train health care providers to recognize the connections between unmet legal needs and health and develop screening questions for patients. Health and legal team members work together to address the identified legal needs. Effective, sustainable MLPs use shared data and expertise to respond to the social determinants of health in 4 ways:

- TRAIN health care, public health, and legal teams to work collaboratively and identify legal and social needs upstream
- TREAT individual patients' health-harming social and legal needs with legal care ranging from triage and consultations to legal representation
- TRANSFORM clinic practice and institutional policies to better respond to patients' health-harming social and legal needs
- PREVENT health-harming legal needs broadly by detecting patterns and improving policies and regulations that have an impact on population health.[13]

MLP uses the acronym I-HELP (Income, Housing and utilities, Education and employment, Legal status, and Personal stability) to identify the most common social determinants of health impacted by legal need and to identify ways in which an MLP can benefit families facing these concerns[5] (**Table 1**).

BENEFITS OF MEDICAL-LEGAL PARTNERSHIP FOR PATIENTS AND FAMILIES
Treatment of Chronic Disease

Asthma
Housing is an important and adverse social condition with legal remedy. In some housing cases, legal advice or representation might be needed to advocate for residents. A primary objective of MLP is to ensure patients have access to the necessary legal expertise to address environmental hazards that, if corrected, would improve the health of the child with asthma. Using legal form letters for clinicians to ask landlords to change conditions is an example of how MLP can address housing conditions.[14]

A New York clinic studied the effect of an MLP intervention to force landlords into providing better living conditions for patients with poorly controlled asthma. Patients with poorly controlled asthma and self-reported household allergen exposure received legal assistance to improve their housing, including fixing leaks, exterminating pests, or providing a different apartment. Of the 12 patients with data available, emergency department visits and hospitalizations decreased by 91% and the use of systemic steroids also decreased. MLP is highly effective in improving the control of inner-city asthmatic patients by effecting improvements in the domestic environment.[15]

In 2008, Cincinnati Children's Hospital Medical Center and the Legal Aid Society of Greater Cincinnati launched the Cincinnati Child Health Law Partnership in 3 pediatric primary care centers that served mostly low-income populations. During the 3-year study period, 1808 referrals were made; those referred were more likely to have asthma. Housing was the most common issue for referrals; 89% of referrals had positive legal outcomes, affected nearly 6000 children and adults, and translated into nearly 200,000 in recovered benefits. Forty-two percent of those followed reported improved housing conditions or prevented homelessness.[16]

Sickle Cell Disease
In Atlanta, a pediatric-based MLP used a legal intervention in pediatric patients with sickle cell disease to determine if legal interventions related to the social determinants of health would positively affect the child's sickle cell disease. Legal problems associated with poverty can potentially affect the health and well-being of the patients and families affected by sickle cell disease who depend on the system of health care to manage their chronic disease and address acute health issues. The Health Law Partnership (HeLP) retrospectively looked at all patients with the diagnosis of sickle cell disease who had been treated by HeLP within 6 years. Seventy-one parents of children with sickle cell disease were referred for legal intervention, and 106 legal needs were identified among these parents. Of these 106 cases, 99 were closed, with 21 resulting in a measurable gain in benefits. In a cohort of families of children with sickle cell disease, access to legal care resulted in a positive impact on patients and parents.[17]

Compliance with Health Care
Patients in a pilot study in California showed increased benefits and better compliance with health care after legal needs were met as part of routine health care in a pediatric practice. A pilot 36-month prospective cohort study of the impact of legal services was

Table 1
I-HELP

	Common Social Determinant of Health	Civil Legal Aid Interventions That Help	Impact of Civil Legal Aid Intervention on Health/Health Care
I-HELP Issue			
Income	Availability of resources to meet daily basic needs	Benefits unit Appeal denials of food stamps, health insurance, cash benefits, and disability benefits	1. Increasing someone's income means she or he makes fewer trade-offs between affording food and health care, including medications. 2. Being able to afford enough healthy food helps people manage chronic diseases and helps children grow and develop.
Housing & utilities	Healthy physical environments	Housing unit Secure housing subsidies, improve substandard conditions, prevent eviction, protect against utility shut off	1. A stable, decent, affordable home helps a person avoid costly emergency department visits related to homelessness. 2. Consistent housing, heat, and electricity helps people follow their medical treatment plans.
Education & employment	Access to the opportunity to learn and work	Education & employment units Secure specialized education services, prevent and remedy employment discrimination and enforce workplace rights	1. A quality education is the single greatest predictor of a person's adult health. 2. Consistent employment helps provide money for food and safe housing, which also helps avoid costly emergency health care services. 3. Access to health insurance is often linked to employment.
Legal status	Access to the opportunity to work	Veterans & immigration units Resolve veteran discharge status, clear criminal/credit histories, assist with asylum applications	1. Clearing a person's criminal history or helping a veteran change their discharge status helps make consistent employment and access to public benefits possible. 2. Consistent employment provides money for food and safe housing, which helps people avoid costly emergency health care services.
Personal & family stability	Exposure to violence	Family law unit Secure restraining orders for domestic violence; secure adoption, custody, and guardianship for children	1. Less violence at home means less need for costly emergency health care services. 2. Stable family relationships significantly reduce stress and allow for better decision making, including decisions related to health care.

From Marple K. Framing legal care as health care from the National Center for Medical-Legal Partnership. Available at: http://medical-legalpartnership.org/new-messaging-guide-helps-frame-legal-care-health-care/. Accessed February 7, 2015; with permission.

conducted to investigate the effectiveness of MLP in pediatrics. The results showed that two-thirds of respondents reported improved child health and well-being caused by increased awareness and use of publicly funded legal aid services resulting in increased access to food and income supports. The study suggests that adding a legal aid attorney to the medical team can increase access to legal and social services and decrease barriers to care.

Sixty-eight percent of participants noted that their issues handled by the legal team were entirely or partially resolved, with those not solved being because of legal restrictions that limited access to successful assistance or slow assistance by referring agencies. There was also a slight increase in well-child checkups.[18]

Reduction of Stress

Chronic stress can be particularly detrimental to health during critical periods, including preconception, maternity, and early childhood development. There is a significant amount of literature describing this mechanism but less literature on how to remedy chronic stress. The MLP approach can effectively and sustainably reduce chronic stressors and their associated negative impact among low-income individuals. Patients in a Tucson study showed decreased stress and improved well-being after receiving legal assistance. Having legal needs met can reduce chronic stress and improve health outcomes in low-income populations.[19]

Beyond Clinics: Healthy Start

The MLP approach has been integrated into Healthy Start initiatives, developed by the US Department of Health and Human Services to address the high infant mortality rate. Healthy Start used community-driven strategies to address the medical, social, behavioral, and cultural needs of high-risk populations with a special focus on maternal and infant care. Recently, 3 Healthy Start projects were awarded funding to collaborate through MLP. Crozer-Keystone Healthy Start (CKHS) is a community-based maternal and child health case management program that is an extension of the Crozer-Keystone Health System.

CKHS staff identify legal needs and appropriately refer CKHS clients to MLP attorneys. Integrating legal services into Healthy Start increases case managers' capacity by alleviating their time and by increasing their capacity to advocate on behalf of clients. Healthy Start case managers and staff provide assistance to program participants in a variety of ways to ensure that their health care and social needs are being met, specifically with regard to having a healthy pregnancy and good birth outcomes. Before MLP integration, Healthy Start case managers would spend an excessive amount of time attempting to resolve participants' complex social needs that often require a legal remedy. Having an attorney on staff allows case managers to refer the most complex issues to the attorney, thereby freeing up time for other participants and issues.

Additionally, through case consultations and trainings, case managers and staff have reported an increase in both knowledge and ability to advocate on behalf of their clients. Being armed with basic information and tools allows them to provide efficient and effective support for their clients.[20]

BENEFITS FOR HEALTH CARE STAFF
Innovative Tools

Increasing fuel costs make it difficult for families to pay for utility services, which can impact health, including children with special health care needs. MLP Boston developed a multistep approach to identify patients in need of comprehensive access to utility service and help them secure utility protection and assistance. MLP developed a training program to help health care staff recognize families in need of utility assistance and provided form letters on the electronic health record to provide patients with necessary documentation. In 2008 and 2009, the number of utility protection letters generated by Boston Medical Center (BMC) Pediatrics Department increased from 193 to 676 letters, a 350% increase. MLP Boston also provided education on utility-related advocacy services to BMC staff and created a utility first aid kit with relevant forms, letters, and policy providing guidance for health care staff regarding their role in ensuring consistent utility access for specific patient populations.[6]

Addressing the health-harming civil legal needs of patients is not the work of attorneys and paralegals alone; it requires involvement from the entire health care team to help screen and treat them. As part of health reform, it is increasingly important that new interventions maximize the effectiveness and efficiency of the existing health care workforce. MLPs need to tell stories and leverage data that show how they (1) increase health care team members' knowledge of social determinants of health; (2) increase the frequency with which health care team members screen for the social determinants of health; (3) allow health care teams to get back to treating medical problems when legal problems are solved; and/or (4) enhance the existing work of case managers, care coordinators, patient navigators, and others.[21]

Improved Health Care Staff Knowledge and Screening Efficacy

MLPs build health care staff knowledge and efficacy through educating health care staff and students about social determinants of health and how they are often intertwined with the law, including advocacy electives, medical school courses, and continuing medical education courses. The MLP approach to health curriculum has been integrated into 29 residency programs nationwide, including pediatric programs, family medicine programs, internal medicine programs, and programs with other specialty programs. In 2009, 25 medical schools participated in MLPs, with 17% having a dedicated MLP course and 20% offering MLP electives. Four partnerships have created joint medical and law student courses.[22–24]

Paul and colleagues[25] evaluated 4 established MLP programs that provided training to health care staff. Ninety-seven of the health care staff in Boston where there is an established MLP reported screening for 2 unmet needs. The Stanford clinic reported reduced concerns about making patients nervous with legal questions (38%–21%), and New York Legal Health reported increasing resident referrals (15%–54%).

A recent study found that after MLP teams trained pediatric residents in Cincinnati, the residents reported increased knowledge and screening for patients' legal issues. A controlled study of an educational intervention whereby the pediatric interns (2008–2009) participated in a new social determinant of health curriculum, with prior-year interns as the control, showed that those who participated in the intervention were more comfortable discussing legal issues (100% vs 71%, $P<.01$) and felt more knowledgeable regarding issues (100% vs 64%). Knowledge was greater in the intervention group post-test in all domains: benefits (72% vs 52%), housing (48% vs 21%), and education (52% vs 33%), with $P<.001$ for all. Intervention interns were more likely to document each issue (benefits 98% vs 60%, housing 93% vs 57%, food 74% vs 56%; $P<.001$ for all). The intervention group had a slightly higher rate of referral to MLP, although the difference did not reach statistical significance.[26]

MLP is at the forefront of training the next generation of health care, public health, and legal professionals to identify and address the root causes of poor health.

SUMMARY

Many of the social determinants of health are rooted in legal problems. MLPs have the potential to positively change clinical systems. This change can be accomplished by integrating legal staff into health care clinics to *educate* staff and residents on social determinants of health and their legal origins, working directly with patients to identify and address legal needs that improve health outcomes and incorporate legal insights and solutions into health care practice where the patient population is overwhelmingly impacted by social determinants of health.

REFERENCES

1. Bachrach D, Pfister H, Wallis K, et al. Addressing patients' social needs: an emerging business case for provider investment. New York: Mannat Health Solutions; 2014.
2. Cook JT, Black M, Chilton M, et al. Are food insecurity's health impacts underestimated in the U.S. population? Marginal food security also predicts adverse health outcomes in young U.S. children and mothers. Adv Nutr 2013;4:51–61.
3. Frank DA, Casey PH, Black MM, et al. Cumulative hardship and wellness of low-income, young children: multisite surveillance study. Pediatrics 2010;5:1115–23.
4. Cutts DB, Meyers AF, Black MM, et al. US housing insecurity and the health of very young children. Am J Public Health 2011;101:1508–14.
5. Kenyon C, Sandel M, Silverstein M, et al. Revisiting the social history for child health. Pediatrics 2007;120:e734–8.
6. Sandel M, Hansen M, Kahn R, et al. Medical-legal partnerships: transforming primary care by addressing the legal needs of vulnerable populations. Health Aff 2010;29:1697–705.
7. United States Department of Commerce, Income, Poverty and Health Insurance in the United States: 2011.
8. Albert H. Cantril, Agenda for access: the American people and civil justice, Am Bar Ass'n '996. AM. BAR ASS'N (May1996).
9. Schulman, Ronca, Bucuvalas, Inc. Massachusetts legal needs survey: findings from a survey of legal needs of low-income households in Massachusetts, vol. 1. New York: Mass Legal Assistance Corp; 2003.
10. Available at: http://www.lsc.gov/sites/lsc.gov/files/LSC/lscgov4/AnnualReports/2012%20Annual%20Report_FINAL-WEB_10.1.pdf. Accessed February 7, 2015.
11. Sandel M, Suther E, Brown C, et al. The MLP vital sign: addressing and managing legal needs in the health care setting. J Leg Med 2014;35(1):41–56.
12. Lawton E, Sandel M. Investing in legal prevention. J Leg Med 2014;35(1):23–39.
13. Available at: http://medical-legalpartnership.org/. Accessed February 7, 2015.
14. Murphy JS, Sandel M. Asthma and social justice: how to get remediation done. Am J Prev Med 2011;41:S57–8.
15. O'Sullivan MM, Brandfield J, Hoskoke SS, et al. Environmental improvements brought by the legal interventions in the homes of poorly controlled inner-city adult asthmatic patients: a proof-of-concept study. J Asthma 2012;49(9):911–7.
16. Klein MD, Beck AF, Henize AW, et al. Doctors and lawyers collaborating to HeLP children-outcomes from a successful partnership between professions. J Health Care Poor Underserved 2013;24:1063–73.

17. Pettignano R, Caley SB, Bliss LR. Medical-legal partnership: impact on patients with sickle cell disease. Pediatrics 2011;128:1482–8.
18. Weintraub D, Rodgers MA, Botcheva L, et al. Pilot study of medical-legal partnership to address social and legal needs of patients. J Health Care Poor Underserved 2010;21:157–68.
19. Ryan AM, Kutob RM, Suther E, et al. Pilot study of impact of medical-legal partnership services on patients' perceived stress and wellbeing. J Health Care Poor Underserved 2012;23:1526–46.
20. Atkins D, Heller SM, DeBartolo E, et al. Medical-legal partnership and healthy start: integrating civil legal aid services into public advocacy. J Leg Med 2014; 35:195–209.
21. Marple, K. Framing legal care as health care: a guide to help civil aid legal practitioners message their work to health care audiences. Available at: http://www.medicalegalpartnership.org. Accessed February 7, 2015.
22. Tobin-Tyler E, Anderson L, Rapport L, et al. Medical-legal partnership in medical education-pathways and opportunities. J Leg Med 2014;35(1):149–77.
23. Benfer EA. Educating the next generation of health leaders: medical-legal partnership and interprofessional graduate education. J Leg Med 2014;35(1):113–48.
24. Tobin-Tyler E, Lawton E, Conroy K, et al, editors. Poverty, health, and law: readings and cases for medical-legal partnership. Durham (NC): Carolina Academic Press; 2011.
25. Paul E, Fortress D, Fullerton BA, et al. Medical-legal partnerships: addressing competency needs through lawyers. J Grad Med Educ 2009;1(2):304–9.
26. Klein MD, Kahn RS, Baker RC, et al. Training in social determinants of health in primary care: does it change resident behavior? Acad Pediatr 2011;11(5): 387–93.

Early Literacy Promotion in the Digital Age

Dipesh Navsaria, MPH, MSLIS, MD[a],*, Lee M. Sanders, MD, MPH[b]

KEYWORDS

- Early literacy • Poverty • Digital media • Reading • Primary care
- Health supervision • Anticipatory guidance

KEY POINTS

- School readiness and educational success is strongly determined by early exposure to print and socioeconomic milieu.
- Early literacy promotion is a key avenue for clinicians to positively influence child development, parenting interactions, and intentional skill building in both child and caregiver.
- Quality children's literature, dialogic reading, and careful support of nurturing relationships in a child's environment are key elements to success.
- Digital media remains an increasingly popular yet not-well-researched exposure starting at younger and younger ages, with a lack of consensus as to how best to advise parents.

The better index of disadvantage for a child is not family income, but how often the child is read to.

—*Nicholas Kristof[1]*

The nation's leading health researchers and public health agencies, not to mention national leaders in economics and national security, have reached consensus on the most cost-effective social factor promoting the nation's health and economic vitality: the quality of early childhood environments before school entry.[2,3] Profound health effects across the life course are strongly and independently associated with home-based exposures during infancy and early childhood, both the negative effects of toxic stress and adverse childhood events as well as the positive and moderating effects of prosocial environments. For pediatric primary care, however, important questions remain. What can the general pediatrician do? What does the pediatrician need to know about these early childhood exposures? What can the pediatrician do to

The authors have nothing to disclose.
[a] Department of Pediatrics, University of Wisconsin School of Medicine and Public Health, 2870 University Avenue, Suite 200, Madison, WI 53705, USA; [b] Department of Pediatrics, Stanford University School of Medicine, 117 Encina Commons, Stanford, CA 94305, USA
* Corresponding author.
E-mail address: dnavsaria@pediatrics.wisc.edu

influence those determinants? What are the implications in the context of expanding income inequality and increasingly early exposure to digital media?

The topic of emergent literacy skills in children has evolved significantly in recent years and has become recognized as not only a vital component of a child's development and early learning but also a marker for other environmental influences, including parent-child engagement. However, that same period has also brought many new questions and challenges with it. How does one ensure that young children living in poverty build literacy skills appropriately so they begin school with skill sets comparable with other children? Across all income groups, how can one advise families well about other forms of media, including interactive digital experiences?

EARLY LITERACY AS A SOCIAL DETERMINANT OF HEALTH

In the United States, more than 1 in 4 children enter kindergarten with poor early literacy skills. These children are not only more likely to live in resource-poor households but also more likely to live in literacy-poor households, among the 17% of children who are not read to on a regular basis.[4] Such disparities in early educational exposures are strongly linked to another dismal fact that has persisted over the past half century: 1 in 4 US children lives in poverty.[5] The American Academy of Pediatrics (AAP) has begun to address child poverty as a key and trenchant determinant of child health.[6] School readiness is strongly associated with the socioeconomic gradient.[7] The language milieu children in lower socioeconomic circumstances inhabit is poorer, with a nearly 30-million-word gap between children being raised in poverty and their more affluent peers (**Table 1**).

Early childhood literacy is one of the proposed mechanisms by which poverty acts as a profound social determinant of child health outcomes, not only to the development of physical health but also to that of cognitive, behavioral, and emotional health. During infancy and early childhood, the physiology of a child in poverty faces toxic stress, defined as prolonged, unremitting stress with limited presence of socioemotional buffering relationships, mediated by disordered cortisol responses. This type of stress is much higher than the typical, normative stress experienced by children in more affluent families.[8] As a result of this toxic stress and associated adverse childhood events, children in poverty are more susceptible to illness and less able to perform adequately in educational settings, where they are more often affected by poor executive functioning, poor short-term memory, anxiety, and other behavioral health conditions.[9] **Fig. 1** shows the sizable difference in reading scores in schools that have a higher percentage of children living in poverty.

Table 1
The difference between low SES and high SES children by age 3 years with respect to vocabulary size, IQ, child-directed utterances, encouragements, and discouragements

1 by Age 3 y	Welfare	Professionals
Vocabulary size	525 words	1100 words
IQ	79	117
Utterances	178/h	487/h
Encouragements	75,000	500,000
Discouragements	200,000	80,000

Abbreviations: IQ, intelligence quotient; SES, socioeconomic status.
From Hart B, Risley TR. Meaningful differences in the everyday experience of young American children. Baltimore: Paul H Brookes Publishing; 1995.

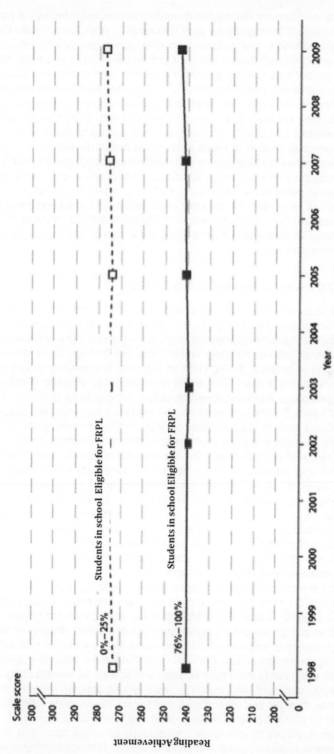

Fig. 1. Average eighth-grade reading achievement scale scores, by percentage of students in school eligible for free or reduced-price lunch: selected years, 1998 through 2009. (*Data from* U.S. Department of Education. National Center for Education Statistics, National Assessment of Educational Progress (NAEP), selected years, 1998 to 2009 Reading Assessments, NAEP Data Explorer.)

Poor early reading skills carry lifelong health consequences, reflected by the continuum from poor emergent literacy during early childhood to poor literacy skills during adolescence and adulthood. The children who enter kindergarten with suboptimal reading skills are at significantly higher risk to be among the children who enter middle school and high school with reading and math skills less than grade level and to be among those who fail to complete high school.[10,11] Children reading less than grade level are at significantly increased risk for serious behavioral and mental health problems.[12] As adults, they are likely to be among the 1 in 3 with limited health literacy, defined as an individual's "capacity to obtain, process and understand basic health information and services needed to make appropriate health decisions."[13,14] Adults with low literacy or low health literacy are at substantially increased risk for poor health outcomes, including poor chronic-illness outcomes, poor physical and mental health status, and increased use of acute health services.[15] In turn, the children of adults with limited literacy are at increased risk for poor child health outcomes, including poor child health access and poor health behaviors.[16] Completing the downward cycle of low literacy, children of adults with limited literacy are also at increased risk themselves for poor emergent literacy.[17]

DIGITAL MEDIA EXPOSURE DURING EARLY CHILDHOOD

During the past decade, early childhood exposure to screen time has rapidly expanded, with disparately greater exposure in low-income, ethnic-minority communities, in which risk for impaired early literacy skills is the greatest. The implications for child health are as of yet incompletely understood, but through some studies, a portrait is beginning to emerge. Young children exposed to greater amounts of unmonitored or unregulated screen time are at increased risk of sleep disturbance and behavioral problems, including attention-deficit hyperactivity disorder, during the school-aged years.[18] Although some limited evidence suggests the possibility of e-books and digital tools to support other early-learning interventions, digital tools alone are unlikely to replace brain's evolutionary reliance on human interaction to develop the full range of early literacy skills. Most digital media does not require or prompt the serve and return adult-child interaction necessary to stimulate brain development.[19] By contrast, well-meaning parents and adult caregivers often use digital media devices as a convenient child sedative or as a timely distractor that allows the adult to disengage from the child without immediate consequences (eg, crying or other demands for attention). Based on prior research regarding the essential nature of adult-child verbal, visual, and tactile interaction during the early years, some are concerned that digital media may be displacing this essential activity and unintentionally impairing normal child development.[20]

Despite the above-mentioned concern, digital media use during infancy has become an increasingly common phenomenon in the last few years and shows no signs of abating.[21] Much of it consists of educational videos, apps, and specialized devices marketed to parents as giving their child a significant edge in learning, despite an almost complete lack of evidence supporting such assertions. When it comes to traditional one-way media (eg, television, DVDs), it is fairly clear that there is little value. Developmentally, children seem not to learn from screens until at least 18 months of age (and some as late as 30 months).[22] Most media aimed at young children rely on a steady diet of quick scene changes and other stimuli that exploit the orienting reflex to keep a child engaged and give the parent the perception that their child is learning.

However, when it comes to interactive media (such as tablet apps and custom devices), there seems to be no evidence in either direction. Although traditional screen media has no educational value and also displaces human interaction and child-directed language,[23] interactive media may or may not have benefit. If interaction with other humans is central to driving development, other forms of interaction may have similar benefits, even if the exchange is not as finely attuned. Nevertheless, no clear evidence exists to support this. Even if such studies emerge, they may be highly specific to particular products and not necessarily generizable to even subclasses of apps or devices.

PARENTS AND ADULT CAREGIVERS: THE GATEKEEPERS TO EMERGENT LITERACY

Promotion of emergent literacy skills, before school entry, is key to supporting the health and development of any child. Literacy is conventionally defined as "the ability to read and write." The subcomponents of literacy include text recognition, text decoding and comprehension, oral language fluency, and numeracy. The educational system is built in large part on an attempt to build these fundamental literacy skills, on which one can build future skills and seek new knowledge.

Emergent literacy, by contrast, is defined as "the skills, knowledge, and attitudes that are presumed to be developmental precursors to conventional forms of reading and writing and the environments that support these developments."[24] The development of literacy skills is not the same as many other aspects of child development. A typical child, if appropriately nurtured, progresses through the stages of gross motor, fine motor, speech, social, and problem-solving domains; in a sense, one can consider these to be mostly hard-wired and primed to develop if given the appropriate scaffolding. Early reading skills, however, are not encoded into a single area of the brain and requires the repurposing and inclusion of other circuits and skills to allow for the process of text decoding that is called reading.[25] Ultimately, it is an amalgamation of oral language, vision, fine-motor skills, memory, and more. Central to this notion of early literacy is a key developmental leap that children make around the concept of print awareness. Before about 3 years of age, most children do not understand that printed text conveys information; after age 3 years, children who have been exposed to print generally understand that print carries meaning to be decoded, even if letter recognition is nil.[26,27]

Positive home environments, rich in the quantity and quality of verbal interactions between adult and child, do have a greater ability, however, to buffer the negative effects of poverty on child health. Decades of research have confirmed the strong independent relationship between a child's emergent literacy skills and a literacy-rich home environment, including accessibility of reading materials in every room of the home, adults' modeling reading by themselves, and dialogic reading. A literacy-rich home environment can moderate social and ethnic disparities in child literacy outcomes.[28]

Adult caregivers are responsible for a key determinant of emergent literacy: child exposure to both print and oral language. Adult-child interaction, which helps children to contextualize words and pictures on a page, is essential to child brain development. An adult who engages in dialogic reading helps the child take on a new role, not merely as a passive recipient of reading, but as a participant, author, and teller of the story.[29] In one study of 382 preschool children,[30] families in which dialogic reading was uncommon were almost twice as likely to have a child with delays.

Adult mediation of emergent literacy also allows for sociocultural diversity in styles of reading, which enhance early child brain development. For example, one study showed that middle-class parents tended to use a more interactive, dialogic style when reading to their children. As the child grew older, they were encouraged to ask questions at appropriate junctures. This situation was in contrast to working-class nonwhite parents, whose style was more centered on drills and skills, naming pictures, counting, and identifying letters but less around narrative and interaction.[31] Children exposed to dialogic reading have higher expressive language scores, have longer and more frequent utterances, and combine words more frequently than their peers whose parents did not use dialogic reading.[32] The use of what is termed nonimmediate talk (conversation that goes beyond the immediate context of the book or story and instead refers the broader world or prior experiences) strongly benefited children. Active engagement with a child via shared book reading was much more beneficial than simply reading at the child.[33] The British Millennium Cohort Study, which followed 12,500 children from birth to age 5 years, observed that early exposure to adults' reading aloud may moderate some of the powerful effect of family income on child reading skills.[34] Although 5-year-old children in the lowest-income homes had expressive vocabularies comparable to 4-year-old children in the most affluent homes, daily reading aloud could reduce that gap by several months.

Adult role modeling is also an evidence-based component of emergent-literacy promotion. A child who observes adults around them reading, writing, and interacting with text on a regular basis are more likely to mimic and adopt those behaviors as they develop and grow.[35] Observational studies in homes of children with advanced early literacy skills commented on the diverse range of adult reading materials found on the floors of bedrooms, kitchens, and bathrooms: from novels to newspapers, from checkbooks to magazines.

Despite this evidence, literacy-rich home environments and adult-child interaction around books remain far from universal during early childhood, particularly in low-income communities. In 2011, the percentage of children aged 1 to 5 years whose family members read to them fewer than 3 days per week was 14%.[36] When examining children ages 3 to 5 years for daily reading, the percentages vary between 35% and 68% (**Fig. 2**). Significant modifiers of reading-aloud frequency are maternal education level (daily reading in 74% of children with college-educated mothers vs only 31% with mothers who had not completed high school) and family income (daily reading in 64% of families living at >200% of the Federal Poverty Line but only 40% in those living under the poverty line) (**Figs. 3** and **4**).

EARLY LITERACY PROMOTION AS STANDARD PEDIATRIC CARE

Attention to the twin facts, the powerful effect of dialogic reading and the trenchant disparities in child exposure to literacy-rich environments, led in 1989 to the conception of the Reach Out and Read (ROR) program. A joint effort of developmental pediatricians Robert Needlman and Barry Zuckerman, alongside early childhood educators Jean Nigro, Kathleen MacLean, and Kathleen Fitzgerald-Rice, the program has 3 components implemented at each well-child visit from 6 months to 5 years:

1. The medical provider discusses book sharing with the parent or adult caregiver, offering age-appropriate tips.
2. The medical provider gives directly to the child a new, developmentally appropriate book, providing for teachable moments about child development.
3. The clinic waiting rooms is literacy rich, with books, posters about reading, and inviting spaces encouraging reading.

More than 15 studies published in peer-reviewed medical journals have shown clear evidence for this model. These studies are summarized in **Box 1**. Since its inception at Boston City Hospital, the program is now implemented in more than 5000 sites nationally, distributing more than 6.5 million books to more than 4 million children.[37] Fidelity to the evidence-based model is assisted by an online CME-offering training, and the impact is reinforced by additional modules adapted to special populations (eg,

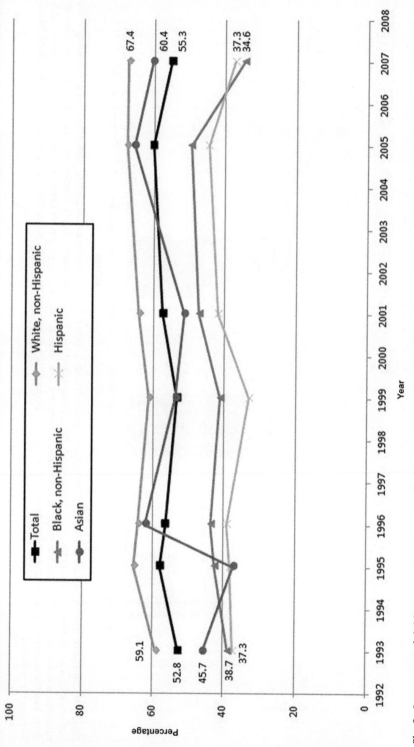

Fig. 2. Percentage of children aged 3 to 5 years (estimates are based on children who have yet to enter kindergarten) who were read to every day in the last week by a family member, by race and Hispanic origin, 1993 to 2007. (*Data from* Child Trends Databank. (2015). Reading to Young Children. Available at: http://www.childtrends.org/?indicators=reading-to-young-children; and the Federal Interagency Forum on Child and Family Statistics. America's Children: Key National Indicators of Well-Being. Washington, DC: U.S. Government Printing Office; 2009. Table ED1. Based on National Household Education Survey analysis.)

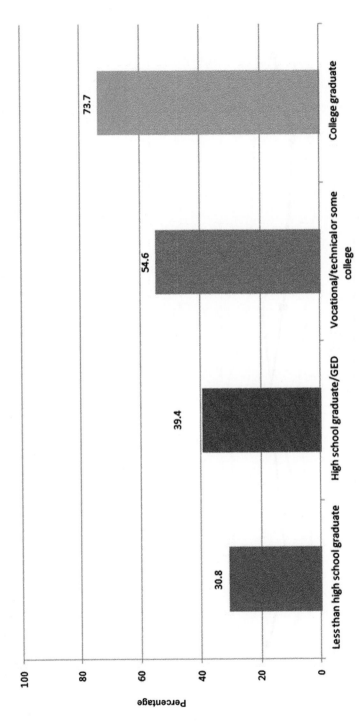

Fig. 3. Percentage of children aged 3 to 5 years (estimates are based on children who have yet to enter kindergarten) who were read to every day in the last week by a family member, by mother's education level, 2007. (*Data from* Child Trends Databank. (2015). Reading to Young Children. Available at: http://www.childtrends.org/?indicators=reading-to-young-children; and the Federal Interagency Forum on Child and Family Statistics. America's Children: Key National Indicators of Well-Being. Washington, DC: U.S. Government Printing Office; 2009. Table ED1. Based on National Household Education Survey analysis.)

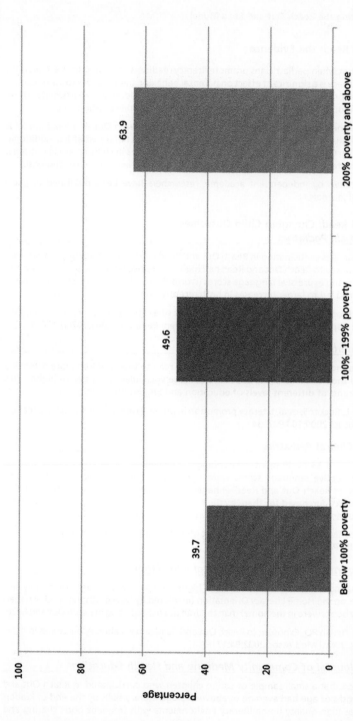

Fig. 4. Percentage of children aged 3 to 5 years (estimates are based on children who have yet to enter kindergarten) who were read to every day in the last week by a family member, by poverty status, 2007. (*Data from* Child Trends Databank. (2015). Reading to Young Children. Available at: http://www.childtrends.org/?indicators=reading-to-young-children; and the Federal Interagency Forum on Child and Family Statistics. America's Children: Key National Indicators of Well-Being. Washington, DC: U.S. Government Printing Office; 2009. Table ED1. Based on National Household Education Survey analysis.)

Box 1
Research supporting the Reach Out and Read Model

Reach Out and Read: the Evidence

Research shows that when pediatricians promote literacy readiness according to the Reach Out and Read model, there is a significant effect on parental behavior and attitudes toward reading aloud, as well as improvements in the language scores of young children who participate. These effects have been found in ethnically and economically diverse families nationwide.

The body of published research supporting the efficacy of the Reach Out and Read model is more extensive than for any other psychosocial intervention in general pediatrics. Additional studies about Reach Out and Read that address language outcomes in children are in progress. To read the complete articles, visit reachoutandread.org/why-we-work/research-findings/.

The following studies by independent academic researchers have been published in peer-reviewed medical journals.

Reach Out and Read: Changing Child Outcomes
Mendelsohn et al., Pediatrics

High-risk urban families participating in Reach Out and Read read more frequently to their children. Children exposed to Reach Out and Read had higher receptive language scores (words the child understands) and expressive language scores (words the child says). Increased exposure to Reach Out and Read led to larger increases in both receptive and expressive language scores.

Mendelsohn AL, Mogiler LN, Dreyer BP, et al. The impact of a clinic-based literacy intervention on language development in inner-city preschool children. Pediatrics 2001;107(1):130–4.

High et al., Pediatrics

Families participating in the Reach Out and Read model read to their children more often (4.3 vs 3.8 d/wk), and their toddlers' receptive and expressive vocabulary scores were higher. This effect held in parents of different levels of education and English proficiency.

High PC, LaGasse L, Becker S, et al. Literacy promotion in primary care pediatrics: can we make a difference? Pediatrics 2000;104:927–34.

Theriot et al., Clinical Pediatrics

Among children aged 33 to 39 months attending a well-child clinic in Louisville, Kentucky, expressive and receptive language scores were significantly and positively associated with both the number of Reach Out and Read–enhanced well-child visits they had attended and the number of books purchased for them by their parents. This finding supports a dose effect for the Reach Out and Read intervention: the more visits, the higher the score.

Theriot JA, Franco SM, Sisson BA, et al. The impact of early literacy guidance on language skills of 3-year-olds. Clin Pediatr 2003;42:165–72.

Sharif et al., Journal of the National Medical Association

Children participating in Reach Out and Read had higher receptive vocabulary scores. They also had higher scores on the Home Literacy Orientation (measured by how much the child was read to and how many books were in the home) than children not participating in Reach Out and Read.

Sharif I, Rieber S, Ozuah PO. Exposure to Reach Out and Read and vocabulary outcomes in inner city preschoolers. J Natl Med Assoc 2002;94:171–7.

Diener et al., Journal of Community Medicine and Health Education

This study showed that a small sample of Latino children who participated in Reach Out and Read from 6 months of age had average or above-average literacy skills by the end of kindergarten, as well as high-quality home literacy environments with frequent book sharing and high book ownership.

Diener ML, Hobson-Rohrer W, Byington CL. Kindergarten readiness and performance of Latino children participating in Reach Out and Read. J Community Med Health Educ 2012;2:133.

Reach Out and Read: Changing Parental Attitudes and Practices
High et al., Archives of Pediatrics and Adolescent Medicine

Parents whose children (<3 years) had received books and educational materials during well-child visits were more likely than parents in a control group to report that they shared books with their children and to cite sharing books as a favorite activity or a child's favorite activity.

High P, Hopmann M, LaGasse L, et al. Evaluation of a clinic-based program to promote book sharing and bedtime routines among low-income urban families with young children. Arch Pediatr Adolesc Med 1998;15:459–65.

Needlman, et al., American Journal of Diseases of Children

Parents who had received a book as part of Reach Out and Read were more likely to report reading books with their children or to say that reading was a favorite activity. The benefits of Reach Out and Read were larger for families receiving Aid to Families with Dependent Children.

Needlman R, Fried LE, Morley DS, et al. Clinic-based intervention to promote literacy. A pilot study. Am J Dis Child 1991;145:881–4.

Weitzman et al., Pediatrics

In a study using direct observation of children's homes, parents were more likely to read aloud to their children and enjoy reading together when their families had more encounters with the Reach Out and Read program.

Weitzman CC, Roy L, Walls T, et al. More evidence for Reach Out and Read: a home-based study. Pediatrics 2004;113:1248–53.

Needlman et al., Ambulatory Pediatrics

In a multicenter study, families exposed to Reach Out and Read were more likely to report reading aloud at bedtime, read aloud 3 or more days per week, mention reading aloud as a favorite activity, and own 10 or more children's books.

Needlman R, Toker KH, Dreyer BP, et al. Effectiveness of a primary care intervention to support reading aloud: a multicenter evaluation. Ambul Pediatr 2005;5:209–15.

Silverstein et al., Pediatrics

English- and non-English-speaking families who participated in the Reach Out and Read model increased their weekly bedtime reading, and more parents reported reading as their own or their child's favorite activity. For non-English-speaking families, the number of children's books in the home also increased as a result of the Reach Out and Read model.

Silverstein M, Iverson L, Lozano P. An English-language clinic-based literacy program is effective for a multilingual population. Pediatrics 2002;109:e76.

Sanders et al., Archives of Pediatrics and Adolescent Medicine

Hispanic parents participating in Reach Out and Read were more likely to report reading to their children than Hispanic parents not participating in Reach Out and Read. When parents read more frequently to their children, they were also more likely to read frequently themselves.

Sanders L, Gershon TD, Huffman LC, et al. Prescribing books for immigrant children. Arch Pediatr Adolesc Med 2000;154:771–7.

Golova et al., Pediatrics

Hispanic parents whose children had received bilingual books, educational materials, and anticipatory guidance about literacy were more likely to report reading books with their child at least 3 d/wk (66% vs 24%) and report that reading books was one of their 3 favorite things to do with their child (43% vs 13%) than parents in a control group. Parents participating in the Reach Out and Read intervention also tended to have more books in the home (for children and adults).

Golova N, Alario AJ, Vivier PM, et al. Literacy promotion for Hispanic families in a primary care setting: a randomized controlled trial. Pediatrics 1998;103:993–7.

Reach Out and Read: Toward Better Primary Care
Jones et al., Clinical Pediatrics

Parents participating in Reach Out and Read were more likely to rate their child's pediatrician as helpful than those not participating. Pediatricians in the Reach Out and Read group were more likely to rate parents as receptive than those in the non–Reach Out and Read group. Mothers in the Reach Out and Read group were 2 times more likely to report enjoyment in reading together with their child than those in the non–Reach Out and Read group.

Jones VF, Franco SM, Metcalf SC, et al. The value of book distribution in a clinic-based literacy intervention program. Clin Pediatr 2000;39:535–41.

King et al., Academic Pediatrics

Successful implementation of the Reach Out and Read program was related to the culture of the clinic. Staff at clinics that struggled to implement Reach Out and Read found their jobs burdensome and reported lacks in communication. Staff at successful Reach Out and Read program sites worked as a team and expressed strong commitments to their communities.

King TM, Muzaffar S, George M. The role of clinic culture in implementation of primary care interventions: the case of Reach Out and Read. Acad Pediatr 2009;9(1):40–6.

Byington et al., Journal of Health Care for the Poor and Underserved

This qualitative study examined the thank-you notes sent to staff at a Reach Out and Read clinic by Hispanic families. Families expressed thanks for the books received, as well as the literacy advice given by doctors and nurses. Many families believed that the books and advice promoted the habit of reading and demonstrated respect the staff felt for the families and their children.

Ortiz KA, Buchi KF. The good habit of reading (el buen habito de la lectura): Parental reactions to an enhanced Reach Out and Read program in a clinic for the underserved. J Health Care Poor Underserved 2008;19:363–8.

For more information, visit www.reachoutandread.org.
From Reach Out and Read: the evidence. Available at: http://www.reachoutandread.org/FileRepository/Research_Summary.pdf; with permission.

multicultural and multilingual communities, children with special health care needs), webinars, and the like. The ROR model has been endorsed in the third edition of the Bright Futures Guidelines for Health Supervision[38] and is slated to have even stronger endorsement in the fourth edition.[39]

The ABCs of Reach Out and Read

Assess: What is the child's response to the book? How does the family react? What is their joint interaction (eg, verbal, body language) around the book? Are books viewed as a positive, negative, or neutral in this family?

Bringing in at the beginning: Bring the book into the visit and hand it to the child at the very beginning to observe the interaction and use it as part of developmental surveillance.

Connect: Does the family need to be referred to community resources such as libraries, adult literacy, home visiting, or other forms of support based on what you learn and enquire about?

As a result of ROR, pediatric providers have also worked with early childhood educators and book publishers to help select developmentally, culturally, and linguistically appropriate books for these pediatric encounters. Individual clinics should include parent and family preferences in book selections. Children of all backgrounds can benefit from seeing depictions of a broad range of diverse people, but children in underrepresented minority groups in particular deserve to see themselves in books. Book selection should attend not only to culturally appropriate faces but also to other practices, such as food, entertainment, clothing, and other aspects of culture. In communities with new immigrants, many families prefer books that include text from their native language, in place of or in addition to English-language text.

Principles of Book Selection

Guiding principles

- Does the book engage the adult? Does the adult find the book interesting?
- Does the book's images (eg, faces) engage the child?
- Beyond age 2 years, does the richness of text relate to rich images and rich textures in a way that encourages the practice of emergent literacy?
- Do the images look like the patients and families you serve?
- Is the language appropriate for those families with limited English proficiency?
- Is the book format appropriate for the child's developmental stage? For example, the thick pages of board books are ideal for a child who has not yet developed a pincer grasp (a pincer grasp is necessary to turn paper pages well) (**Table 2**).
- Is the intention for the book to be read aloud to the child or primarily for the child to explore the book on their own? A picture book with paper pages may be fine for an adult or older child to read aloud to a toddler but may not be appropriate for that child to explore on their own.

Although books to avoid can be found in many genres, when considering appropriate choices, there are some key features to steer clear of:

- Books that market products or characters; these are often no more than thinly veiled advertisements
- Message books, including those that promote health themes
- Some pop-up books or other books with mechanical or electronic gimmicks

Considerations on Digital Media

Although there is little research helping us delineate what qualities of electronic media might be preferable, there are some principles that can assist parents in selecting quality electronic books:

- Just as in traditional books, is there clear narrative flow and are the illustrations done with care?
- When the reader is invited to tap or touch something to elicit a response, does that interaction further the narrative or distract from it?
- Does the program/book/app create links to outside (Internet-based) content that distracts, markets, or otherwise diverts attention away from the narrative?

BEYOND REACH OUT AND READ

In 2014, the AAP provided national recommendations and a policy statement, effectively directing that the ROR model become a routine part of standard pediatric practice at all health supervision visits, with reinforcement of the need for cultural sensitivity

Table 2
Milestones of early literacy development

Newborn to 6 months
Talk, Read, Sing, Play: Right from birth, babies are listening, looking, and learning.
So find, and enjoy, those everyday moments when you can talk, read, sing, and play together with your baby.

	6–12 mo	12–24 mo	2–3 y	3–4 y	4–5 y
Motor Development What your child is doing	Holds head steady Sits in lap without support Grasps book, puts in mouth Drops, throws book	Holds and walks with book No longer puts book in mouth right away Turns board book pages	Learns to turn paper pages, 2–3 pages at a time Starts to scribble	Turns pages one at a time, and from left to right Sits still for longer stories Scribbles and draws	Starts to copy letters and numbers Sits still for even longer stories
Communication and Cognition What your child is saying and learning	Smiles, babbles, coos Likes and wants your voice Likes pictures of baby faces Begins to say "ma," "ba," "da" Responds to own name Pats picture to show interest	Says single words, then 2- to 4-word phrases Gives book to adult to read Points at pictures Turns book right-side up Names pictures, follows simple stories	Adds 2–4 new words per day Names familiar objects Likes the same book again and again Completes sentences and rhymes in familiar stories	Recites whole phrases from books Moves toward letter recognition Begins to detect rhyme Pretends to read to dolls and stuffed animals	Can listen longer Recognizes numbers, letters Can retell familiar stories Can make rhymes Learning letter names and sounds

Anticipatory Guidance					
What parents can do	Talk back and forth with your baby; make eye contact	Smile and answer when your child speaks or points	Ask "Where's the dog?" or "What is that?"	Ask "What happens next?" in familiar stories	Relate the story to your child's own experiences
	Cuddle, sing, talk, play, read	Let your child help turn the pages; keep naming things	Be willing to read the same book again and again	Point out letters, numbers	Let your child see *you* read
Ask questions and wait for your child to answer	Point at and name things, eg, nose, ball, baby, dog	Use books in family routines: naptime, playtime, bedtime; on the potty; in the car, bus	As you read, talk about the pictures	Point out words and pictures that begin with the same sound	Ask your child to tell the story
Read and speak in your first language	Follow baby's cues for "more" or "stop"	Use books to calm or distract your child while waiting	Keep using books in daily routines	Together, make up stories about the pictures	Encourage writing, drawing
	Play games such as "peek-a-boo" or "pat-a-cake"				Point out the letters in your child's name
			Let your child choose which book to read. Find stories about things your child likes		
What to Read	Board and cloth books; books with baby faces; nursery rhymes	Board books; rhyming books; picture books; books that name things	Rhyming books; picture books that tell stories; search and find books	Picture books that tell longer stories; counting and alphabet books	Fairy tales and legends; books with longer stories, fewer pictures

Babies learn best from caring adults. From birth, it's important for parents to notice and respond to what interests their child. Reading aloud and talking together every day creates secure relationships and a strong foundation for learning. Books should be part of every family's naptime, playtime, and bedtime routines.
Available at: http://www.reachoutandread.org/resource-center/literacy-materials/literacy-milestones/. Accessed June 29, 2015.

and community advocacy in advancing early childhood literacy.[40] Although ROR is the most commonly used pediatric intervention to promote emergent literacy, other programs have promise, utilizing a higher intensity or different modalities to have an effect.

Among them are programs such as Alan Mendelsohn's Bellevue Project for Early Language, Literacy and Education Success (BELLE) project, which combines early literacy promotion with video feedback to build parental skills around interaction[41]; Raising a Reader, which engages caregivers around book sharing with their children from birth through age 8 years.[42] Advocacy efforts are characterized by initiatives such as the Clinton Foundation's Too Small to Fail initiative.[43]

The Early Brain and Child Development Leadership Group at the AAP developed a table (**Table 3**) providing themes and suggestions for promoting early brain and child development within the context of the Bright Futures visit. Early literacy promotion is part of these suggestions, but the suggestions are broader than that, encompassing other elements of supporting high-quality parent-child interaction and using intentional skill building as an approach to enhancing parental capacities and capabilities.

A PRESCRIPTION FOR INNOVATIVE PEDIATRIC PRIMARY CARE

To address the social determinants of child health, including emergent literacy, one needs innovative new models for future systems of pediatric primary care. Such innovation, already begun in primary care practices and communities nationwide, should be open to entirely new models of care. Short, inexpensive interventions such as ROR are one, but wholesale structural change in the very model of how health care is delivered should be considered as well, taking the principles outlined earlier to scale. These types of innovations could include the following:

- Professional development for clinic staff, including non-MDs and non-RNs, to provide early-literacy guidance
- Short videos, led by parents and endorsed by pediatric providers, that provide culturally sensitive modeling and messaging around early literacy and developmental guidance
- Group well-child visits, that allow both parents and developmental experts to share what works in their diverse home environments
- Leveraging mobile technology to improve social support for parents around their infants' play and early cognitive environment
- Active partnerships between primary care practices and neighboring preschools and early childhood care environments
- Population-based monitoring of early-childhood indicators to provide real-time feedback and geomapped hot-spotting to pediatric practices

Certainly, other innovative ideas abound. A new generation of pediatric providers and child-health systems are necessary to meet the health and developmental needs of all children, starting in early childhood. What ideas do you have? What ideas can you test with your families in clinic, beginning tomorrow?

While schools can do much to raise achievement among children who initially lag behind their peers, all too often pre-school gaps set in train a pattern of ever increasing inequality during school years and beyond. Any drive to improve social mobility must begin with an effective strategy to nurture the fledgling talent in young children so often lost before it has had a chance to flourish.
—*The Sutton Trust[44]*

Table 3
The first 1000 days: bright Futures examples for promoting EBCD

Pediatricians Are Encouraged to→ General Principles → Brief Description Well Child Care Visit	Explore the Child's Environment What Pediatricians Might Briefly Assess During Well Child Care	Build Relationships/Reciprocity How Pediatricians Might Strengthen the Parent-Child Bond or Attachment	Cultivate Development What Pediatricians Might Teach Parents About Development	Develop Parenting Confidence How Pediatricians Might Support Parents as They Nurture Their Child's Development
	Assess foundational needs: • Food and sleep • Safety • Social and emotional supports • Strengths and barriers to success	Describe (or notice) parent-child interactions, emphasize the importance of responsive caregiving, and support the parent-child relationship (dyadic dance)	Explain current and emerging developmental skills	1. Praise and encourage age-appropriate but responsive caregiving 2. Praise and encourage parental self-care and the nurturing of social supports
Prenatal/Newborn/Week 1	Assess for food (plans to breastfeed?), safety, and parental supports	Explain that relationships and everyday interactions build the baby's brain	Explain the importance of parent-baby interaction during the infant's quiet-alert state	Encourage parents to consider he way they were parented. Explore what they plan to do and not to do as parents
2–4 wk	Assess overall parental well-being (maternal depression or substance use?)	Encourage responsive caregiving (responding promptly to cries of distress builds trust)	Prepare parent for the emerging social smile	Find opportunities to reassure and praise the parents, and encourage them to support each other
2 mo	Assess for family adjustment—parent self-care, return to work/childcare, time with partner, impact of new infant on siblings	Encourage smiling back at the baby's social smile (the beginning of the parent-child interaction, or dyadic dance, that	Anticipate cooing conversations	Enjoy interactions with an increasingly social baby

(continued on next page)

Table 3
(continued)

General Principles →	Explore the Child's Environment	Build Relationships/Reciprocity	Cultivate Development	Develop Parenting Confidence
Pediatricians Are Encouraged to →	What Pediatricians Might Briefly Assess During Well Child Care	How Pediatricians Might Strengthen the Parent-Child Bond or Attachment	What Pediatricians Might Teach Parents About Development	How Pediatricians Might Support Parents as They Nurture Their Child's Development
		leads to cooing, feeding, and speaking)		
4 mo	Assess the parent's perception of the baby's temperament	Encourage attention to the baby's coos and cues—irritability may indicate boredom	Encourage reaching for objects that are safe and easy to hold	Recommend regular bedtime routine
6 mo	Ask if there is a quiet, predictable, and safe sleep environment with bedtime routines	Support fun feeding interactions (use feeding time as a happy, interactive time with the baby)	Anticipate the development of social-emotional distress (eg, separation anxiety, stranger anxiety)	Support the enjoyment of books
9 mo	Ask if the environment is safe for exploration (crawling)	Respond to the child's emotional cues (eg, stranger anxiety) and offer brief reassurance. When the child is seeking your reaction to strangers (social referencing), note it and smile	Acknowledge the continued development of strong emotions like frustration, anger, and fear	Be aware of your facial expressions. Social referencing indicates that your child is reading your emotions and feeling your stress
12 mo	Ask about in-person face time vs virtual screen time	Never sneak away—give the baby clear cues before separating from them	Encourage language by responding to child's nonverbal cues or asking child to point ("where is ...?")	Recognize and praise child's good behavior, providing time in and using redirection for negative behaviors

Age				
15 mo	Ask about beliefs and practices concerning discipline (eg, use of yelling or spanking)	Acknowledge all attempts by the child to communicate and respond to the child's use of language and sound	Capitalize on safe exploration of the physical world by encouraging labeling ("what is that?")	Praise parents for allowing exploration and welcoming child when he/she seeks comfort and security
18 mo	Assess for consistency in setting limits for unsafe (eg, electrical outlets) or impulsive (eg, hitting or biting) behaviors	Encourage playful learning through pointing, naming, and labeling. Providing positive attention for desired behaviors is time-in	Explain that emotions can be overwhelming; support efforts to teach self-soothing, like time-out	Support parents in selectively ignoring negative attentionseeking behaviors
24 mo	Ask about parents' plans for or progress with potty training	Encourage pretend play by following the child's lead during play	Support self-dressing and feeding, but avoid forcing potty training	Support parents' ability to calmly and safely respond to a child's frustrations by acknowledging all the child's attempts to communicate using words
30 mo	Assess parents' social supports and ability to cope with tantrums, toilet training, and other challenging behaviors	Try to take strong emotions out of conflicts and remain calm and safe	Provide and supervise playtime with others	Support parents by recognizing that many parents find this age challenging, and encourage parents to resist the temptation to use electronic devices (eg, TV) as a means of avoiding challenging behaviors

(continued on next page)

Table 3
(continued)

Pediatricians Are Encouraged to →	Explore the Child's Environment	Build Relationships/Reciprocity	Cultivate Development	Develop Parenting Confidence
General Principles →	What Pediatricians Might Briefly Assess During Well Child Care	How Pediatricians Might Strengthen the Parent-Child Bond or Attachment	What Pediatricians Might Teach Parents About Development	How Pediatricians Might Support Parents as They Nurture Their Child's Development
36 mo	Assess for quality early childhood education experiences	Support the recognizing, normalizing, and labeling of emotions to promote the child's use of basic emotional language	Children are focused on themselves (egocentric), making play with others difficult. Play dates and opportunities to play with peers build foundational social-emotional skills	Support parental attempts to recognize and encourage/praise the child's positive behaviors (eg, playing nicely)

The promotion of early brain and child development (EBCD) is an essential element of pediatric care. Coupled with supporting the development of a positive, nurturing relationship between the parent and child, health professionals must foster a strong foundation for children's lifelong learning, behavior, and health. The basic science is clear: during the first few years of life, safe, stable, and nurturing relationships promote healthy brains by decreasing toxic stress and encouraging foundational mental skills.

Because translating this science within the busy medical home can be a challenge, the following grid was developed. This grid, developed by the American Academy of Pediatrics Early Brain and Child Development Leadership Workgroup, distills the information from a wide array of resources into a practice-friendly framework for pediatricians. This grid is not intended to be a comprehensive resource but rather provides examples of some evidence-informed actions consistent with the Bright Futures guidelines that proactively address the child-parent/caregiver relationship and the child's development.

EBCD is used in this grid as a mnemonic device for actions health professionals should take to support early brain development: *explore* the quality of the child's socioemotional home environment, *build* relationships, *cultivate* development, and *develop* parent confidence and competence.

For more EBCD information and resources, visit the EBCD Web site at www.aap.org/ebcd and the Bright Futures Web site at www.brightfutures.aap.org.

Data from Refs.[45–56]

REFERENCES

1. Kristof N. Is a hard life inherited? New York: The New York Times; 2014.
2. Campbell F, Conti G, Heckman JJ, et al. Early childhood investments substantially boost adult health. Science 2014;343(6178):1478–85.
3. Shonkoff JP. Changing the narrative for early childhood investment. JAMA Pediatr 2014;168(2):105–6.
4. U.S. Department of Education, National Center for Education Statistics, School Readiness Survey, Early Childhood Program Participation Survey, and Parent and Family Involvement in Education Survey of the National Household Education Surveys Program (SR-NHES:1993, ECPP-NHES:2001, and PFI-NHES:2007).
5. Population Reference Bureau, analysis of data from the U.S. Census Bureau, Census 2000 Supplementary Survey, 2001 Supplementary Survey, 2002 through 2013 American Community Survey. Available at: http://datacenter.kidscount.org/data/tables/43-children-in-poverty-100-percent-poverty?loc=1&loct=1#detailed/1/any/false/36,868,867,133,38/any/321,322 and http://datacenter.kidscount.org/data/tables/47-children-below-200-percent-poverty?loc=1&loct=1#detailed/1/any/false/36,868,867,133,38/any/329,330. Accessed June 29, 2015.
6. AAP Agenda for Children 2013: Child Poverty Strategic Priority. Available at: http://www.aap.org/en-us/about-the-aap/aap-facts/AAP-Agenda-for-Children-Strategic-Plan/Pages/AAP-Agenda-for-Children-Strategic-Plan-Poverty-Child-Health.aspx. Accessed June 29, 2015.
7. Larson K, Russ SA, Nelson BB, et al. Cognitive ability at kindergarten entry and socioeconomic status. Pediatrics 2015;135(2):e440–8.
8. Garner AS, Shonkoff JP, Siegel BS, et al. Early Childhood Adversity, Toxic Stress, and the Role of the Pediatrician: Translating Developmental Science into Lifelong Health. PEDIATRICS 2012;129(1):e224–31.
9. Slopen N, McLaughlin KA, Shonkoff JP. Interventions to improve cortisol regulation in children: a systematic review. Pediatrics 2014;133(2):312–26.
10. Watts TW, Duncan GJ, Siegler RS, et al. What's past is prologue: relations between early mathematics knowledge and high school achievement. Educ Res 2014;43(7):352–60.
11. Hernandez DJ. Double Jeopardy: how third-grade reading skills and poverty influence high school graduation. Baltimore, MD: Annie E. Casey Foundation; 2011.
12. Montes G, Lotyczewski BS, Halterman JS, et al. School readiness among children with behavior problems at entrance into kindergarten: results from a US national study. Eur J Pediatr 2012;171(3):541–8.
13. Kindig DA, Panzer AM, Nielsen-Bohlman L. Health literacy: a prescription to end confusion. Washington, DC: National Academies Press; 2004.
14. Kutner M, Greenburg E, Jin Y, et al. The health literacy of America's adults: results from the 2003 National Assessment of Adult Literacy. Washington, DC: National Center for Education Statistics; 2006. NCES 2006-483.
15. DeWalt DA, Berkman ND, Sheridan S, et al. Literacy and health outcomes. J Gen Intern Med 2004;19(12):1228–39.
16. Sanders LM, Federico S, Klass P, et al. Literacy and child health: a systematic review. Arch Pediatr Adolesc Med 2009;163(2):131–40.
17. Op. cit. Kutner 2006.
18. Garrison MM, Christakis DA. The impact of a healthy media use intervention on sleep in preschool children. Pediatrics 2012;130(3):492–9.

19. Christakis DA. Interactive Media Use at Younger Than the Age of 2 Years: Time to Rethink the American Academy of Pediatrics Guideline? JAMA Pediatr 2014; 168(5):399–400.
20. Radesky JS, Schumacher J, Zuckerman B. Mobile and interactive media use by young children: the good, the bad, and the unknown. Pediatrics 2015; 135(1):1–3.
21. Common Sense Media. Zero to eight: children's media use in America 2013. Available at: https://www.commonsensemedia.org/research/zero-to-eight-childrens-media-use-in-america-2013. Accessed June 29, 2015.
22. Schmidt ME, Rich M, Rifas-Shiman SL, et al. Television viewing in infancy and child cognition at 3 years of age in a US cohort. Pediatrics 2009;123(3): e370–5.
23. Christakis DA, Gilkerson J, Richards JA, et al. Audible television and decreased adult words, infant vocalizations and conversational turns: a population-based study. Arch Pediatr Adolesc Med 2009;163(6):554–8.
24. Whitehurst GJ, Lonigan CJ. Child development and emergent literacy. Child Dev 1998;69(3):848–72.
25. Wolf M. Proust and the squid. New York: Harper Perennial; 2008.
26. Mason JM. When do children begin to read: an exploration of four year old children's letter and word reading competencies. Read Res Q 1980;15:203–27.
27. Adams MJ. Beginning to read: thinking and learning about print. Cambridge (MA): MIT Press; 1990.
28. Baker CE. Mexican mothers' English proficiency and children's school readiness: mediation through home literacy involvement. Early Education and Development 2014;25(3):338–55.
29. Zevenbergen AA, Whitehurst GJ. Dialogic reading: a shared picture book reading intervention for preschoolers. on reading books to children: parents and teachers. London: Routledge; 2003.
30. Glascoe FP, Leew S. Parenting behaviors, perceptions, and psychosocial risk: impacts on young children's development. Pediatrics 2010;125(2):313–9.
31. Heath SB. What no bedtime story means: narrative skills at home and school. Lang Soc 1982;11:49–76.
32. Whitehurst G, Falco FL, Lonigan CJ, et al. Accelerating language development through picture book reading. Dev Psychol 1988;24(4):552–9.
33. Reese E, Cox A. Quality of adult book reading affects children's emergent literacy. Dev Psychol 1999;35(1):20–8.
34. The Sutton Trust. Cognitive gaps in the early years: a summary of findings from the report 'Low Income and Early Cognitive Development in the UK'. 2010. Available at: http://learning.wales.gov.uk/docs/learningwales/publications/140211-sutton-trust-en.pdf. Accessed June 29, 2015.
35. Weigel DJ, Martin SS, Bennett KK. Ecological influences of the home and the child-care center on preschool-age children's literacy development. Read Res Q 2005;40(2):204–33.
36. Child and Adolescent Health Measurement Initiative, National Survey of Children's Health 2011. http://childhealthdata.org/learn/NSCH. Accessed June 29, 2015.
37. Reach Out and Read National Center. History of Reach Out and Read. 2014. Available at: https://www.reachoutandread.org/FileRepository/History_of_ReachOutAndRead.pdf. Accessed June 29, 2015.
38. Hagan JF, Shaw JS, Duncan PM, editors. Bright futures: guidelines for health supervision of infants, children, and adolescents. 3rd edition. Elk Grove Village (IL): American Academy of Pediatrics; 2008.

39. Hagan JF, Shaw JS, Duncan PM, editors. Bright futures: guidelines for health supervision of infants, children, and adolescents. 4th edition. Elk Grove Village (IL): American Academy of Pediatrics, in press.

40. High PC, Klass P, Donoghue E, et al. Literacy promotion: an essential component of primary care pediatric practice. Pediatrics 2014;134(2):404–9.

41. Mendelsohn AL, Huberman HS, Berkule SB, et al. Primary care strategies for promoting parent-child interactions and school readiness in at-risk families: early findings from the Bellevue Project for Early Language, Literacy and Education Success (BELLE). Arch Pediatr Adolesc Med 2011;165(1):33–41.

42. Raising a reader: independent evaluations. Available at: http://www.raisingareader.org/site/PageNavigator/Impact/PerformanceOutcomes.html. Accessed June 29, 2015.

43. Too Small to Fail. Available at: http://toosmall.org. Accessed June 29, 2015.

44. op.cit, The Sutton Trust, 2010.

45. Bright Futures guidelines, 3rd edition. Promoting family support. Available at: http://brightfutures.aap.org/pdfs/Guidelines_PDF/2-BF_Promoting_Family_Support.pdf. Accessed June 29, 2015.

46. Circle of Security Parenting Video. Available at: http://www.youtube.com/watch?v=cW2BfxsWguc. Accessed June 29, 2015.

47. Connected Kids. Available at: http://www2.aap.org/connectedkids/. Accessed June 29, 2015.

48. Early Brain and Child Development. Available at: http://www.aap.org/ebcd. Accessed June 29, 2015.

49. Incorporating recognition and management of perinatal and postpartum into pediatric practice. Available at: http://pediatrics.aappublications.org/content/126/5/1032.full.pdf+html?sid=40e5dde5-3c2d-486d-8d07-59bea786c0a7. Accessed June 29, 2015.

50. Partnering with parents: apps for raising happy, healthy children (Institute for Safe Families). Available at: http://www.instituteforsafefamilies.org/materials/partnering-with-parents. Accessed June 29, 2015.

51. Promoting First Relationships. Available at: http://pfrprogram.org/. Accessed June 29, 2015.

52. Reach Out and Read (strategies to promote early literacy). Available at: http://www.reachoutandread.org/. Accessed June 29, 2015.

53. References for evidence-based programs for young children. Available at: http://pediatrics.aappublications.org/content/125/Supplement_3/S155.full.pdf+html?sid=80ab934d-c265-40d6-99ed-ff83d1553136. Accessed June 29, 2015.

54. "Still Face" experiment video. Available at: http://www.youtube.com/watch?v=apzXGEbZht0. Accessed June 29, 2015.

55. Zero to Three. Available at: http://www.zerotothree.org/. Accessed June 29, 2015.

56. Available at: http://www.aap.org/en-us/advocacy-and-policy/aap-health-initiatives/EBCD/Documents/EBCD_Well_Child_Grid.pdf. Accessed June 29, 2015.

Children, Families, and Disparities

Pediatric Provisions in the Affordable Care Act

Aimee M. Grace, MD, MPH[a,b,*], Ivor Horn, MD, MPH[c,d],
Robert Hall, JD, MPAff[e], Tina L. Cheng, MD, MPH[f,g]

KEYWORDS

- Affordable Care Act • Health insurance • Health reform • Child health policy

KEY POINTS

- The impact of the Affordable Care Act (ACA) will be far-reaching for children and families, and has the potential to significantly decrease disparities.
- The ACA aims to improve Access to coverage, provide Better care, and ensure Consumer protections (ABC).
- The ACA faces multiple challenges to come, including a Congress whose leaders have repeatedly stated their intention to alter or repeal the legislation.

The Affordable Care Act (ACA; "Obamacare") "has the potential to do more to meet the health needs of America's racial and ethnic minorities, and more to reduce racial and ethnic health disparities, than any other law in living memory," wrote Dr John

Funding: This publication was supported by the DC-Baltimore Research Center on Child Health Disparities P20 MD000198 from the National Institute on Minority Health and Health Disparities (IH, TLC) and Centro SOL: Johns Hopkins Center for Salud/(Health) and Opportunity for Latinos (TLC). The content is solely the responsibility of the authors and does not necessarily represent the official views of the funding agencies.
Financial Disclosures: None.
Conflict of Interest: None.
[a] Office of US Senator Brian Schatz, 722 Hart Senate Office Building, Washington, DC 20510, USA; [b] George Washington University School of Medicine and Health Sciences, 2150 Pennsylvania Ave NW, Washington, DC 20037, USA; [c] Center for Diversity and Health Equity, Seattle Children's Hospital, 4800 Sand Point Way NE, Seattle, WA 98105, USA; [d] Department of Pediatrics, University of Washington School of Medicine, 4333 Brooklyn Ave NE, Seattle, WA 98105, USA; [e] Department of Federal Affairs, American Academy of Pediatrics, 601 13th Street NW #400N, Washington, DC 20005, USA; [f] General Pediatrics and Adolescent Medicine, Johns Hopkins School of Medicine, 200 N Wolfe Street, Baltimore, MD 21287, USA; [g] Department of Population, Family and Reproductive Health, Bloomberg School of Public Health, 615 N Wolfe Street, Baltimore, MD 21205, USA
* Corresponding author. Children's National Health System, 111 Michigan Avenue NW, Washington, DC 20010.
E-mail address: agrace@stanfordalumni.org

Pediatr Clin N Am 62 (2015) 1297–1311
http://dx.doi.org/10.1016/j.pcl.2015.06.003
0031-3955/15/$ – see front matter Published by Elsevier Inc.

McDonough, former Senior Advisor on National Health Reform to the US Senate Committee on Health, Education, Labor, and Pensions.[1] Indeed, US Representative James Clyburn (D-SC) called the ACA "the civil rights act of the 21st century."[1] Others have challenged the constitutionality of the ACA and have been concerned about its implementation. The ACA has caused and continues to catalyze sweeping changes throughout the health system in the United States. Poorly explained, complex, controversial, confusing, and subject to continuous legal challenge and regulatory definition, the law stands as a hallmark piece of legislation that will change the health sector in America for decades. What is the ACA, and how does it affect children and families? This article summarizes this significant law, with a focus on children, families, and disparities. Also provided is the context of the current system of health care coverage in the United States.

SETTING THE STAGE: A REVIEW OF CHILDREN'S HEALTH INSURANCE PROGRAMS

In the United States in 2011, 18% of the total population younger than 65 (Medicare noneligible) was uninsured; within this group, 16% were children, 25% were parents, and 59% were adults without dependent children.[2] As outlined next, children in the United States have various primary health insurance options (whose scope and provisions are changing with implementation of the ACA, as later described).

Private Insurance

Private insurance is available to children and families through employer-based insurance and through buying insurance on one's own (in the individual market). In 2011, 49% of all Americans were covered through employer-sponsored insurance, and 5% had private nongroup insurance.[3] In 2009, 51% of children ages birth to 18 in the United States had employer-sponsored insurance, 33% had Medicaid or Children's Health Insurance Program (CHIP), 4% had individual coverage, 1% had other public insurance, and 10% were uninsured.[4]

The growth of employer-sponsored insurance in the United States emerged after World War II. Price controls limited the amount of wages that employers could provide; thus, such benefits as health care became the incentives that lured workers to jobs. Over the decades, employer-sponsored insurance has become a standard in the United States. Covered benefits, cost sharing, and treatment limitations/exclusions tend to be at the discretion of insurers, under applicable state and/or federal law.

Historically, when parents have enrolled in private insurance, either through their employer or in the individual market, children have also been covered according to plan specifications as dependents. Before the ACA, children aged out of parents' private insurance plans at age 19, or possibly age 22 if they were full-time students.

Medicaid

Established in 1965, Medicaid has historically covered pregnant women, low- and middle-income children, and poor elderly and disabled people in the United States. In 2011, 68 million people were enrolled in Medicaid, including 48% children, 27% adults, 9% elderly, and 15% disabled.[5] In general, only citizens and lawfully residing residents in the United States for 5 years are eligible. Medicaid is a joint federal-state program, with states with lower incomes receiving a higher percentage of federal payments in what is called the Federal Matching Assistance Percentage (FMAP).

Contrary to common public understanding, Medicaid has not historically covered all people below the federal poverty level (FPL; $11,670 per year for individuals and $23,850 per year for a family of four in 2014). Federal law establishes minimum federal eligibility criteria, which states may choose to exceed at their option. These minimum criteria include coverage of all pregnant women under 133% FPL, all children up to 6 years old under 133% FPL, and all children aged 6 to 18 under 100% FPL.[6] However, state-by-state variations in Medicaid coverage thresholds make the current system patchy and inconsistent. One saying goes, "If you've seen one Medicaid program, you've seen one Medicaid program." Medicaid programs in different states may also have different names (ie, MediCal in California), and/or may be combined with their CHIP program. Additionally, many children and their parents may be eligible but not enrolled,[7] or may "churn" between Medicaid and other insurance coverage because of eligibility changes.[8] By statute, Medicaid covers the Early and Periodic Screening, Diagnostic, and Treatment (EPSDT) program, considered a comprehensive standard of benefits for pediatric care.[9]

Children's Health Insurance Program

Established in 1997 as part of the Balanced Budget Act, CHIP covers children in low- and middle-income households who are not eligible for Medicaid as another joint federal-state program (with higher federal reimbursement than Medicaid).[10] States have flexibility to design their CHIP programs. For example, states can use CHIP funds to expand their Medicaid programs, create separate CHIP programs, or offer a mix of both types. In separate CHIP programs, states have flexibility, within federal rules and guidelines, to determine benefit packages and cost-sharing requirements. CHIP covers nearly 8 million children, and has helped to protect children against declining private coverage that has left many adults without adequate insurance in the past two decades.[11] Indeed, since the enactment of CHIP in 1997, the share of children who are uninsured has fallen by half—from 13.9% to 6.6%.[12]

The CHIP Reauthorization Act in 2009 increased appropriations for the program and included funding to encourage enrollment of children eligible but not enrolled, such as Express Lane eligibility (whereby states can use administrative data from other programs, such as Supplemental Nutrition Assistance Program or food stamps, to enroll individuals in Medicaid), 12-month continuous eligibility,[13] and state bonuses for reaching enrollment goals. It also improved benefits, enhanced data collection, and created a new emphasis on measuring the quality of care that children received.[11]

Military

TRICARE, which provides health benefits for eligible uniformed service members and dependents, covers unmarried children of active duty service members and eligible other members up to age 21, or 23 if in college. TRICARE serves 9.7 million Active Duty Service members, National Guard and Reserve members, retirees, their families, survivors, and certain former spouses worldwide,[14] including approximately 2 million children.[15] The program provides direct care through military treatment facilities and also incorporates network and non-network participating civilian health care professionals, institutions, pharmacies, and suppliers. TRICARE offers three primary options of health plans: (1) TRICARE Standard (the non-network benefit), (2) TRICARE Extra (a preferred provider organization–type benefit), and (3) TRICARE Prime (a health maintenance organization–type option). Other plan options may include dental or pharmacy benefits. The basic TRICARE package includes a well-baby and well-child care benefit modeled after the basic CHIP requirements for children, and includes routine newborn care, health supervision examinations, routine immunizations, periodic health screenings, and developmental assessments delivered in accordance with the American Academy of Pediatrics guidelines.[15] Medicaid covers 1 in 12 military children, and also serves as an important supplemental insurer for one in nine military children with special health care needs.[15]

Indian Health Service

The Indian Health Service (IHS) provides health care and disease prevention services to approximately 2.2 million American Indians (IA) and Alaska Natives (AN) through a network of hospitals, clinics, and health stations.[16] It is not a portable insurance system. IHS provides direct services through IHS-operated and tribally operated facilities that are generally limited to members or descendents of members of federally recognized tribes who live on or near federal reservations.[16] Medicaid is also an important source of health insurance coverage for AIs and ANs.

A BRIEF HISTORY OF HEALTH REFORM

Medicare and Medicaid were enacted in 1965 under President Lyndon B. Johnson, and were the largest sweeping changes to the health sector in US history. In the 1970s, efforts by Senator Ted Kennedy to establish a national health insurance program, and by President Richard Nixon to establish universal coverage, were ultimately unsuccessful.[17] President Bill and First Lady Hillary Clinton in the 1990s also worked for health reform; however, their efforts also eventually failed. In 2006, Massachusetts passed significant health reform under Governor Mitt Romney, designed to provide near-universal health insurance coverage for the state's residents.

President Barack Obama made health reform a large part of his 2008 presidential campaign. An early victory for President Obama was the passage of the CHIP Reauthorization Act in 2009. After tremendous Congressional efforts, the Patient Protection and Affordable Care Act was signed into law on March 23, 2010. It was further amended by the Health Care and Education Reconciliation Act (also known as the reconciliation sidecar) on March 30, 2010, and this amended law is referred to as the Affordable Care Act.

Although the ACA has faced numerous legal challenges since its enactment, its constitutionality was most directly challenged in the Supreme Court case of *National Federation of Independent Business v Sebelius*. In 2012, the Supreme Court ruled that the ACA was indeed constitutional, because it determined that the penalty for not having insurance (the "individual mandate") was within the government's ability to tax. However, it ruled that mandatory Medicaid expansion (to be addressed later) was unconstitutional because it was overly coercive to states. As such, most provisions of the ACA stood, other than a significant crux of the law's design: Medicaid expansion to the poorest of the poor in America. A second Supreme Court challenge in *King v Burwell*, decided in June 2015, upheld the legality of federal subsidies regardless of whether the insurance Marketplace is run by the state or the federal government.

AN OVERVIEW OF THE AFFORDABLE CARE ACT

The ACA's 900+ pages, not including its amendments and implementing regulations, create legislation that is complex, powerful, and at times overwhelming. The ACA has 10 parts, or titles, and each is packed with numerous reforms. An excellent, comprehensive overview of each title and its reforms is found elsewhere.[1] Notably, Title I changes insurance rules and sets up Marketplaces ("Exchanges", see later). Title II modifies public programs, focusing on Medicaid. Title III focuses on quality improvement across the health system, modifies Medicare's drug benefit, and creates a new preventive benefit in the program. Title IV focuses on prevention, establishes a prevention and public health trust fund, and establishes new menu labeling rules.

Title V creates a significant investment in the health care workforce. Title VI invests in program integrity, with strategies to decrease so-called "fraud and abuse," and modifies a patient-centered outcomes research body. The sidecar legislation added important improvements that addressed access in Medicaid by funding states to improve Medicaid payments for primary care services to Medicare levels, and also smoothed income and tax credit rules while closing the Medicare Part D "donut hole."[18]

Many of the ACA's provisions work to address racial/ethnic and socioeconomic status disparities in the United States. The "ABC's" of the ACA include *Access* to coverage, *Better* insurance, and *Consumer* protections (**Table 1**).

AFFORDABLE CARE ACT PROVISIONS AFFECTING CHILDREN AND FAMILIES

Numerous provisions within the ACA affect children, whether directly or via reforms that impact their parents and family members. Many have the potential to be very successful in improving health coverage and care for children.

Access to Coverage

Medicaid

Title II of the ACA mandates the most comprehensive and far-reaching set of changes to Medicaid since its establishment in 1965.[1] Although states have had a significant

Table 1
"ABC" acronym to describe the Affordable Care Act

	Keywords	Description	Details
A	Access to coverage	More individuals with insurance coverage	Expansion of health insurance to cover nearly 32 million more children, parents, and other individuals.
			Creation of health insurance marketplaces ("exchanges") for individuals to shop for affordable health insurance.
			Expansion of Medicaid to those up to 138% FPL, with strengthening of both Medicaid and CHIP.
			Provision of insurance subsidies on a sliding scale for those with incomes up to 400% FPL.
			Individual mandate to purchase health insurance, or pay a small penalty.
			Young adults can stay on their parents' plans until age 26.
B	Better insurance	Higher quality, lower cost	Preventive care covered with no cost sharing.
			Essential health benefits requirements.
			Medical loss ratio requirements: insurance companies must spend at least 80%–85% of beneficiaries' premiums on medical care (not administrative costs), or else pay a rebate.
			Decrease fraud and abuse.
C	Consumer protections	Beneficial market reforms	No pre-existing condition exclusions.
			No annual or lifetime limits on insurance coverage.

Abbreviation: FPL, Federal Poverty Level.

degree of freedom in implementing Medicaid (in accordance with some set federal principles), the ACA makes Medicaid into a more federally-directed program. Many ACA changes affect children and families.

By 2014, Medicaid coverage was available for all individuals not previously eligible (ie, childless, nonpregnant, nonelderly adults) with household incomes at or below 133% of FPL; however, because the first 5% of every enrollee's income is not counted, the new national eligibility standard for Medicaid is 138% FPL.[1] The federal government pays states for the costs of services to newly Medicaid-eligible individuals at 100% in 2014, 2015, and 2016; 95% in 2017; 94% in 2018; 93% in 2019; and 90% thereafter.[1] Although this sweeping Medicaid eligibility expansion was the intent of the ACA as passed originally, the Supreme Court's 2012 ruling established that the Medicaid expansion is now optional for states. At the time of this writing, only 31 states (including the District of Columbia) have actually adopted the Medicaid expansion.[19] Because federal subsidies in the Marketplaces take effect for individuals above the Medicaid eligibility threshold, effectively the poorest of the poor in the United States may continue without reliable and affordable access to coverage.

The ACA also establishes requirements to streamline and coordinate enrollment processes and provides federal support to establish "navigators" to assist with public education and enrollment.

Medicaid has much lower rates of reimbursement to providers compared with private insurance (generally highest reimbursement) and Medicare (Medicaid rates have historically been approximately 70% of Medicare's rates[20]). This lower reimbursement has resulted in practices limiting or not taking Medicaid patients, thus limiting access to care for Medicaid enrollees. Under the ACA, Medicaid reimbursement rates for many primary care services (including the administration of vaccines) were increased to at least Medicare rates for calendar years 2013 and 2014, and were available to physicians with a primary specialty designation of internal medicine, family medicine, or pediatrics. Although this 2-year funding increase has expired at the time of this writing, advocacy efforts persist for Congress to continue Medicaid payment parity for pediatric providers, and many states have decided to extend the provision using state funds.

Young adults and foster youth

Under the ACA, young adults may stay as dependents on their parents' health plans until age 26. Recent evidence suggested that 3 million young adults have gained coverage as a result.[21] A 2013 study based on data from two nationally representative surveys compared young adults who gained access to dependent coverage under the ACA with a control group (ages 26–34) who were not affected by the new policy. The study found strong evidence of increased access to care because of the law, with significant reductions in the number of young adults who delayed getting care and in those who did not receive needed care because of cost.[21] Two studies have demonstrated that enactment of the dependent-coverage provision was associated with financial protection from medical costs.[22,23] However, a November 2014 study that evaluated nationally representative data surrounding the implementation of the ACA confirmed that health care coverage for young adults increased but that young adults do not report improved health status, affordability of health care, or use of flu vaccination, compared with their older counterparts.[24] Persons aged 19 to 25 years were more likely to have a usual source of care than those aged 26 to 34 years, but both age groups saw declines in this measure of access to care. The authors inferred that efforts must continue to address access and quality in addition to coverage for young adults, because insurance may be necessary but not sufficient to alter health care use and overall health.[24] Children who were covered by Medicaid or CHIP and become young adults may or may not be eligible for Medicaid depending on their state's eligibility levels. However, foster youth may stay on Medicaid up to age 26.

Parents

Research shows that expanding coverage for parents leads to significant increases in coverage for children and more stable coverage for children over time; studies also show that, when parents are covered, children are more likely to receive needed care.[13] As such, insurance expansions for both adults and children can help to improve children's health.

Children with special health care needs

The ACA creates a Medicaid state option to provide medical assistance in a medical home ("health home" in the law's provision) to individuals with chronic conditions (ie, a mental health condition, a substance use disorder, asthma, diabetes, heart disease, and obesity) or one chronic condition and the likelihood of contracting at least one additional chronic condition.[25] Implementation of this provision offers states a higher federal match to fund their health homes program, although few states have taken this option. In this program, an enrollee may select, as his or her designated health home, a physician, a team of health care professionals operating with a physician, or a health team. The payment methodology for the program can be determined by states and may be tiered to reflect the severity or number of a patient's chronic conditions and the specific capabilities of the health home.[25]

Better Insurance

Preventive care without cost sharing

Section 2713 of the ACA requires the coverage of specific preventive care benefits for adults and children in all nongrandfathered individual and group health care plans without cost sharing. For children, the following must be provided without cost sharing[26]:

1. Immunizations for routine use that are recommended by the Advisory Committee on Immunization Practices of the Centers for Disease Control and Prevention[27];
2. Evidence-informed preventive care and screenings provided for in the comprehensive guidelines supported by the Health Resources and Services Administration. These guidelines specifically include the periodicity schedule and screenings of the Bright Futures Recommendations for Preventive Pediatric Health Care[28] and the Uniform Panel of the Secretary's Advisory Committee on Heritable Disorders in Newborns and Children.[29]

Essential health benefits

The ACA defined an "essential health benefits" provision, which specifies three primary elements[30]:

1. A list of benefit categories that must be provided in nongrandfathered insurance policies in the small group market (grandfathered plans are those existing at the time of ACA passage [March 23, 2010]);
2. A requirement that the scope of plans subject to the standard be equal to the scope of a "typical employer plan" currently existing in the marketplace; and
3. Rules regarding actuarial value (the percentage that the average person can expect the plan to cover) and cost sharing. (The actuarial value is expressed through "metal" tiers: platinum [90%], gold [80%], silver [70%], and bronze [60%], with a separate cost-sharing calculation for some participants in silver plans[30]).

The categories of essential health benefits that apply to plans inside and outside the Marketplace include ambulatory patient services; emergency services; hospitalization; maternity and newborn care; mental health and substance use disorder services, including behavioral health treatment; prescription drugs; rehabilitative and habilitative services and devices; laboratory services; preventive and wellness services and chronic disease management; and pediatric services, including oral and vision care.[31] ACA coverage of certain benefit categories that were not always covered by insurance plans, such as mental health/substance use disorder treatment, maternity and newborn care, and habilitative services, is a significant step forward. "Habilitative" services are "health care services that help a person keep, learn or improve skills and functioning for daily living,"[32] such as physical therapy to help a child with cerebral palsy function maximally, versus rehabilitative services that help to restore a child to previous functioning. Additionally, the fact that "pediatric services" was defined as an essential health benefit was considered a great win for children.

However, the law was implemented as a "benchmark plan approach" (where the essential health benefits were defined based on existing commercial norms in selected state benchmark plans) instead of as a national standard (using a model, such as Medicaid's Early and Periodic Screening, Diagnostic, and Treatment Program, or recommendations from the American Academy of Pediatrics). A recent study sought to determine how states address pediatric coverage in their benchmark plans, specifically which pediatric services were explicitly included or excluded. The study found that the benchmark plan approach to the definition of essential health benefits, particularly pediatric services, has resulted in a state-by-state patchwork of coverage with exclusions.[30] Because the U.S. Department of Health and Human Services (HHS) has indicated the intention to review its approach to essential health benefits regulation for the 2016 year, the study authors recommended that HHS revise its regulations to address both covered services and actuarial value; bar pediatric treatment limits and exclusions, particularly exclusions based on mental retardation, mental disability, or other developmental conditions; incorporate the concept of medical necessity into a defined pediatric benefit; and permit CHIP plans to be used as a benchmark for pediatric services.[30]

Consumer Protections

Insurance market reforms

Significant private insurance market reforms seek to decrease discrimination and improve consumer protections. Many of these reforms impact children and families, and they include, among others:

- Guaranteed issue and prohibition on pre-existing condition exclusions. Health plans must permit all comers to enroll regardless of age, gender, health status, or other factors that would otherwise predict the use of health services. Plans also cannot deny coverage for those with pre-existing conditions.
- Ban on medical underwriting (the practice of covering, or refusing to cover, someone or pricing premiums based on the applicant's medical history).[1] Insurers are allowed to vary premiums within a geographic region by only three categories: (1) age (older enrollees must pay no more than three times the premium of the youngest participants; the current practice in most states is much higher), (2) use of tobacco products, and (3) whether the enrollee is part of an employer or insurer program that rewards them for participating in certain wellness activities.[1]

- Coverage of young adults. The law allows young adults to stay on their parents' health insurance plans until age 26, and foster care youth to stay in Medicaid up to age 26.
- Ban on rescissions. A rescission is a retroactive termination of health coverage. Health care plans can generally no longer retroactively cancel individuals' health insurance coverage if they get sick.
- Ban on annual or lifetime dollar limits on health insurance coverage.
- Limits on out-of-pocket expenditures. The maximum out-of-pocket cost limit for any individual Marketplace plan for 2015 can be no more than $6,600 for an individual plan and $13,200 for a family plan.[33]

EFFORTS TO ADDRESS RACIAL AND ETHNIC HEALTH DISPARITIES

The ACA invests in increased data collection and research about health disparities, and initiatives to increase the racial and ethnic diversity of health care providers and provide them with strengthened cultural competency training.[34] The law also demonstrates an increased focus on minority health, because it elevates the National Institute on Minority Health and Health Disparities at the National Institutes of Health to a full Institute.[34] The ACA's impact on selected special populations is discussed next.

American Indians and Alaska Natives

AIs and ANs experience significant health disparities, including an infant mortality rate 1.7 times the non-Hispanic white population, the highest rate of sudden infant death syndrome of any population group, and suicide rates for AI/AN youth that were three times greater than rates for whites of similar age.[35] The ACA strengthens the IHS and benefits AI/AN populations through multiple avenues[36]:

1. Permanent reauthorization of the Indian Health Care Improvement Act, which prescribes the duties and responsibilities that allow IHS to improve its health care delivery systems and permit tribal governments to make technical changes in the future.
2. Support of comprehensive Native American youth suicide prevention efforts by streamlining the Substance Abuse and Mental Health Services Administration grants for Indian youth suicide prevention including demonstration projects on telemental health and youth suicide prevention curriculum programs in schools serving AI youth.[37]
3. Increases in clinician recruitment and retention in tribally operated health programs.
4. Structures that increase revenue through third-party payments to the IHS that support direct care and contract health services.
5. Elimination of premiums and deductibles for AI/ANs who receive IHS, tribal programming, or urban IHS.
6. Elimination of cost sharing for AIs with incomes at or below 300% FPL enrolled in coverage through a state exchange.[38]
7. Enrollment in Marketplace coverage any time of year, with no limited enrollment period. AI/AN populations can also change plans up to once per month.[39]

Home Visiting for Communities at Risk

The ACA established the Maternal, Infant, and Early Childhood Home Visiting program, which "facilitates collaboration and partnership at the federal, state, and community levels to improve the health of at-risk children through evidence-based home visiting programs."[40] The programs for home visiting reach pregnant women, expectant fathers, and parents and caregivers of children younger than the age of 5. The Maternal, Infant, and Early Childhood Home Visiting program is administered by the Health Resources and Services Administration in collaboration with HHS' Administration for Children and Families.[40] In particular, the statute specifies that at-risk communities include those with concentrations of premature birth, low-birth-weight infants, and infant mortality, including infant death caused by neglect, or other indicators of at-risk prenatal, maternal, newborn, or child health; poverty; crime; domestic violence; high rates of high school drop-outs; substance abuse; unemployment; or child maltreatment.

ONGOING CHALLENGES

Despite the ACA's progress, multiple challenges remain in the post-ACA landscape for children and families.

Children's Health Insurance Program Funding Extension

CHIP is at a crossroads under the new ACA landscape. CHIP has historically had bipartisan support and has helped to improve insurance coverage for low-moderate income children in the United States. With the ACA, multiple questions arise: How do CHIP plans compare with plans in the Marketplace? Should CHIP continue to exist, and if so, for how long? The ACA included important provisions for CHIP, including a "maintenance of effort" provision such that all states must maintain their CHIP eligibility levels at least through September 30, 2019. Funding for CHIP was set to expire by October 2015, but Congress acted to extend it for two more years with the passage of the Medicare Access and CHIP Reauthorization Act in April 2015. As such, whether CHIP should remain funded after 2017 will remain a subject of debate.

Several studies have demonstrated that CHIP plans offered better financial protection (with less cost sharing and minimal premiums) and similar or more comprehensive benefits[41–43] compared with plans in the Marketplace. Another study focused on separate CHIP plans found that they provide robust coverage of pediatric benefits, and substantial financial protection for families, reinforcing that CHIP is a "strong model for ensuring comprehensive and affordable coverage for children."[44]

Pediatric Dental Care

Although "pediatric services," including oral and vision care, is considered one of the essential health benefits, the dental benefit for children has actually become a "loophole."[45] The ACA specifies that, if a separate stand-alone dental plan also exists in the Marketplace, then qualified health plans (QHPs) in the Marketplace do not also have to offer a pediatric dental benefit. However, there is no requirement for families to purchase these stand-alone plans. Additionally, families face affordability issues for dental coverage when it is not embedded in a Marketplace plan, because those non-QHPs may not have the same assistance in terms of subsidies, cost-sharing reduction, or out-of-pocket limits as do QHPs.[46] Finding dental plans in some Marketplaces has also proved difficult.[45] Outside the Marketplace, plans have to ensure that their customers have access to all of the essential health benefits, including pediatric dental coverage, and be "reasonably assured" that their customers have purchased dental coverage. As such, many children within and outside the Marketplace may go without dental coverage, despite it being an essential health benefit.

The "Family" or "Kid" Glitch

Many parents continue to receive coverage through their employers. Under the ACA, employer-sponsored insurance is considered unaffordable if the employee contribution to the premium costs more than 9.5% of the employee's annual household income - at which point the employee would be eligible to purchase insurance in the Marketplace, possibly with subsidies.[13] Families not able to afford family employer-based coverage are not eligible for exchange subsidies. This situation, referred to as the "kid glitch" or "family glitch," has the potential to leave more children uninsured, particularly if CHIP is not extended past 2017 (discussed previously).

Network Adequacy

Network adequacy refers to a health plan's ability to deliver the benefits promised by providing reasonable access to a sufficient number of in-network primary care and specialty clinicians, and other health care services included under the terms of the contract.[47] The ACA requires that QHP issuers maintain provider networks that are "sufficient in number and type of providers" and include essential community providers, such as Federally Qualified Health Centers, family planning providers, and school-based health centers, many of which serve large numbers of children and

Table 2	
ACA action steps for pediatric clinicians	
Advocacy	Collect stories about how the ACA has impacted your patients or your practice and share them with your members of Congress. If there are unanticipated negative consequences of health reform experienced by your patients, bring them to the attention of your American Academy of Pediatrics chapter, medical society, public health officials, and/or Congressional representatives.
	Be aware of opportunities to advocate for child health policy issues that arise, such as reauthorization of CHIP, Medicaid payment parity, strengthening of essential health benefits standards, and dental coverage.
	Consider joining the American Academy of Pediatrics Key Contact network by e-mailing kids1st@aap.org.
Research	Much more pediatric-specific research is needed to assess the impact of the ACA on children, families, disparities, and pediatric practitioners.
	Potential research topics include monitoring changes in insurance coverage, enrollment, benefits, and network adequacy for children, adolescents, young adults and parents, and monitoring quality of care, sentinel health outcomes, cost, and socioeconomic and racial/ethnic disparities related to implementation of the ACA.
Clinical care	Inform families about the law, and encourage parents to sign up for insurance if they are uninsured.
	Pediatric clinicians can offer resources to patients and families in the clinical setting to help them navigate the insurance marketplaces and help in the decision-making regarding the most appropriate plan to meet the needs of the child and family. The American Academy of Pediatrics' public-facing Web site (healthychildren.org/ACAmarketplace) has information for families, and is also available in Spanish. The federal government has also launched the HealthCare.gov Web site and a 24-h call center at 1–800–318–2596 to provide educational information and enrollment assistance.[50]
	Ensure that children have a dental home and are receiving care in light of dental care loopholes in the ACA.
	Connect families and collaborate with home visiting programs in your area.

youth in many communities.[48] However, concerns have arisen regarding the adequacy of provider networks under Marketplace plans for children. For example, it was reported that Seattle Children's Hospital was initially excluded from some health plans in the state's exchange, prompting legal challenges based on network adequacy to ensure that children in Washington State have access to this important pediatric hospital.[49]

IMPLICATIONS: WHAT SHOULD PEDIATRIC CLINICIANS DO?

It is important for pediatric clinicians to understand the basics of the ACA, as discussed in this article. Moving forward, specific action steps for pediatricians include those discussed in **Table 2**.

SUMMARY

The ACA faces multiple challenges, including a Congress whose leaders have repeatedly stated their intention to hobble or repeal the legislation. However, the ACA's many successes remain: because of better access to insurance, there are 25% fewer uninsured people in the United States.[51] Additionally, countless Americans have better insurance and new consumer protections. We expect the impact of the ACA to be far-reaching for children and families, and to decrease disparities. Time will tell.

REFERENCES

1. McDonough JE. Inside national health reform. Berkeley (CA): University of California Press; 2011.
2. The Henry J. The uninsured — As a share of the nonelderly population, by poverty levels and family type. Kaiser Family Foundation; 2011. Available at: http://kff.org/uninsured/slide/the-uninsured-as-a-share-of-the-nonelderly-population-by-poverty-levels-and-family-type-2011/. Accessed January 31, 2015.
3. The Henry J. Health care coverage and personal health care expenditures in the U.S. Kaiser Family Foundation; 2011. Available at: http://kff.org/health-costs/slide/health-care-coverage-and-personal-health-care-expenditures-in-the-u-s-2011/. Accessed January 31, 2015.
4. National Conference of State Legislatures. Health insurance coverage of children ages birth to 18 in the United States, 2009. 2009. Available at: http://www.ncsl.org/research/health/children-without-health-insurance-coverage.aspx. Accessed January 31, 2015.
5. Paradise J. Medicaid moving forward. The Henry J. Kaiser Family Foundation, March 9, 2015. Available at: http://kff.org/health-reform/issue-brief/medicaid-moving-forward/. Accessed June 30, 2015.
6. Medicaid: an overview of spending on mandatory vs optional populations and services. The Henry J. Kaiser Family Foundation, 2005. Available at: http://kff.org/medicaid/issue-brief/medicaid-an-overview-of-spending-on-mandatory/. Accessed June 30, 2015.
7. Kenney GM, Lynch V, Huntress M, et al. Medicaid/CHIP participation among children and parents. Washington, DC: Robert Wood Johnson Foundation/Urban Institute; 2012.
8. Sommers B, Rosenbaum S. Issues in health reform: how changes in eligibility may move millions back and forth between Medicaid and insurance exchanges. Health Aff 2011;30(2):228–36.

9. Rosenbaum S, Wise PH. Crossing the Medicaid-private insurance divide: the case of EPSDT. Health Aff 2007;26(2):382–93.

10. Medicaid.gov. Children's Health Insurance Program Financing. Available at: http://www.medicaid.gov/medicaid-chip-program-information/by-topics/financing-and-reimbursement/childrens-health-insurance-program-financing.html. Accessed January 31, 2015.

11. Racine AD, Long TF, Helm ME, et al. Children's Health Insurance Program (CHIP): accomplishments, challenges, and policy recommendations. Pediatrics 2014; 133(3):e784–93.

12. Martinez ME, Cohen RA. Health insurance coverage: early release of estimates from the national health interview survey. Centers for Disease Control and Prevention: National Center for Health Statistics, Hyattsville, MD; 2012.

13. Rudowitz R, Artiga A, Arguello R. Children's Health Coverage: Medicaid, CHIP, and the ACA. The Henry J. Kaiser Family Foundation; 2014. Available at: http://kff.org/health-reform/issue-brief/childrens-health-coverage-medicaid-chip-and-the-aca/. Accessed June 30, 2015.

14. United States Department of Defense. Evaluation of the TRICARE Program: access, cost, and quality: Fiscal Year 2012 report to Congress. 2012. Available at: http://www.tricare.mil/hpae/_docs/TRICARE2012_02_28v5.pdf. Accessed May 31, 2015.

15. Shin P, Rosenbaum S, Mauery DR. Medicaid's role in treating children in military families. Washington, DC: The George Washington University School of Public Health and Health Sciences Center for Health Services Research and Policy; 2005. Available at: https://publichealth.gwu.edu/departments/healthpolicy/DHP_Publications/pub_uploads/dhpPublication_3A51C30E-5056-9D20-3DBA521960F44B1A.pdf. Accessed May 31, 2015.

16. Artiga S, Arguello R, Duckett P. Health coverage and care for American Indians and Alaska Natives. The Henry J. Kaiser Family Foundation; 2013. Available at: http://kff.org/disparities-policy/issue-brief/health-coverage-and-care-for-american-indians-and-alaska-natives/. Accessed June 30, 2015.

17. National health insurance: a brief history of reform efforts in the U.S. The Henry J. Kaiser Family Foundation; 2009. Available at: https://kaiserfamilyfoundation.files.wordpress.com/2013/01/7871.pdf. Accessed June 30, 2015.

18. The Health Care and Education Reconciliation Act: section-by-section analysis. Available at: http://www.dpc.senate.gov/healthreformbill/healthbill63.pdf. Accessed January 31, 2015.

19. Status of state action on the Medicaid expansion decision. The Henry J. Kaiser Family Foundation; 2015. Available at: http://kff.org/health-reform/state-indicator/state-activity-around-expanding-medicaid-under-the-affordable-care-act/. Accessed July 26, 2015.

20. American Academy of Pediatrics. Keep Medicaid strong for children. 2014. Available at: http://www.aap.org/en-us/advocacy-and-policy/federal-advocacy/Documents/MPIOne-PagerOct2014AdvocacyDay.pdf. Accessed January 31, 2015.

21. Sommers BD, Buchmueller T, Decker SL, et al. The affordable care act has led to significant gains in health insurance and access to care for young adults. Health Aff 2013;32(1):165–74.

22. Mulcahy A, Harris K, Finegold K, et al. Insurance coverage of emergency care for young adults under health reform. N Engl J Med 2013;368:2105–12.

23. Chua K, Sommers BD. Changes in health and medical spending among young adults under health reform. JAMA 2014;311(23):2437–8.

24. Kotagal M, Carle AC, Kessler LG, et al. Limited impact on health and access to care for 19- to 25-year-olds following the Patient Protection and Affordable Care Act. JAMA Pediatr 2014;168(11):1023–9.

25. Children and the Medical Home. American Academy of Pediatrics. Available at: https://www.aap.org/en-us/advocacy-and-policy/federal-advocacy/Documents/ACAmedicalhomefactsheet.pdf. Accessed June 30, 2015.

26. American Academy of Pediatrics. Achieving bright futures: implementation of the ACA Pediatric Preventive Services Provision. Available at: http://www.aap.org/en-us/professional-resources/practice-support/Periodicity/BF%20Introduction%20F010914.pdf. Accessed January 31, 2015.

27. Red Book Online. Immunization schedules for 2015. 2015. Available at: http://redbook.solutions.aap.org/SS/Immunization_Schedules.aspx. Accessed January 31, 2015.

28. American Academy of Pediatrics/Bright Futures. Recommendations for preventive pediatric health care. 2014. Available at: http://www.aap.org/en-us/professional-resources/practice-support/Periodicity/Periodicity%20Schedule_FINAL.pdf, Accessed January 31, 2015.

29. U.S. Department of Health and Human Services Secretary's Advisory Committee on Heritable Disorders in Newborns and Children. 2013 Annual Report. 2013. Available at: http://www.hrsa.gov/advisorycommittees/mchbadvisory/heritabledisorders/reportsrecommendations/reports/heritdisordersnewbornschildrenannualrpt13.pdf. Accessed January 31, 2015.

30. Grace AM, Noonan KG, Cheng TL, et al. The ACA's pediatric essential health benefit has resulted in a state-by-state patchwork of coverage with exclusions. Health Aff 2014;33(12):2136–43.

31. 42 U.S.C. 18022.

32. Rosenbaum S. Habilitative services coverage for children under the essential health benefit provisions of the Affordable Care Act. Issue Brief. Palo Alto (CA): Lucile Packard Foundation for Children's Health; 2013.

33. Healthcare.gov. Out-of-pocket maximum. Available at: https://www.healthcare.gov/glossary/out-of-pocket-maximum-limit/. Accessed January 31, 2015.

34. Whitehouse.gov. The Affordable Care Act helps American Indians and Alaska Natives. Available at: http://www.whitehouse.gov/sites/default/files/docs/the_aca_helps_ai_an.pdf. Accessed January 31, 2015.

35. Centers for Disease Control and Prevention, Office of Minority Health and Health Disparities. Health disparities affecting minorities. Available at: http://www.cdc.gov/minorityhealth/brochures/AIAN.pdf. Accessed January 31, 2015.

36. Coley D, Hale A. Affordable Care Act (ACA) and Native Youth. Available at: http://www.ihs.gov/aca/includes/themes/newihstheme/display_objects/documents/AffordableCareActandNativeYouth.pdf. Accessed June 30, 2015.

37. Indian Health Care Improvement Reauthorization and Extension Act of 2009.

38. 25 U.S.C. 1623.

39. Healthcare.gov. Health coverage for American Indians & Alaska Natives. Available at: https://www.healthcare.gov/american-indians-alaska-natives/. Accessed January 31, 2015.

40. US Department of Health & Human Services, Administration for Children & Families, Early Childhood Development. Home Visiting. Available at: http://www.acf.hhs.gov/programs/ecd/home-visiting. Accessed January 31, 2015.

41. Bly A, Lerche J, Rustagi K. Comparison of Benefits and Cost Sharing in Children's Health Insurance Programs to Qualified Health Plans. Wakely Consulting Group. 2014.

42. Report to the Chairman, Subcommittee on Health Care, Committee on Finance, U.S. Senate: Children's Health Insurance: Information on Coverage of Services, Costs to Consumers, and Access to Care in CHIP and Other Sources of Insurance. US Government Accountability Office. 2013.
43. Medicaid and CHIP Payment and Access Commission (MACPAC). Report to the Congress on Medicaid and CHIP. MACPAC. 2014.
44. Cardwell A, Jee J, Hess C, et al. Benefits and cost sharing in separate CHIP programs. Washington, DC: National Academy for State Health Policy and Georgetown University Health Policy Institute Center for Children and Families; 2014.
45. Rovner J. Legal loopholes leave some kids without dental insurance. Washington, DC: NPR; 2014.
46. Touschner J. Emerging policies on dental coverage for kids: a children's health policy blog. Washington, DC: Georgetown University Health Policy Institute Center for Children and Families; 2013. Available at: http://ccf.georgetown.edu/all/emerging-policies-on-dental-coverage-for-kids/. Accessed January 31, 2015.
47. McCarty S, Farris M. ACA implications for state network adequacy standards. Princeton (NJ): State Health Reform Assistance Network/Robert Wood Johnson Foundation; 2013.
48. National Academy for State Health Policy. Key implementation issues: network adequacy. Available at: http://www.nashp.org/children-in-vanguard/network-adequacy. Accessed January 31, 2015.
49. Landa A. WA: Seattle Children's Still Pressing Case Against OIC on Network Adequacy. State of Reform. 2014. Available at: http://stateofreform.com/news/states/washington/2014/03/oic-judge-turns-insurers-motion-dismiss-seattle-childrens-case/. Accessed January 31, 2015.
50. Grace A, Bucciarelli R. Pediatricians and affordable care act open enrollment: an opportunity to assist families in navigating health insurance. Clin Pediatr 2014;53(1).
51. Ungar L. Uninsured rates drop dramatically under Obamacare. USA Today; 2015. Available at: http://www.usatoday.com/story/news/nation/2015/03/16/uninsured-rates-drop-sharply-under-obamacare/24852325/. Accessed June 30, 2015.

Community Health Workers as a Component of the Health Care Team

Sheri L. Johnson, PhD[a], Veronica L. Gunn, MD, MPH[a,b,*]

KEYWORDS

- Community health worker • PCMH • Health care access • Care continuum
- Care coordination • Navigators • Promoters

KEY POINTS

- Evidence supports the positive impact of community health workers (CHWs) on some pediatric health care outcomes.
- Opportunities for continued integration of CHWs into the pediatric health care delivery system are expanding.
- Continued rigorous research demonstrating reduction in health care disparities and improved health outcomes is warranted.

INTRODUCTION

Community health workers (CHWs) create connections between health care systems, local community residents, and community-based organizations to increase health care access, promote appropriate levels of care utilization, and improve health outcomes for individuals and populations. In the United States, CHWs are defined as "frontline public health workers who are trusted members of and/or have an unusually close understanding of the community they serve."[1] CHWs often focus on reaching socially and economically disadvantaged groups and bridging cultural divides between patients, communities, health care providers, and health care systems.[2–4] CHWs also engage in policy advocacy[5,6] and community-based research[7] aimed at improving conditions necessary for health.

Ideally, a bidirectional flow of knowledge and resources enables CHWs and health systems to improve how health care services are delivered to specific populations.

Disclosure: The authors have no conflicts of interest to disclose.
[a] Department of Pediatrics, Center for the Advancement of Underserved Children, Medical College of Wisconsin, 8701 Watertown Plank Road, Milwaukee, WI 53226, USA;
[b] Department of Pediatrics, Medical College of Wisconsin, Population Health Management, Children's Hospital of Wisconsin, PO Box 1997, C525, Milwaukee, WI 53201-1997, USA
* Corresponding author.
E-mail address: vgunn@chw.org

Pediatr Clin N Am 62 (2015) 1313–1328
http://dx.doi.org/10.1016/j.pcl.2015.06.004
0031-3955/15/$ – see front matter © 2015 Elsevier Inc. All rights reserved.

Abbreviations	
CHR	Community Health Representative
CHW	Community Health Worker
FHW	Frontline Health Worker
LHW	Lay Health Worker
PN	Patient Navigator
PS	Promotoras

Knowledge of local health beliefs and practices can contribute to the development of culturally relevant health care service delivery. In addition, CHWs' perspectives regarding community-level assets and needs can inform the structure of responsive, patient- and community-centered medical homes.[8,9]

Variation exists in the level and type of training that CHWs receive.[10] Job titles and roles also differ across settings.[11] A 2002 integrative literature review reported evidence of CHW effectiveness in increasing access to care, particularly among underserved populations.[12] A more recent systematic review found mixed evidence demonstrating the impact of CHW interventions on behavior change and health outcomes and low to moderate strength of evidence regarding health care utilization. The authors concluded that more rigorous research is needed.[13] A systematic review of lay health worker interventions in pediatric chronic disease concluded modest improvement in urgent care use, symptoms, and caregiver quality of life.[14] No reviews were located that focused specifically on the comparative effectiveness of pediatric CHW interventions across ethnic groups or geographic settings. However, selected studies in the United States have reported that programs using some variation of a CHW increased public insurance enrollment and insurance continuity for Latino children,[15] improved childcare knowledge among American Indian adolescent mothers,[16] and demonstrated the potential to impact early caries prevention among American Indian and Alaska Native children.[17] Improved breastfeeding initiation and exclusivity, childhood immunization rates, and pulmonary tuberculosis cure rates as compared with usual care have been reported in the international literature.[18] Less convincing evidence for the impact of lay health worker interventions on child morbidity and increases in pediatric health care seeking behavior were reported.[18] A qualitative review of barriers and facilitators to lay health worker program implementation found that trusting relationships between lay health workers and participants are a hallmark of program strength.[19]

HISTORICAL PERSPECTIVE

CHWs were recognized as critical to the success of the primary health care system by the World Health Organizations' Alma-Ata declaration in 1978. To achieve optimal population health, the declaration emphasized the importance of "bringing health care as close as possible to where people live and work."[20] Thus, investing in CHWs emerged as a key strategy. Although the initial implementation emphasis focused on low- to moderate-income countries, acknowledgment of the importance of CHWs in the primary health care system spread across the globe.

Before the formal recognition of Alma-Ata, CHWs served in a range of formal and informal caregiving roles, defined by local needs, culture, and law. Health promotion roles for natural helpers are traced back at least 300 years.[21] In China, "barefoot doctors" were deployed to rural areas to improve health in the 1940s.[21] In Mexico and Latin America, *promotores de salud*" have provided health-related services for decades. Importantly, other nations including Cuba and Iran have long invested in systems that link local health councils, CHWs and facility-based care.[22,23]

Community Health Workers in the United States

Between 1966 and 2006, significant progress in CHW workforce development occurred in the United States.[21] Initial community health work programs focused on addressing poverty, social problems, and their relationship to health. By the early 1970s, CHWs were used in short-term public and privately funded special projects, such as the Resource Mothers curriculum for CHWs developed by the Virginia Task Force on Infant Mortality.[21] State and federal initiatives to incorporate CHWs emerged in the 1990s. In 1992, the Arizona Department of Health Services received state general funds to implement the Health Start Program, which continues to use CHWs to educate, support, and advocate for pregnant/postpartum women and their families.[24]

By the end of the 1990s, state legislation calling for study of training standards and certification of CHWs was passed in Texas, followed by legislation authorizing a CHW certification program in Ohio in 2003.[21] The Patient Navigator Outreach and Chronic Disease Prevention Act passed in 2005, codified a specific role for CHWs in the US health care delivery system.[25]

The Patient Protection and Affordable Care Act (ACA) provides increased policy-level support for the community health workforce in the United States.[26] The law allows services provided by CHWs to be reimbursed by Medicaid under specific conditions; grant funding for CHWs through the ACA is earmarked for outreach to medically underserved communities, health behavior promotion, health insurance enrollment, home visitation for maternal and child health, and referral to health care and community-based resources.[27]

TRAINING AND CERTIFICATION

Federal labor policy recognizes and tracks the CHW workforce. Duties are related broadly to outreach, support, informal counseling, and referral to improve health.[28] In 2013, the Bureau of Labor Statistics estimated that 45,800 individuals were employed as CHWs nationally. States with the highest employment level for the occupation included California, Texas, Illinois, New York, and Florida. The median hourly wage reported in 2013 was $16.64, and CHWs were employed in a variety of settings including individual and family services, local government, and outpatient care centers. Some workforce studies estimate that between 25% and 35% of CHWs are volunteers, suggesting that a greater number of individuals function in this capacity.[29]

Some states have legislated training and certification standards for CHW practice.[10] Qualitative data reported by Kash and colleagues[10] indicates that the impetus for CHW training and certification initiatives grew from recognition of unmet needs among cultural, economic, or geographic populations. Well-organized networks of CHWs are involved in advocacy for the profession, and for the people and communities they serve. Other states are less formalized. Training is offered via a variety of venues including community colleges, area health education centers, and workforce development agencies. Local nonprofit organizations and academic researchers also develop training specific to the health concern identified. Variation in criteria for selecting CHWs, and in the length and content of training impedes comparison of outcomes across studies.[11] O'Brien and colleagues[11] report that only 41% of intervention studies using CHWs described selection criteria for CHWs, and 59% included description of CHW training.

Debate regarding the benefits and potential negative impacts of formalized training and certification continues. Formalized training runs the risk of sapping CHWs of the interpersonal qualities that have been identified as necessary for success, such as empathy, warmth, nonjudgment, and acceptance. In health care professions, it is well-documented that as formal education proceeds future health care providers report declines in empathy over time.[30,31] Exposure to the culture of medicine and development of an "insider" identity for CHWs may increase the potential for explicit and implicit bias toward marginalized social groups, despite shared identity. Provider bias can be a contributing factor to health care disparities.[32] Thus, although integration of CHW as members of the health care team is recommended specifically as an important strategy to address health care disparities,[33] continued attention to the potential for unintended negative consequences of professionalization is warranted.

EVIDENCE OF EFFECTIVENESS
Facilitating Access to Health Care: Patient Navigators

Patient navigators (PN) help to facilitate successful progression through the health care delivery system, to achieve optimal outcomes.[34] Early PN interventions focused on reducing social disparities in cancer outcomes among adult women. Evidence for PN effectiveness with pediatric populations is emerging. Szilagyi and colleagues[35] reported increased preventive care visits and immunization rates among an urban adolescent, largely low-income population, using a PN intervention. Hambidge and colleagues[36] used master's level PNs who lived in the predominantly Spanish-speaking urban community being served to deliver a tiered intervention aimed at increasing pediatric immunization and well-child visits. Improvements in public insurance enrollment and underimmunization in the first 15 months of life were achieved. Conversely, Schuster and colleagues[37] reported no improvement in well-child care visits for low-income African-American children using a case management/home visiting intervention. Of note, the case managers and home visitors were experienced, had college degrees or more, and were described as African American. They were trained and tasked to address barriers to access by providing health education and advocacy, but did not have direct access to resources within a health care system. The authors do not discuss interpersonal qualities related to trust building, which are often cited as critical for success in typical PN interventions.

Improving Health Care Quality and Outcomes by Community Health Workers

Well-child care redesign research indicates that adding nonmedical providers to the health care team has the potential to improve the experience and outcomes of low income-children and caregivers with developmental and behavioral concerns.[38] Farber[39] reported that incorporation into the well-child care of bilingual, college-educated parent coaches with specific training in parent–child interaction resulted in positive developmental outcomes. Brown and colleagues[40] provided brief communication training to bilingual, paraprofessional medical assistants to improve identification of mental health concerns in a pediatric primary care setting. Improvement in parents' perceptions of care and willingness to discuss mental health concerns was reported. No studies specifically focused on CHWs addressing emotional and behavioral concerns in the pediatric primary care setting were located. However, Wissow and colleagues[41] tested a common factors approach, which emphasized a range of relationship-based factors associated with child and adolescent mental health outcomes. Children of color randomized to pediatric primary care providers trained in these skills experienced significant decreases in impairment as measured by the

Strengths and Difficulties Questionnaire, a brief validated measure of emotional and behavioral problems in children. Of note, the common factors model specifically scopes a role for paraprofessionals. Recommendations related to practice organization highlight recruitment of "aides" from the community served by the practice. Although the authors do not use the CHW job title, the job description mirrors the responsibilities often associated with CHW roles. Key functions include "creating expectations about care, influencing the kinds of concerns for which patients seek help, and supporting patients in carrying out treatment recommendations."[41]

Lessons learned from efforts to incorporate CHWs in the adult primary care setting can inform efforts to improve management of emotional and behavioral disorders in pediatric care. Waitzkin and colleagues[42] tested a collaborative model of depression care, pairing *promotoras* who focused on social and contextual influences, with primary care providers. No significant differences between the *promotora*-enhanced intervention and control group were found. However, qualitative data indicated strong agreement across primary care physicians, administrators, and nonprofessional support staff regarding the value of the promotoras. Challenges to implementation of a clinic-based *promotora* intervention included identifying adequate space, primary care physician and *promotora* turnover, and balancing multiple workplace demands.[43]

Stronger results from CHW interventions are reported for physical health outcomes. A 2009 systematic review by Postma and colleagues[44] of CHW interventions for children with asthma indicated consistent positive outcomes. In a sample of low-income, ethnically diverse pediatric patients, home-based asthma self-management delivered by CHWs combined with clinic-based nurse education resulted in better self-reported caretaker quality of life and more patient's symptom-free days, compared with only clinic-based care.[45] Study authors concluded that CHWs were successful in promoting effective asthma-related behavior changes because trusting relationships with families built on shared experiences and community identity. Margellos-Anast and colleagues[46] also reported significant improvement in asthma control and caregiver quality of life resulting from a CHW health education intervention delivered to African-American children and caregivers living in low-income communities. Authors noted that selection criteria for CHWs emphasized the importance of having a "cultural connection" to the target communities, and passion for positively impacting the health of neighborhood residents. Prior disease specific experience or knowledge was not necessary.

Community Health Workers Enable Culturally Relevant Medical Care Through Patient-Centered Medical Homes and Accountable Care Organizations

CHWs who may share experiences, language, and culture can be well-equipped to help patient families (particularly those with complex conditions) coordinate care across health care delivery systems in patient-centric and culturally effective ways, critical attributes of the patient-centered medical home (PCMH).[47] Pediatric health systems now appreciate the benefits of a "medical home" for patients, and the ACA incentivizes the development of patient centered medical homes.[48] The Agency for Healthcare Research and Quality describes 5 attributes and functions of the PCMH: (1) comprehensive care, (2) patient centered, (3) coordinated, (4) accessible services, and (5) quality and safety.[49] The American Academy of Pediatrics promotes a slightly expanded definition of medical home for the pediatric population, which includes care that is accessible, continuous, comprehensive, patient- and family-centered, coordinated, compassionate, and culturally effective.[50] Each definition acknowledges the influence of myriad factors on health outcomes – including individual factors, the influence of family norms and behaviors, access to health systems, the influence of communities, and larger societal and global influences – and the PCMH's role in facil-itating health across all domains (**Fig. 1**).[51] A population-based model of patient-centered care recognizes that physicians and patients each bring cultural experience and values into the care process. In many cases, the lived experience of providers and patients is vastly different. To facilitate the provision of comprehensive, patient-centered care that meaningfully engages patients in ways that respect their unique needs, culture, values, and family norms, PCMHs may effectively incorporate CHWs as a component of the care delivery team.[47]

Financial Impact of Community Health Workers

The cost effectiveness of CHWs has been explored in many different settings including in the emergency department,[52] and as extensions of primary care in the United States and abroad to increase access to care and manage chronic conditions.[53–56] However, there are few studies assessing the cost effectiveness of CHWs serving a pediatric population in the United States. Many well-designed analyses of CHW programs for pediatric populations in the United States have focused on asthma-based interven-tions, and few of these included some cost analysis.[57–60] A high-intensity, CHW-based intervention to decrease exposure to indoor asthma triggers in Seattle-King County projected a 4-year net savings of $189 to $721 per participant relative to a low-intensity group.[57] Study authors estimated that if the reductions in urgent care costs persisted among the high-intensity group, the potential savings per child could range from $1316 to $1849 discounted at 3% per year. Similarly, a crossover study of a

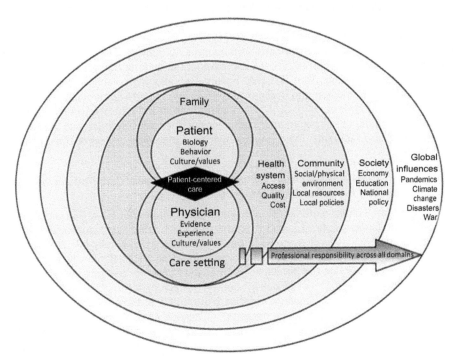

Fig. 1. Medical College of Wisconsin population-based model of a patient-centered care. (*From* Meurer LN, Young SA, Meurer JR, et al. The urban and community health pathway: preparing socially responsive physicians through community-engaged learning. Am J Prev Med 2011;41(4S3):S228–36; with permission.)

home-based environmental asthma management intervention delivered by lay health workers resulted in significant decreases in asthma-related emergency department visits and inpatient stays, at a relatively low per-family cost of $450 to $500.[58] A cost analysis of a community-based asthma management initiative in Boston showed an adjusted return on investment of 1.33 after controlling for changes in a comparison population, and a social return on investment of 1.85, which accounted for improvements in missed school and missed work days[60] (**Box 1**).

A community-based pediatric asthma initiative provided by outreach workers in Tacoma, Washington, resulted in significant improvements in caregiver quality of life, completed asthma management plans, and self-reported asthma hospitalizations. A formal cost-effectiveness analysis was not performed owing to the self-reported nature of health care utilization; however, study authors opined that – based on the estimated $840 cost per hospitalization day (in 2002 dollars), and the average program cost of $200 per family – the reported reduction in hospitalizations suggested that the intervention could decrease overall health care costs.[59] Although target populations for CHW-based interventions and outcome measures often differ, a systematic review of the economic value of home-based interventions to improve asthma morbidity concluded that the benefits of such programs – including interventions delivered by CHWs – exceeded the program costs.[62]

CHALLENGES AND FUTURE MODELS
Expanded Scope from a Disease Focus to Include Social Influences on Health Outcomes

As insurers and consumers in the United States are beginning to hold health care delivery systems accountable for population-based outcomes, providers are exploring ways to address social influences on health outcomes. Public health data have long demonstrated that health-related behaviors and environmental, cultural, and social influences impact population health outcomes collectively more than the actual delivery of health care services[63,64] (**Fig. 2**).

Box 1

Case study 1: Community health workers in community-based asthma management at Children's Hospital of Boston

Since 2005, the Community Asthma Initiative (CAI) of Boston Children's Hospital has used community health workers (CHWs), along with nurse case managers, to deploy a community-based asthma initiative to improve disease management.[60] CHWs conduct a series of home visits with enrolled children, educate families on asthma prevention and treatment (including identifying asthma triggers such as pests, dust, smoke, and mold), and provide demonstrations on how to reduce or eliminate exposure to specific triggers. CHWs provide families with supplies to address environmental triggers, such as pillow covers, plastic storage bins, and HEPA vacuum cleaners, and also facilitate family connection with local home inspectors to ensure that landlords address environmental hazards, such as leaking pipes or pests, which can exacerbate asthma. The CAI is a partnership between families of children with asthma, CHWs, primary care providers, schools, and community-based organizations to ensure that children with asthma receive the appropriate interventions to improve asthma outcomes. An evaluation of the CAI demonstrated significant decreases in asthma-related emergency department visits, hospitalizations, patient missed school days, parent missed work days, and limitations of physical activity owing to asthma.[61]

Data from Woods ER, Bhaumik U, Sommer SJ, et al. Community asthma initiative: evaluation of a quality improvement program for comprehensive asthma care. Pediatrics 2012;129(3):465–72.

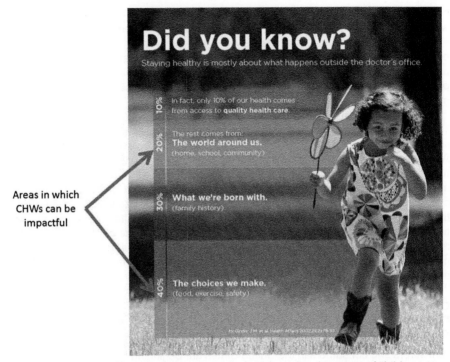

Fig. 2. Determinants of health. CHW, community health worker. (*Courtesy of* Children's Hospital and Health System of Wisconsin, Milwaukee, WI; with permission; and *Data from* McGinnis JM, Williams-Russo P, Knickman JR. The case for more active policy attention to health promotion. Health Aff (Millwood) 2002;21(2):78–93.)

These findings are consistent with the population-based model of patient centered care, and the social ecological model of health. Each model acknowledges the influence of multiple determinants of health, including family norms and beliefs, community influences, and the influence of larger society. These factors are particularly relevant for a pediatric population that depends on adults to meet basic needs, and who typically learn health behaviors from influential adults.

As such, efforts to improve pediatric health outcomes must address the social determinants of health in culturally and socially acceptable ways.[64] Goepp and colleagues[65] uncovered powerful psychosocial factors driving low-acuity pediatric emergency department utilization using a participatory ethnographic research approach. CHWs were instrumental in identifying deterrents to primary care utilization that were previously misunderstood as willful abuse of the system. The incorporation of CHWs into a care delivery team may remove barriers to care that impede improvements in child health outcomes. The Community Rx program being piloted in Chicago links patients with an e-prescription for social support services in their community and a CHW who facilitates communication between the patient, community-based service, and clinic provider.[66] Although the CHW role in pediatric health service delivery has been focused historically on disease management, there may be an important role for CHWs to support development of caregiver skills to address social influences on health outcomes. Pediatric health systems investing in efforts to address the social determinants of health can consider training CHWs in individual-level capacity building and change management techniques, such as motivational interviewing, to facilitate sustainable behavior change among pediatric patient families (**Box 2**).

Use of Community Health Workers as a Component of the Care Delivery Team

Efforts to formalize the use of CHWs to improve the continuity and coordination of care between health care delivery infrastructures (ie, between hospitals and primary care settings) have met with mixed success to date. Burns and colleagues[70] described a hospital-based quality improvement initiative that used in-person and telephonic support by CHWs to decrease readmission rates among an adult population at high risk of readmission. Although the intervention patients had lower readmission rates compared with usual care, there was no improvement in follow-up with a primary care provider among the intervention patients, and the decrease in readmissions did not attain significance. Importantly, the authors described several challenges to CHWs implementation of the improvement, including inconsistent notification of CHWs of an eligible patient before discharge and CHWs not having ready access to information regarding patient appointments. In contrast, the Camden Coalition of Healthcare Providers has effectively used CHWs as integral members of the care delivery team to facilitate understanding of chronic health conditions, support health

---

Box 2

Case study 2: Community health workers addressing social determinants of health outcomes as a component of primary care services at Children's Hospital of Wisconsin

Children's Hospital of Wisconsin uses community health navigators as part of a comprehensive, capacity-building initiative to improve the health of communities in which children live, learn, and grow. The navigators, trusted residents of the communities in which they work, use a strengths-based approach to caregiver skill building to enable caregivers to successfully address social influences on health outcomes. The models that inform navigator training include Prochaska's transtheoretical (Stages of Change) model,[67] social cognitive theory,[68] and the health belief model.[69] Lucy's story is illustrative of the way Children's Hospital of Wisconsin's navigators serve as a critical extension of the care delivery team whose focus on social determinants of health provides an important complement to the clinical services, and enables a comprehensive approach to health.

Lucy is an 8-year-old girl with a history of poorly controlled type I diabetes mellitus, who has been hospitalized multiple times for diabetic ketoacidosis. Lucy and her mother have worked with clinicians in the Children's Hospital Diabetes Clinic and with her Children's Medical Group primary care pediatrician to manager her disease. After several months of sporadically attended clinic appointments at which Lucy's blood sugar readings were frequently elevated, Lucy's pediatrician became concerned that Lucy's mother may have low health literacy, and engaged the community health navigator who serves Lucy's neighborhood. The navigator met Lucy and her mother at their residence, and learned that they were effectively homeless, moving from willing friend or family member as able, and squatting in abandoned buildings when they could not stay with friends. As a result, they were often without electricity. Insulin must be refrigerated to maintain its effectiveness, and Lucy often was without electricity (much less a refrigerator), making it impossible to manage her diabetes well. The community health navigator worked with Lucy's mother in a capacity-building manner, assessing her familiarity with housing resources and comfort in completing the application process, even engaging in role play to facilitate her readiness to change and to build her confidence in navigating the often intimidating process for securing housing and energy assistance utility relief. After working with the navigator, Lucy's mother was able to secure stable housing with appliances and utilities. In addition, the diabetes clinic staff, primary care provider, and community health navigator all worked collaboratively to support Lucy and her mother in effectively managing her diabetes.

behavior change, and keep patients connected with their primary care providers, reducing the need for higher acuity health care settings, and ultimately decreasing the total cost of care.[71]

Inclusion of CHWs as an integral member of a care delivery team requires buy-in from providers and staff alike for success, although not all health care professionals perceive the value of CHWs in improving health outcomes. Mobula and colleagues[72] demonstrated that primary care providers and clinic staff with greater cultural competence, preparedness, and motivation were more likely to perceive CHWs as helpful in reducing health care disparities. Attention to building organizational cultural competency may be needed to successfully implement team-based care. Effectively leveraged, CHWs' knowledge of local assets and credibility within the community could facilitate an enhanced relationship among patients and provider care teams. This in turn, could foster greater provider appreciation for the relevance of CHWs, resulting in improvement of internal cultural competencies.

Practice Considerations

Health care systems will need to consider a variety of factors when incorporating CHWs in the care delivery team (**Box 3**). Roles among team members will need to be clarified, ensuring that all team members are enabled to practice at the top of their license or training (because CHWs are not always licensed). Discussions regarding scope of practice can often create tension among provider groups, and may be particularly challenging when incorporating nonlicensed team members into the care delivery continuum. Systems that acknowledge and appreciate the value of CHWs in effectively engaging patients and families in unique ways that are cost effective and result in improved outcomes will be willing to work through these difficult conversations. Sargeant and colleagues[73] describe 5 elements of interprofessional primary care teamwork related to effectiveness – understanding and respect of roles, awareness that team building requires effort, understanding primary care principles, practical "know how," and communication. Findings from Solheim and colleagues[74] emphasize that effective primary health care practice requires attentiveness to community complexity, and the capacity to integrate perspectives from individuals and families. CHWs are a logical conduit for bidirectional flow of information to and from the health care delivery system. When CHWs are incorporated into a care delivery team to enable local and authentic means of supporting patient families in community and home-based health improvement, providers should recognize that differences in vernacular and style of engagement may exist. Misunderstanding and distrust among the care delivery team can occur. Clear role definition, frequent opportunities for collaboration, training in cultural humility,[75] and development of operational structures

---

Box 3
Practice considerations for integrating community health workers

- Create culture supportive of community health workers (CHW) role in care delivery team.
- Define CHW role (eg, health education, access, clinical support, etc) and associated workflow adjustments among care team.
- Determine training required for CHWs.
- Establish metrics of CHW effectiveness.
- Develop mechanism for CHW documentation in the electronic health record.
- Implement mechanism to bill for CHW services.

to facilitate information exchange and validation will be instrumental in developing an effective care continuum.

An important enabler to meaningfully use CHWs as members of a care delivery team is developing means of including CHW documentation in the electronic health record. Because US health care delivery systems historically were not established to manage population health, electronic health records have not typically been designed to document social determinants of health and the interventions used by health care systems to address them.[76] Documentation in the medical record helps to ensure clear communication among care delivery team members, and may be necessary to secure reimbursement for CHWs service. However, practical, ethical, and legal considerations regarding documentation in the medical record require careful attention. Despite these challenges, some systems have enabled CHWs to effectively leverage their EHRs to meet patient needs and document progress toward goals. The Heart of TX Community Health Center has enabled CHWs to use reports from their electronic health record to recall diabetic patients due for examinations.[77] The Children's Hospital of Wisconsin's employed CHWs receive referrals from primary care providers, school nurses, inpatient providers, and other colleagues within the system, and are working to formalize this referral process in the electronic health record (Gunn VL, personal communication, January 12, 2015). Other barriers to integrating CHWs into the care delivery team include lack of clarity in mechanisms for reimbursement for services, and lack of metrics to measure CHW contribution to improving health outcomes, enhancing the quality of care and decreasing the total cost of care.[78]

Outcomes from policy- and systems-level approaches implemented in Massachusetts are beginning to emerge; early signs of success related to sustaining the CHW workforce through recognition, training, and funding are reported.[79] Texas advanced Medicaid policy to formally include CHWs as members of the health care team. Minnesota has established a comprehensive infrastructure, and enacted policy that allows Medicaid reimbursement for CHWs who complete certification and serve under approved supervisory staff in the primary care setting.[80] Several other states have enacted policy relative to CHW scope of practice, training, and certification.[10] Health care systems and providers can benefit from lessons learned thus far, and proceed with more informed implementation. Continued attention to recruitment, training, and supervision criteria is warranted to achieve improved health outcomes and cost effectiveness. Consideration of potential roles for CHWs along the prevention and health promotion continuum may complement the contributions that CHWs make to chronic disease management. The CHW workforce in pediatric patient-centered medical homes could be used to promote physical activity, fresh fruit and vegetable consumption, literacy, and positive parenting skills, among other strategies to positively impact the health of the population.

SUMMARY

CHWs are increasingly recognized as key to local and national efforts aimed at reducing health care disparities and advancing health equity. For decades, CHWs have been important components of health care service delivery to vulnerable and underserved populations throughout the world. CHWs have demonstrated ability to improve access to health care, facilitate care coordination, and support improved health outcomes; and have shown a reduction in health care costs and increases in quality of living. Recent federal policies clarifying reimbursable services by CHWs and the development of several evidence-based CHW interventions to improve pediatric health outcomes create a favorable environment for pediatric systems to thoughtfully incorporate CHWs into the health care continuum. Continued rigorous research demonstrating reduction in health care disparities and improved health outcomes is warranted.

REFERENCES

1. American Public Health Association. Community Health Workers. In: American Public Health Association. 2014. Available at: http://www.apha.org/apha-communities/member-sections/community-health-workers. Accessed January 18, 2015.
2. Haines A, Sanders D, Lehmann U, et al. Achieving child survival goals: potential contribution of community health workers. Lancet 2007;369:2121–31.
3. Love MB, Gardner K, Legion V. Community health workers: who they are and what they do. Health Educ Behav 1997;24(4):510–22.
4. Brownstein JN, Hirsch GR, Rosenthal EL, et al. Community health workers "101" for primary care providers and other stakeholders in health care systems. J Ambul Care Manage 2011;34(3):210–20.
5. Charles-Azure J, Lette E. Promotion of healthier beverages in Indian communities. IHS Prim Care Provid 2005;30:143–7.
6. McGill J. What can one program do? Energy drinks regulated in Montana thanks to efforts of Blackfeet CHRs. In: Indian Health Service. n.d. Available at: http://www.ihs.gov/chr/index.cfm?module=oneProgram. Accessed January 2, 2015.
7. Arredondo E, Mueller K, Mejia E, et al. Advocating for environmental changes to increase access to parks: engaging promotoras and youth leaders. Health Promot Pract 2013;14(5):759–66.
8. Findley S, Matos S, Hicks A, et al. Community health worker integration into the health care team accomplishes the triple aim in a patient-centered medical home: a Bronx tale. J Ambul Care Manage 2014;37(1):82–91.
9. Wennerstrom A, Bui T, Harden-Barrios J, et al. Integrating community health workers into a patient-centered medical home to support disease self-management among Vietnamese Americans: lessons learned. Health Promot Pract 2015;16(1):72–83.
10. Kash BA, May ML, Tai-Seale M. Community health worker training and certification programs in the United States: findings from a national survey. Health Policy 2007;80(1):32–42.
11. O'Brien MJ, Squires AP, Bixby RA, et al. Role development of community health workers: an examination of selection and training processes in the intervention literature. Am J Prev Med 2009;37(6S1):S262–9.
12. Swider SM. Outcome effectiveness of community health workers: an integrative literature review. Public Health Nurs 2002;19(1):11–20.
13. Viswanathan M, Kraschnewski JL, Nishikawa B, et al. Outcomes and costs of community health worker interventions: a systematic review. Med Care 2010;48(9):792–808.
14. Raphael JL, Rueda A, Lion KC, et al. The role of lay health workers in pediatric chronic disease: a systematic review. Acad Pediatr 2013;13(5):408–20.
15. Flores G, Abreu M, Chaisson CE, et al. A randomized, controlled trial of the effectiveness of community-based case management in insuring uninsured Latino children. Pediatrics 2005;116(6):1433–41.
16. Barlow A, Varipatis-Baker E, Speakman K, et al. Home-visiting intervention to improve child care among American Indian adolescent mothers: a randomized trial. Arch Pediatr Adolesc Med 2006;160(11):1101–7.
17. Albino JE, Orlando VA. Promising directions for caries prevention with American Indian and Alaska Native children. Int Dent J 2010;60(3S2):216–22.

18. Lewin S, Munabi-Babigumira S, Glenton C, et al. Lay health workers in primary and community health care for maternal and child health and the management of infectious diseases. Cochrane Database Syst Rev 2010;(3):CD004015.
19. Glenton C, Colvin CJ, Carlsen B, et al. Barriers and facilitators to the implementation of lay health worker programmes to improve access to maternal and child health: qualitative evidence synthesis. Cochrane Database Syst Rev 2013;(10):CD010414.
20. World Health Organization. Declaration of Alma-Ata International Conference on Primary Health Care, Alma-Ata, USSR, 6–12 September 1978. In: Primary Health Care. 2008. Available at: http://www.who.int/publications/almaata_declaration_en.pdf?ua=1. Accessed January 26, 2015.
21. U.S. Department of Health and Human Services. Community Health Worker National Workforce Study. In: Health Resources and Services Administration, Bureau of Health Professions. 2007. Available at: http://bhpr.hrsa.gov/healthworkforce/reports/chwstudy2007.pdf. Accessed December 3, 2014.
22. Drain PK, Barry M. Global health: 50 years of U.S. embargo: Cuba's health consequences and lessons. Science 2010;328(5978):572–3.
23. Javanparast S, Baum F, Labonte R, et al. The experience of community health workers training in Iran: a qualitative study. BMC Health Serv Res 2012;12:291.
24. Arizona Department of Health Services. Health Start Program. In: Office of Women's Health. Available at: http://www.azdhs.gov/phs/owch/women/healthstart.htm. Accessed January 21, 2015.
25. U.S. Government Publishing Office. Public Law 109-18-Patient Navigator Outreach and Chronic Disease Prevention Act of 2005. In: Public and Private Laws. 109th Congress. H.R. 1812. 2005. Available at: http://www.gpo.gov/fdsys/pkg/PLAW-109publ18/pdf/PLAW-109publ18.pdf. Accessed January 26, 2015.
26. U.S. Government Publishing Office. Public Law 111-148-Patient Protection and Affordable Care Act. In: Public and Private Laws. 111th Congress. H.R. 3590. 2010. Available at: http://www.gpo.gov/fdsys/pkg/PLAW-111publ148/pdf/PLAW-111publ148.pdf. Accessed January 26, 2015.
27. Islam N, Nadkarni SK, Zahn D, et al. Integrating community health workers within patient protection and Affordable Care Act implementation. J Public Health Manag Pract 2015;21(1):42–50.
28. United States Department of Labor. Occupational employment and wages, May 2013: 21–1094 Community Health Workers. In: Bureau of Labor Statistics. 2014. Available at: http://www.bls.gov/oes/current/oes211094.htm. Accessed January 21, 2015.
29. Rosenthal EL, Wiggins N, Ingram M, et al. Community health workers then and now: an overview of national studies aimed at defining the field. J Ambul Care Manage 2011;34(3):247–59.
30. Bellini LM, Shea JA. Mood change and empathy decline persist during three years of internal medicine training. Acad Med 2005;80(2):164–7.
31. Hojat M, Mangione S, Nasca TJ, et al. An empirical study of decline in empathy in medical school. Med Educ 2004;38(9):934–41.
32. Institute of Medicine. Unequal treatment: confronting racial and ethnic disparities in health care. Washington, DC: The National Academies Press; 2003.
33. Ingram M, Reinschmidt KM, Schachter KA, et al. Establishing a professional profile of community health workers: results from a national study of roles, activities and training. J Community Health 2012;37(2):529–37.
34. Freeman HP, Rodriguez RL. History and principles of patient navigation. Cancer 2011;117:3537–40.

35. Szilagyi PG, Humiston SG, Gallivan S, et al. Effectiveness of a citywide patient immunization navigator program on improving adolescent immunizations and preventive care visit rates. Arch Pediatr Adolesc Med 2011;165(6):547–53.

36. Hambidge SJ, Phibbs SL, Chandramouli V, et al. A stepped intervention increases well-child care and immunization rates in a disadvantaged population. Pediatrics 2009;124(2):455–64.

37. Schuster MA, Wood DL, Duan N, et al. Utilization of well-child care services for African-American infants in a low-income community: results of a randomized, controlled case management/home visitation intervention. Pediatrics 1998; 101(6):999–1005.

38. Coker TR, Windon A, Moreno C, et al. Well-child care clinical practice redesign for young children: a systematic review of strategies and tools. Pediatrics 2013;131(S1):S5–25.

39. Farber ML. Parent mentoring and child anticipatory guidance with Latino and African American families. Health Soc Work 2009;34(3):179–89.

40. Brown JD, Wissow LS, Cook BL, et al. Mental health communications skills training for medical assistants in pediatric primary care. J Behav Health Serv Res 2013;40(1):20–35.

41. Wissow LS, Gadomski A, Roter D, et al. Improving child and parent mental health in primary care: a cluster-randomized trial of communication skills training. Pediatrics 2008;121(2):266–75.

42. Waitzkin H, Getrich C, Heying S, et al. Promotoras as mental health practitioners in primary care: a multi-method study of an intervention to address contextual sources of depression. J Community Health 2001;36(2):316–31.

43. Getrich C, Heying S, Willging C, et al. An ethnography of clinic "noise" in a community-based, promotora-centered mental health intervention. Soc Sci Med 2007;65(2):319–30.

44. Postma J, Karr C, Kieckhefer G. Community health workers and environmental interventions for children with asthma: a systematic review. J Asthma 2009;46(6):564–76.

45. Krieger J, Takaro TK, Song L, et al. A randomized controlled trial of asthma self-management support comparing clinic-based nurses and in-home community health workers: the Seattle-King County Healthy Homes II Project. Arch Pediatr Adolesc Med 2009;163(2):141–9.

46. Margellos-Anast H, Gutierrez MA, Whitman S. Improving asthma management among African American children via a community health worker model: findings from a Chicago-based pilot intervention. J Asthma 2012;49(4):380–9.

47. Martinez J, Ro M, Villa NW, et al. Transforming the delivery of care in the post-health reform era: what role will community health workers play? Am J Public Health 2011;101(12):e1–5.

48. Patient Centered Primary Care Collaborative. Joint Principles of the Patient-Centered Medical Home. 2007. Available at: http://www.pcpcc.net/joint-principles. Accessed December 8, 2014.

49. U.S. Department of Health and Human Services. Defining the Patient Centered Medical Home. In: Agency for Healthcare Research and Quality. n.d. Available at: http://pcmh.ahrq.gov/page/defining-pcmh. Accessed December 8, 2014.

50. American Academy of Pediatrics. Family-Centered Medical Home Overview. In: National Center for Medical Home Implementation. n.d. Available at: http://medicalhomeinfo.org/about/medical_home/. Accessed December 8, 2014.

51. Meurer LN, Young SA, Meurer JR, et al. The urban and community health pathway: preparing socially responsive physicians through community-engaged learning. Am J Prev Med 2011;41(4S3):S228–36.

52. Enard KR, Ganelin DM. Reducing preventable emergency department utilization and costs by using community health workers as patient navigators. J Healthc Manag 2013;58(6):412–28.

53. Whitley EM, Everhart RM, Wright RA. Measuring return on investment for outreach by community health workers. J Health Care Poor Underserved 2006; 17(1 Suppl):6–15.

54. Gilmer TP, Rose S, Valentine WJ, et al. Cost-effectiveness of diabetes care management for low-income populations. Health Serv Res 2007;42(5):1943–59.

55. Prinja S, Jeet G, Verma R, et al. Economic analysis of delivering primary health care services through community health workers in 3 North Indian states. PLos One 2014;9(3):e91781.

56. Gaziano TA, Bertram M, Tollman SM, et al. Hypertension education and adherence in South Africa: a cost-effectiveness analysis of community health workers. BMC Public Health 2014;14:240.

57. Krieger JW, Takaro TK, Song L, et al. The Seattle-King County Healthy Homes Project: a randomized, controlled trial of a community health worker intervention to decrease exposure to indoor asthma triggers. Am J Public Health 2005;95(4): 652–9.

58. Bryant-Stephens T, Kurian C, Guo R, et al. Impact of a household environmental intervention delivered by lay health workers on asthma symptom control in urban, disadvantaged children with asthma. Am J Public Health 2009;99(S3): S657–65.

59. Primomo J, Johnston S, DiBiase F, et al. Evaluation of a community-based outreach worker program for children with asthma. Public Health Nurs 2006; 23(3):234–41.

60. Bhaumik U, Norris K, Charron G, et al. A cost analysis for a community-based case management intervention program for pediatric asthma. J Asthma 2013; 50(3):310–7.

61. Woods ER, Bhaumik U, Sommer SJ, et al. Community asthma initiative: evaluation of a quality improvement program for comprehensive asthma care. Pediatrics 2012;129(3):465–72.

62. Nurmagambetov TA, Barnett SB, Jacob V, et al. Economic value of home-based, multi-trigger, multicomponent interventions with an environmental focus for reducing asthma morbidity a community guide systematic review. Am J Prev Med 2011;41(2S1):S33–47.

63. McGinnis JM, Foege WH. Actual causes of death in the United States. JAMA 1993;270(18):2207–12.

64. McGinnis JM, Williams-Russo P, Knickman JR. The case for more active policy attention to health promotion. Health Aff (Millwood) 2002;21(2):78–93.

65. Goepp JG, Chin NP, Massad J, et al. Pediatric emergency department outreach: solving medical problems or revealing community solutions? J Health Care Poor Underserved 2004;15(4):522–9.

66. Parekh A. Clinical-community linkages: a step towards better health. In: U.S. Department of Health and Human Services. 2013. Available at: http://obgyn. bsd.uchicago.edu/FacultyResearch/Lindaulab/hhs%20blog%20post%20(2).pdf. Accessed January 17, 2015.

67. Prochaska JO. Systems of psychotherapy: a transtheoretical analysis. 2nd edition. Pacific Grove (CA): Brooks-Cole; 1984 (Originally published 1979).

68. Bandura A. Social learning theory. Englewood Cliffs (NJ): Prentice Hall; 1977.

69. Rosenstock IM, Strecher VJ, Becker MH. Social Learning Theory and the Health Belief Model. Health Educ Q 1988;15(2):175–83.

70. Burns ME, Galbraith AA, Ross-Degnan D, et al. Feasibility and evaluation of a pilot community health worker intervention to reduce hospital readmissions. Int J Qual Health Care 2014;26(4):358–65.

71. Gawande A. The hot spotters. In: The New Yorker. 2011. Available at: http://www.newyorker.com/magazine/2011/01/24/the-hot-spotters. Accessed January 18, 2015.

72. Mobula LM, Okoye MT, Boulware LE, et al. Cultural competence and perceptions of community health workers' effectiveness for reducing health care disparities. J Prim Care Community Health 2015;6(1):10–5.

73. Sargeant J, Loney E, Murphy G. Effective interpersonal teams: "contact is not enough" to build a team. J Contin Educ Health Prof 2008;28(4):228–34.

74. Solheim K, McElmurry BJ, Kim MJ. Multidisciplinary teamwork in US primary health care. Soc Sci Med 2007;65(3):622–34.

75. Tervalon M, Murray-Garcia J. Cultural humility versus cultural competence: a critical distinction in definition physician training outcomes in multicultural education. J Health Care Poor Underserved 1998;9(2):117–25.

76. Phalen J, Paradis R. How Community health workers can reinvent health care delivery in the US. In: Health Affairs Blog. 2015. Available at: http://healthaffairs.org/blog/2015/01/16/how-community-health-workers-can-reinvent-health-care-delivery-in-the-us/. Accessed January 18, 2015.

77. Gard AM, FNP-BC. Anatomy of implementation: the structural framework for meaningful use of electronic health records. In: National Health Care for the Homeless Council. 2012. Available at: http://www.nhchc.org/wp-content/uploads/2012/01/Anatomy-of-Implementation-The-Structural-Framework-for-MU-of-EHR.pdf. Accessed January 17, 2015.

78. California Health Workforce Alliance. Taking innovation to scale: community health workers, promotores, and the triple aim. In: California Health and Human Services Agency. 2013. Available at: http://www.chhs.ca.gov/PRI/_Taking%20Innovation%20to%20Scale%20-%20CHWs,%20Promotores%20and%20the%20Triple%20Aim%20-%20CHWA%20Report%2012-22-13%20(1).pdf. Accessed January 19, 2015.

79. U.S. Department of Health and Human Services. State legislation supports professional development of community health workers, leading to greater professional recognition, enhancements in training, and funding. In: Agency for Healthcare Research and Quality. 2013. Available at: https://innovations.ahrq.gov/profiles/state-legislation-supports-professional-development-community-health-workers-leading. Accessed January 21, 2015.

80. Rosenthal EL, Brownstein JN, Rush CH, et al. Community health workers: part of the solution. Health Aff (Millwood) 2010;29(7):1338–42.

Foster Care and Child Health

Lolita M. McDavid, MD, MPA

KEYWORDS

- Foster care • Adverse conditions of childhood • Child health

KEY POINTS

- Children in foster care have needs beyond routine well-child care.
- The importance of adverse early life experiences can extend into adulthood.
- It is important to design services and care delivery that meet the needs of foster children and their families.

The term "foster care" has many connotations: crisis situations, endangered children, families unable to carry out parental responsibilities due to substance dependency, poverty, death, or abandonment. For this article, a working definition includes children in the custody of the following:

- A county or state welfare system
- A tribal court
- Children who may live in a foster home, group home, kinship care, or residential treatment center
- Children who will return home
- Those for whom a permanent plan will be made[1]

FOSTER CARE IN THE UNITED STATES

From the English Poor Laws in the sixteenth century, it was common for poor children and adults to be indentured into service. Unlike slavery, this had a term, usually 7 years, after which time the indentured servant was free of the master who was providing board and keep for labor. Children were usually placed because they

The author has nothing to disclose.
Child Advocacy and Protection, Rainbow Babies and Children's Hospital, Case Western Reserve University School of Medicine, 11100 Euclid Avenue, Mailstop 6003, Cleveland, OH 44106, USA
E-mail address: lolita.mcdavid@uhhospitals.org

Pediatr Clin N Am 62 (2015) 1329–1348
http://dx.doi.org/10.1016/j.pcl.2015.06.005
0031-3955/15/$ – see front matter © 2015 Elsevier Inc. All rights reserved.
pediatric.theclinics.com

were orphans, not because of abuse or neglect, which was considered acceptable. The first foster "system" is considered the Children's Aid Society in New York in 1853. The founder, Charles Loring Brace, conceived a unique solution to the thousands of orphan children on the streets of New York: putting them on "orphan trains" and sending them to farms. The results varied from loving homes to cruel treatment, but it gave the children placement.[2] Societies were formed to protect children and then the supervision came under governmental auspices. In the twentieth century, the movement was from orphanages to foster care and, more recently, kinship care. In the 1960s, with the recognition of the prevalence of child abuse, laws were enacted in all states to mandate the reporting of child abuse and neglect. In 1974, the Child Abuse Prevention and Treatment Act, which provided funding to states, was passed by Congress. I993, the Family Preservation and Family Support Program (P.L.103-66), provided funding to states to help children either be returned to families or placed for adoption. The days of orphanages were becoming history. In 1997, the law was reauthorized and the law stressed time-limited reunification efforts and promoted adoption in an effort children would not linger in foster care.[3,4]

Children enter the foster care system for many reasons: abuse, neglect, abandonment, or parental inability to care for them. Being in the system and separating them from their family/caregivers can accentuate the stress they experience.

THE NUMBERS

There has been a marked decline in children entering the foster care system over the past decade, with black children in care declining 47.1% between 2002 and 2012. Blacks represent 12% of the US population, but black children represent almost one-quarter of all children in foster care.[5]

The number of children in foster care varies; it is annually approximately 400,000, down from 524,000 in 2002[6,7] (**Box 1**, **Tables 1** and **2**).

Box 1
Exiting foster care 2013

Children exiting foster care during FY 2013

Mean *age at exit* 9.1 years

Mean *time in care* is 20 months

  Less than 1 month 11%

  1–11 months 35%

  12 months to 35 months 40%

  3–4 years 9%

  5 years or more 5%[7]

From Children's Bureau, Administration on Children Youth and Families, Administration for Children and Families, US Department of Health and Human Services. Analysis and Reporting System, Preliminary FY 2013 Estimates as of July 2014. The AFCARS Report. 2014. Available at: http://www.acf.hhs.gov/programs/cb.

Table 1
Annual numbers 2009–2013

Trends in Foster Care and Adoption	2009	2010	2011	2012	2013
Number *in foster care* on September 30 of the FY	418,672	404,878	397,827	396,892	402,378
Number *entered* foster care during FY	254,896	256,092	251,365	251,539	254,904
Number *awaiting adoption* on September 30 of FY	113,798	108,746	106,352	101,737	101,840
Number with *parental rights terminated* during FY	71,381	65,747	62,786	59,063	58,887
Number *adopted* with public agency involvement	57,187	53,547	50,901	52,042	50,608

Children in Foster Care on September 30, 2013: 52% boys; 48% girls; Mean age 8.9 years; 45% younger than 6 years.

Table 2
Children in foster care by race/ethnicity 2013

	N = 254,904	
Children Entering Foster Care During FY2013 Race/Ethnicity	Percent	Number
American Indian/Alaskan Native	2	5465
Asian	1	1620
Black or African American	22	54,835
Native Hawaiian/Pacific Islander	0	534
Hispanic (of any race)	21	53,786
White	45	114,666
Unknown/Unable to determine	3	7936
Two or more races	6	15,240

THE PEDIATRICIAN'S ROLE

The role of the pediatrician is to advocate for the child, not only in matters of physical health but also in mental health, educational, and social settings. Although medical providers educate parents and serve as their resource, we must also help the family, both birth parents and foster parents, navigate the health and welfare mazes they face; this is even more important when dealing with foster children. It is the responsibility of the pediatrician to assist the foster parent in understanding the child's behaviors, where they may have originated, and how to work with the child to overcome negative behaviors.

THE CHILD ENTERING THE FOSTER CARE SYSTEM

Most children in the foster care system are eligible for Medicaid or a state child health plan. It is incumbent on health care providers, in cooperation with social service agencies, to ensure that children are enrolled in a medical plan, either managed care or fee-for-service. Children in foster care represent a twofold Medicaid expenditure; they account for between 1% and 3% of children receiving Medicaid but between 4% and 8% of Medicaid expenditures.[8]

When possible, children in the foster care system should continue to receive care at the same facility, if not from the same provider. This may be the only continuity in the child's life while in foster care. The health provider serves as a repository of the child's health information as well as history of the child's development and behavior.[9] In an ideal world, the child would continue with the same provider who has cared for the child since birth. Unfortunately, children who enter the system may not have an established relationship with a provider or clinic.

In the *Textbook of Pediatric Care*, Szilagyi and Jee[10] provide comprehensive guidelines for children entering foster or kinship care as follows:

Health screen within 72 hours of placement to assess and document the following:

- Symptoms or signs of child abuse and neglect, with referral as needed
- Growth parameters
- Symptoms or signs of acute illness
- Symptoms or signs of chronic illness
- Developmental screening results and referral for evaluation
- Behavioral and mental health screening results and referral for evaluation
- Appropriate referral for emergent health issues or sexual abuse evaluation
- Appropriate treatment of identified issues
- Health education of foster or kinship caregiver

Health information gathering: an ongoing process that recognizes the importance of knowing the birth history, including maternal drug and alcohol use, prenatal care, and birth events, as well as prematurity and hospitalization.

Comprehensive health evaluation within 30 days of placement to

- Review all available health history
- Address health concerns
- Assess adjustment to foster or kinship care, child care, school, and visitation
- Address behavior concerns and daily schedule
- Assess growth parameters
- Perform a mental health evaluation or review evaluation or make referral
- Perform a complete physical examination
- Screen for signs and symptoms of child abuse and neglect
- Perform all recommended routine screening tests per American Academy of Pediatrics guidelines for age and tests for at-risk children including hearing, vision, lead, complete blood count with differential, sexually transmitted diseases, hepatitis B and C
- Review and administer needed immunizations
- Provide age-appropriate anticipatory guidance with emphasis on transition issues
- Provide appropriate or indicated treatment and referrals, including vision, hearing, and dental
- Provide communication in writing of health plan to foster care agency

Follow-up admission assessment within 90 days of placement to

- Review all the available history, assessments, and plans
- Address interval concerns
- Document growth parameters
- Assess child and foster parent(s)' concerns for adjustment
- Screen for emerging signs of child abuse and neglect that may not have been observed earlier

- Perform focused physical examination for any previously identified issues, including growth parameters, failure to thrive, or obesity
- Review applicable school information, including the need for individual education plans (IEP)
- Ensure that all referrals and recommended treatments are in progress or completed[10]

Although the American Academy of Pediatrics' schedule for pediatric preventive care can be followed if the child has had regular care, Szilagyi and Jee[10] propose the following modified periodic preventive care schedule:

- Children younger than 6 months should be seen monthly if considered high risk: developmental, growth, prematurity, prenatal drug/alcohol exposure
- Children age 12 to 24 months should been seen every 3 months
- Children between 2 and 21 years should be seen every 6 months[10]

It is possible to allow a longer spacing if the child has been in the foster home a length of time for which the foster parent feels comfortable with any identified issues. It is important to be cognizant of the time demands on the foster family.

Approximately 70% of children in foster placement will return to the birth parents or relatives and thus it is desirable to allow birth families to participate in the initial screening whenever possible.[11]

NEED FOR MENTAL HEALTH SERVICES

Children are most likely to enter the foster system in the first year of life.[12] Developmentally this is when children form attachment bonds to caregivers. Because many children have more than 1 foster care placement only magnifies attachment disorders. In a study looking at the prevalence of psychiatric disorders among older youth in the foster care system, 61% of the 17-year-olds interviewed had at least 1 psychiatric disorder and 62% of those reported the onset before entering the foster care system.[13] Whether the child or young adult comes with a diagnosis, it is important to evaluate all children entering the system to determine the need for mental health services.

Children in the foster care system have more mental heath concerns than children in the general population, but the magnitude of mental health issues is alarming, consuming 25% to 41% of the mental health expenditures.[14] In one national sample, it was found that 48% of children in the child welfare system have mental health concerns, but only one-quarter receive services.[15] With suicide being the leading cause of death in all youth 12 to 17 years old, it is not surprising that children in the foster care system are at risk for behavioral and mental health diagnoses.[16] In an Australian study that looked at the prevalence of emotional and behavior problems, children in home-based foster care had rates of behavior and mental health issues 3 to 4 times that of children in the community. In this study, 53.4% of the children in home-based foster care needed professional help by caregiver report, but only 26.9% received it in the preceding 6 months.[17]

Children who have multiple placements and those who have placements interrupted by a return home, are disproportionately high users of mental health service use. These children also are responsible for increased medical costs.[18]

Foster parents should be involved in understanding what the child's prior environment means to current functioning. A child who hoards and hides food when in a foster placement that provides routine meals is not "stealing," but instead may be acting out a fear that food will not be available. The foster parent may have limited information about the child and thus may see the hoarding of food as devious behavior. The child will not express such behavior through an analytical lens and it may frustrate a new foster parent. It is the role of the medical and mental health providers to help foster parents interpret and react to such behaviors.

ADVERSE CHILDHOOD EXPERIENCE

Unlike "What Happens in Vegas Stays in Vegas," what happens in childhood does not stay in childhood. The original adverse childhood experience (ACE) study in 1995 surveyed more that 17,000 adults enrolled in Kaiser Permanente. The investigators looked at 7 categories of adverse child experiences:

- Abuse by category: psychological, physical, sexual
- Household dysfunction by category: substance abuse, mental illness, mother treated violently, criminal behavior in the household

The study showed that ACEs are common; 52.1% of those surveyed had at least 1 exposure and one-fourth had 2 or more exposures. The striking findings by the researchers were the relationship between ACEs and adult disease and death.[19]

Of significance, the study focused on a population in which most of the participants were white, educated, and middle class, not the population that usually ends up in foster care (Appendix 1).

Additional studies have shown that life stresses and psychological burdens carry well beyond childhood and into adulthood. In a survey of 101 women age 18 to 71 years (mean 36.83), on a 10-item ACE questionnaire (ACE),

97% reported at least 1 ACE,
70% reported more than 5 ACEs
33% reported more than 8 ACEs.[20]

Although we would like to believe that removing children from a negative setting and placing them in a more nurturing setting will ensure a healthy adult outcome, research shows that not to be so. ACE studies demonstrate that negative child experiences are cumulative and carry on into adult life.[21]

CENTERING CARE

Collaborations exist in many cities between public children's bureaus, child-serving agencies, and departments of pediatrics and/or children's hospitals. The benefit of these partnerships is to provide the "medical home" for a particularly vulnerable population. Often a care coordinator ensures that the evaluations are timely and that the patients can access medical, mental health, and dental services. Forms can be completed, school issues addressed, and needs identified not only for the foster family but also for the family to which the child returns.

EXITING THE FOSTER CARE SYSTEM

Most children entering the foster care system are eligible for Medicaid; when young adults exit the foster care system they are often without medical or dental coverage. Studies show that approximately half of all youth who "age out" of the system have no health insurance. This is in a population that often has chronic health conditions and behavior/mental health diagnoses.[22]

The Affordable Care Act extends Medicaid coverage for youth leaving foster care, regardless of income, until the age of 26. It is important that pediatricians, foster families, and most importantly, foster youth, are aware and enrolled.[23]

DOCUMENTATION

Cooperation between the public agency and the health care community (physicians, mental health professions, and dentists) is crucial. It is important that the agency that has custody of the child attempts to obtain as much medical history as possible about the child. In the era of electronic medical records (EMR), there is still a place for paper records that can accompany the child. It negates the problem of interface between different EMRs and the ability to compile all the information needed.

It may be useful to have a dedicated paper record that not only addresses the special information needed for the foster child, but that is portable and allows the foster parent to have information readily available. **Figs. 1–11** show a template designed to be used with any child, but is particularly relevant to children who have out-of-home placements with multiple caregivers. The document accompanies the child.

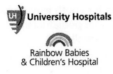

University Hospitals

Rainbow Babies
& Children's Hospital

Child's Data Page

Photo
(change annually)

_____
Child's full name

_____
Nickname

_____
Other last names used

_____
SS #

_____   _____
Birthplace   Birthdate

_____   _____   _____   _____
Gender   Race   Height   Weight

_____   _____   _____
Eye color   Hair color   Birthmark

_____
Blood type

_____
Biological mother's name

_____
Biological father's name

Additional comments:

_____

_____

_____

Fig. 1. Cover page. (*Courtesy of* M. Boutry, MD; with permission.)

Child's name

Address   City/ZIP

Insurance   Group #

Police   Poison Control   Fire

Hospital   Telephone

Pediatrician   Telephone

Pharmacy   Telephone

Dentist   Telephone

Specialist   Telephone

Specialist   Telephone

Specialist   Telephone

Emergency Contact: If parent cannot be reached

Name   Relationship

                                                 Telephone

Fig. 2. Emergency information. (*Courtesy of* M. Boutry, MD; with permission.)

Agency	Name/Role	Telephone
Help Me Grow Program		
– Help Me Grow Worker (Service Coordinator)		
– Developmental Specialist		
OT/PT/Speech		
University Hospitals – Social Worker		
County Social Worker		
Case Worker		
Board of Mental Retardation/ Developmental Disabilities (MRDD)		
Visiting Nurse		
WIC		

Fig. 3. Important telephone numbers. (*Courtesy of* M. Boutry, MD; with permission.)

Birth weight: lbs/oz

Birth length: inches

My baby was delivered in week _____ of pregnancy.

Problems at birth

Surgeries

Date   Surgery

Date   Surgery

Allergies

Allergy   Reaction

Allergy   Reaction

Allergy   Reaction

Admissions (Hospital Stays)

From   To   Reason Admitted

From   To   Reason Admitted

From   To   Reason Admitted

Fig. 4. Medical history. (*Courtesy of* M. Boutry, MD; with permission.)

Chronic (Long-Term) Problems
Ask the doctor to complete this form

Date Entered	Description

Fig. 5. Chronic problems. (*Courtesy of* M. Boutry, MD; with permission.)

Chronic (Long-Term) Medications

Date Ordered	Name of Medication	Why am I giving this medication to my child?	Dose/ Amount

Fig. 6. Chronic medications. (*Courtesy of* M. Boutry, MD; with permission.)

Date Ordered	Name of Medication	Why am I giving this medication to my child?	Dose/ Amount

Fig. 7. Other medications. (*Courtesy of* M. Boutry, MD; with permission.)

Date	Time	Test/X-rays	Results

Fig. 8. Tests and X-rays. (*Courtesy of* M. Boutry, MD; with permission.)

Date: _____

Type of Visit: _____ Well _____ Sick _____ Follow-Up

Pediatrician (this visit): _____

Age: _____ Height: _____ Weight: _____ BMI: _____

Today we discussed: _____

_____

_____

_____

_____

Please mark if the following were discussed:

_____ Hearing   _____ Relationship issues (foster family, birth family)

_____ Vision   _____ Adjustment to placement, visitation, etc.

_____ Dental   _____ Developmental/school needs

_____ Nutrition   _____ Behavioral/emotional issues

_____ Immunizations   _____ Permanency plan

Plan:

Medication: _____

Nutrition recommendations: _____

_____

Today's immunizations: _____

Labs to be drawn: _____

Other tests: _____

Specialist referrals: _____

My next appointment is: _____

Fig. 9. Visit summary (to be completed at each visit). (*Courtesy of* M. Boutry, MD; with permission.)

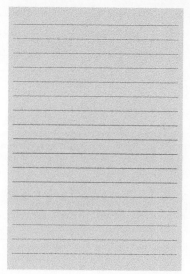

Fig. 10. Notes. (*Courtesy of* M. Boutry, MD; with permission.)

Child's Name: _____   Birthdate: _____

Hepatitis B (HEP B)

1. _____

2. _____

3. _____

Diphtheria, Tetanus, Pertussis (DTaP)

1. _____

2. _____

3. _____

4. _____

5. _____

Tetanus/Diphtheria (Td)

1. _____

Pneumococcal Conjugate (PVC)

1. _____

2. _____

3. _____

4. _____

H. influenza Type b (Hib)

1. _____

2. _____

3. _____

4. _____

Influenza Vaccine (Flu)

1. _____

2. _____

Varicella (VAR)

1. _____

2. _____

Hepatitis A (HEP A)

1. _____

2. _____

Interactive Polio (IPV)

1. _____

2. _____

3. _____

4. _____

Measles, Mumps, Rubella (MMR)

1. _____

2. _____

Meningococcal Vaccine

1. _____

2. _____

Human Papilloma Virus (HPV)

1. _____

2. _____

3. _____

Rotavirus

1. _____

2. _____

3. _____

**Make a copy of this form.
This form is for your records.**

Fig. 11. Immunization record. (*Courtesy of* M. Boutry, MD; with permission.)

ACKNOWLEDGMENTS

I thank Mireille Boutry, MD, for permission to use the University Hospitals Rainbow Parent Network Medical Journal, and Nathan Elekonich, Rainbow Babies and Children's Hospital, Public Relations and Development, for assistance with graphics and formatting.

REFERENCES

1. McCarthy J. Meeting the health care needs of children in the foster care system: summary of state and community efforts key findings. Washington, DC: Georgetown University Child Development Center; 2002.
2. Foster care: background and history. Available at: http://family.findlaw.com/foster-care/foster-care-background-and-history.html. Accessed January 7, 2005.
3. Barbell K, Freundlich M. Foster care today. Washington, DC: Casey Family Programs; 2001.
4. Encyclopedia of children and childhood in history and society. Foster care. 2008. Available at: http://www.faqs.org/childhood/Fa-Gr/Foster-Care.html. Accessed January 13, 2015.
5. Office of Data, Analysis, Research, and Evaluation, Administration on Children Youth and Families, Administration for Children and Families, US Department of Health and Human Services. Recent demographic trends in foster care. Data Brief 2013-1, September 2013.
6. Children's Bureau, Administration on Children Youth and Families, Administration for Children and Families, US Department of Health and Human Services. Trends in foster care and adoption: FFY 2002-2013. 2014. Available at: http://www.acf.hhs.gov/programs/cb. Accessed January 7, 2015.
7. Children's Bureau, Administration on Children Youth and Families, Administration for Children and Families, US Department of Health and Human Services. The AFCARS Report. 2014. http://www.acf.hhs.gov/programs/cb. Accessed December 2, 2014.
8. Rosenbach M. Children in foster care: challenges in meeting their health care needs through Medicaid. Policy Brief - Mathematica Policy Research, Inc 2001. Available at: http://aspe.hhs.gov/hsp/fostercare-health00/. Accessed December 2, 2014.
9. The Children's Partnership. Improving health outcomes for children in foster care: the role of the electronic medical record systems. Number 5. 2009. Available at: www.chiildrenspartnership.org. Accessed January 13, 2015.
10. Szilagyi M, Jee SH. Children in foster and kinship care. In: American Academy of Pediatrics textbook of pediatric care. American Academy of Pediatrics; 2009.
11. American Academy of Pediatrics, Committee on Early Childhood, Adoption, and Dependent Care. Health care of young children in foster care. Pediatrics 2002; 109:536–41.
12. Jones Harden. B. Infants in the child welfare system: a developmental perspective on policy and practice. Zero to Three. 2007. Available at: www.zerotothree.org. Accessed January 13, 2015.
13. McMillen JC, Zima BT, Scott LD Jr, et al. Prevalence of psychiatric disorders among older youths in the foster care system. J Am Acad Child Adolesc Psychiatry 2005;44(1):88–95.
14. Mekonnen R, Noonan K, Rubin D. Achieving better health care outcomes for children in foster care. Pediatr Clin North Am 2009;56:405–15.

15. Burns BJ, Phillips SD, Wagner R, et al. Mental health need and access to mental health services by youths involved in child welfare: a national survey. J Am Acad Child Adolesc Psychiatry 2004;43(8):960–70.
16. Flores G, Lesley B. Children and US federal policy on health and health care seen but not heard. JAMA Pediatr 2014;168(12):1155–63.
17. Sawyer MG, Carbone JA, Searle AK, et al. The mental health and wellbeing of children and adolescents in home-based foster care. Med J Aust 2007;186(4): 181–4.
18. Rubin DM, Alessandrini EA, Freudtner C, et al. Placement stability and mental health costs for children in foster care. Pediatrics 2004;113:1336–41.
19. Felitti VJ, Anda RF, Nordenberg D, et al. Relationship of childhood abuse and household dysfunction to many of the leading causes of death in adults—the adverse childhood experiences (ACE) study. Am J Prev Med 1998;14(4): 245–58.
20. Bruskas D, Tessin DH. Adverse childhood experiences and psychosocial well-being of women who were in foster care as children. Permanente J 2013;17(3): e131–41.
21. Dube SR, Fellitti VJ, Dong M, et al. The impact of adverse childhood experiences on health problems: evidence from four birth cohorts dating back to 1900. Prev Med 2003;37:268–77.
22. American Academy of Pediatrics, Council on Foster Care, Adoption, and Kinship Care and Committee on Early Childhood. Health care of youth aging out of foster care. Pediatrics 2012;130:1170–3.
23. Allen KD, Hendricks T. Medicaid and children in foster care. Hamilton (NJ): State Policy Advocacy and Reform Center; 2013.

APPENDIX 1: POTENTIAL INFLUENCES THROUGHOUT THE LIFE SPAN OF ADVERSE CHILDHOOD EXPERIENCES

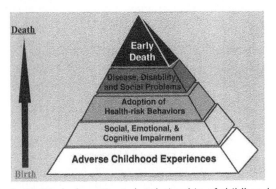

From Felitti VJ, Anda RF, Nordenberg D, et al. Relationship of childhood abuse and house-hold dysfunction to many of the leading causes of death in adults. The Adverse Childhood Experiences (ACE) Study. Am J Prev Med 1998;14(4):245–58; with permission.

Index

Note: Page numbers of article titles are in **boldface.**

A

ABC acronym, for Affordable Care Act, 1301
ACA. *See* Affordable Care Act.
Acetaminophen hypothesis, for asthma, 1202
Add Health characteristics, 1143
Adolescents
    environmental toxicant effects on, 1177
    obesity in, 1247–1248
    tobacco smoke effects on, 1179
Adverse childhood experiences
    foster care and, 1141
    in poverty, 1118
Advocacy
    for Affordable Care Act, 1307
    for obesity prevention, 1249
    for poverty prevention, 1120, 1122
    for utility services, 1268–1269
    for youth violence prevention, 1155
Affordable Care Act, **1297–1311**
    breastfeeding provisions in, **1701–1091**
    community health workers in, 1315
    ongoing challenges in, 1306–1308
    overview of, 1300–1305
    pediatrician role in, 1307–1308
    radial and ethnic disparities and, 1305–1306
    versus children's health insurance programs, 1298–1300
AFIX (assessment, feedback, incentives, exchange) program, 1101
Air pollution, 1176–1177
Alcohol use, 1179–1181
Aldrin, 1186, 1189
Allostatic load, in poverty, 1119
Alma-Alta declaration, of World Health Organization, 1314–1315
Alternative Benefit Plans, Medicaid, for breastfeeding, 1078–1079
American Academy of Pediatric Dentistry, 1217–1218
American Academy of Pediatrics, recommendations for early literacy, 1285, 1288–1292
Amorphous calcium phosphates, for caries prevention, 1220
Anticipatory guidance, for obesity prevention, 1249–1250
Apatite, in teeth, fluoride treatment for, 1219
Arsenic exposure, 1182–1184
Assault, statistics on, 1138–1139
Asthma, **1199–1214**
    epidemiology of, 1200–1202

Pediatr Clin N Am 62 (2015) 1349–1362
http://dx.doi.org/10.1016/S0031-3955(15)00124-8
0031-3955/15/$ – see front matter © 2015 Elsevier Inc. All rights reserved.

I

I-HELP acronym, for legal needs, 1266–1267
Immunization, **1093–1109**
    barriers to, 1095–1105
    cost-effectiveness of, 1093
    disparities in, 1095
    exemptions for, 1098–1099, 1103
    information systems for, 1102–1103
    missed opportunities for, 1101–1104
    parent acceptance of, 1104–1105
    quality improvement in, 1101–1102
    recommendations for, 1099–1105
    reminder interventions for, 1102
    statistics on, 1093–1095
    vaccine shortages in, 1097
Income, insufficient. *See* Poverty.
Indian Health Care Improvement Act, 1305
Indian Health Service, 1300
Indirect pulp cap procedure, 1221
Infants
    early brain and child development promotion in, 1289–1290
    environmental toxicants effects on, 1176
    literacy development in, 1286–1287
    obesity in, 1245–1246
    tobacco smoke effects on, 1179
Inflammation, in asthma, 1202–1203
Information systems, immunization, 1102–1103
Integrated pest management, 1207

J

Jacobi, Abraham, as founder of pediatrics, 1111–1112

L

Lactation programs. *See* Breastfeeding.
Lay health workers. *See* Community health workers.
Lead exposure, 1182–1184
Learning, poverty effects on, 1115, 1117–1118
Legal issues, **1263–1271**
    accessing support, 1265
    in immunization, 1103
    in low-income populations, 1264
    in passing Affordable Care Act, 1300
    medical-legal partnership approach to, 1265–1270
    social determinants as, 1263–1264
Life expectancy, poverty effects on, 1119
LIFT program, 1125
Lindane, 1189
Literacy

Tobacco use, smoke exposure in, 1177–1179, 1204, 1206–1207. *See also* Dual tobacco use.
Toddlers
early brain and child development promotion in, 1291
environmental toxicants effects on, 1176
literacy development in, 1286–1287
obesity in, 1246–1247
Too Small to Fail initiative, 1288
Tooth decay, 1215–1226
Toxaphene, 1187
Toxic stress
in poverty, 1118–1119, 1274
youth violence in, 1143
Toxicants, environmental. *See* Dual tobacco use; Environmental toxicants.
Trauma
from youth violence, 1138–1139
in poverty, 1118
TRICARE military health insurance program, 1299–1300

U

Urban Indian Youth Health Survey, 1143
Urban Institute report, on poverty, 1120
Utility services, legal aid for, 1268–1269

V

Vaccination. *See* Immunization.
Vaccines for Children program, 1095, 1099
VetoViolence, 1153
Victimization, in youth violence, 1140–1141
Video Interaction Project, 1125
Violence. *See* Youth violence.
Vitamin D hypothesis, for asthma, 1202
Volatile organic compounds, 1187–1188

W

Weapon carrying, 1149
Well-being, poverty effects on, 1115–1126
Wheezing, in asthma, 1203
WHO M-POWER campaign, for smoking cessation, 1178
WIC program
breastfeeding provisions in, 1078–1082, 1084
immunization promotion in, 1103–1104
obesity education in, 1251
Witnessing, of youth violence, 1140–1141
Women, Infants, and Children (WIC) program
breastfeeding provisions in, 1078–1082, 1084
immunization promotion in, 1103–1104
obesity education in, 1251

United States Postal Service

Statement of Ownership, Management, and Circulation
(All Periodicals Publications Except Requestor Publications)

1. Publication Title	2. Publication Number	3. Filing Date
Pediatric Clinics of North America	4 2 4 - 6 6 0 0	9/18/15

4. Issue Frequency	5. Number of Issues Published Annually	6. Annual Subscription Price
Feb, Apr, Jun, Aug, Oct, Dec	6	$200.00

7. Complete Mailing Address of Known Office of Publication *(Not printer)* *(Street, city, county, state, and ZIP+4®)*

Elsevier Inc.
360 Park Avenue South
New York, NY 10010-1710

Contact Person
Stephen R. Bushing

Telephone *(Include area code)*
215-239-3688

8. Complete Mailing Address of Headquarters or General Business Office of Publisher *(Not printer)*

Elsevier Inc., 360 Park Avenue South, New York, NY 10010-1710

9. Full Names and Complete Mailing Addresses of Publisher, Editor, and Managing Editor *(Do not leave blank)*

Publisher *(Name and complete mailing address)*

Linda Belfus, Elsevier Inc., 1600 John F. Kennedy Blvd., Ste. 1800, Philadelphia, PA 19103-2899

Editor *(Name and complete mailing address)*

Kerry Holland, Elsevier Inc., 1600 John F. Kennedy Blvd., Ste. 1800, Philadelphia, PA 19103-2899

Managing Editor *(Name and complete mailing address)*

Adrianne Brigido, Elsevier Inc., 1600 John F. Kennedy Blvd., Ste. 1800, Philadelphia, PA 19103-2899

10. Owner *(Do not leave blank. If the publication is owned by a corporation, give the name and address of the corporation immediately followed by the names and addresses of all stockholders owning or holding 1 percent or more of the total amount of stock. If not owned by a corporation, give the names and addresses of the individual owners. If owned by a partnership or other unincorporated firm, give its name and address as well as those of each individual owner. If the publication is published by a nonprofit organization, give its name and address.)*

Full Name	Complete Mailing Address
Wholly owned subsidiary of	1600 John F. Kennedy Blvd., Ste. 1800
Reed/Elsevier, US holdings	Philadelphia, PA 19103-2899

11. Known Bondholders, Mortgagees, and Other Security Holders Owning or Holding 1 Percent or More of Total Amount of Bonds, Mortgages, or Other Securities. If none, check box ☐ None

Full Name	Complete Mailing Address
N/A	

12. Tax Status *(For completion by nonprofit organizations authorized to mail at nonprofit rates)* *(Check one)*
The purpose, function, and nonprofit status of this organization and the exempt status for federal income tax purposes:
☐ Has Not Changed During Preceding 12 Months
☐ Has Changed During Preceding 12 Months *(Publisher must submit explanation of change with this statement)*

13. Publication Title	14. Issue Date for Circulation Data Below
Pediatric Clinics of North America	August 2015

PS Form 3526, July 2014 [Page 1 of 3 (Instruction Page 3)] PSN 7530-01-000-9931 PRIVACY NOTICE: See our Privacy policy in www.usps.com

15. Extent and Nature of Circulation			Average No. Copies Each Issue During Preceding 12 Months	No. Copies of Single Issue Published Nearest to Filing Date
a. Total Number of Copies *(Net press run)*			1899	1557
b. Legitimate Paid and/or Requested Distribution (By Mail and Outside the Mail)	(1)	Mailed Outside County Paid/Requested Mail Subscriptions stated on PS Form 3541. *(Include paid distribution above nominal rate, advertiser's proof copies and exchange copies)*	884	674
	(2)	Mailed In-County Paid/Requested Mail Subscriptions stated on PS Form 3541. *(Include paid distribution above nominal rate, advertiser's proof copies and exchange copies)*		
	(3)	Paid Distribution Outside the Mails Including Sales Through Dealers And Carriers, Street Vendors, Counter Sales, and Other Paid Distribution Outside USPS®	522	585
	(4)	Paid Distribution by Other Classes of Mail Through the USPS (e.g. First-Class Mail®)		
c. Total Paid and/or Requested Circulation *(Sum of 15b (1), (2), (3), and (4))*			1406	1259
d. Free or Nominal Rate Distribution (By Mail and Outside the Mail)	(1)	Free or Nominal Rate Outside-County Copies included on PS Form 3541	73	67
	(2)	Free or Nominal Rate In-County Copies Included on PS Form 3541		
	(3)	Free or Nominal Rate Copies mailed at Other classes Through the USPS (e.g. First-Class Mail)		
	(4)	Free or Nominal Rate Distribution Outside the Mail *(Carriers or Other means)*		
e. Total Nonrequested Distribution *(Sum of 15d (1), (2), (3) and (4))*			73	67
f. Total Distribution *(Sum of 15c and 15e)*			1479	1326
g. Copies not Distributed *(See instructions to publishers #4 (page #3))*			420	231
h. Total *(Sum of 15f and g)*			1899	1557
i. Percent Paid and/or Requested Circulation *(15c divided by 15f times 100)*			95.06%	94.95%

* If you are claiming electronic copies go to line 16 on page 3. If you are not claiming Electronic copies, skip to line 17 on page 3.

16. Electronic Copy Circulation	Average No. Copies Each Issue During Preceding 12 Months	No. Copies of Single Issue Published Nearest to Filing Date
a. Paid Electronic Copies		
b. Total paid Print Copies (Line 15c) + Paid Electronic copies (Line 16a)		
c. Total Print Distribution (Line 15f) + Paid Electronic Copies (Line 16a)		
d. Percent Paid (Both Print & Electronic copies) (16b divided by 16c X 100)		

☐ I certify that 50% of all my distributed copies (electronic and print) are paid above a nominal price

17. Publication of Statement of Ownership
☐ If the publication is a general publication, publication of this statement is required. Will be printed in the **October 2015** issue of this publication.

Date

18. Signature and Title of Editor, Publisher, Business Manager, or Owner

Stephen R. Bushing
Stephen R. Bushing – Inventory/Distribution Coordinator

September 18, 2015

I certify that all information furnished on this form is true and complete. I understand that anyone who furnishes false or misleading information on this form or who omits material or information requested on the form may be subject to criminal sanctions (including fines and imprisonment) and/or civil sanctions (including civil penalties).

PS Form 3526, July 2014 (Page 2 of 3)

Printed and bound by CPI Group (UK) Ltd, Croydon, CR0 4YY

08/06/2025

01896873-0003